Obstetric Ultrasound

Obstetric Ultrasound: Artistry in Practice

John C. Hobbins, MD
Professor of Obstetrics and Gynecology
University of Colorado Health Sciences Center
Denver, Colorado

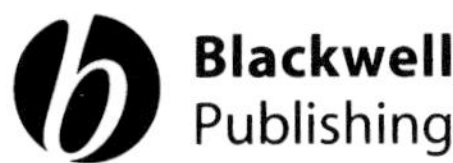

Published by Blackwell Publishing
Blackwell Publishing, Inc., 350 Main Street, Malden, Massachusetts 02148-5020, USA
Blackwell Publishing Ltd, 9600 Garsington Road, Oxford OX4 2DQ, UK
Blackwell Publishing Asia Pty Ltd, 550 Swanston Street, Carlton, Victoria 3053, Australia

First published 2008

1 2008

Library of Congress Cataloging-in-Publication Data

Hobbins, John C., 1936-
Obstetric ultrasound : artistry in practice / John C. Hobbins.
p. ; cm.
Includes bibliographical references and index.
ISBN 978-1-4051-5815-2
1. Ultrasonics in obstetrics. I. Title.
[DNLM: 1. Ultrasonography, Prenatal–methods. 2. Embryonic Development.
3. Fetal Development. 4. Fetal Diseases–ultrasonography. 5. Pregnancy–physiology.
6. Pregnancy Complications–ultrasonography. WQ 209 H682o 2007]
RG527.5.U48H59 2007
618.2′07543–dc22

2007008365

ISBN: 978-1-4051-5815-2

A catalogue record for this title is available from the British Library

Set in 9.25/11.5 Minion by Aptara Inc., New Delhi, India
Printed and bound in Singapore by Markono Print Media Pte Ltd

Commissioning Editor: Martin Sugden
Editorial Assistant: Jennifer Seward
Development Editor: Elisabeth Dodds
Production Controller: Debbie Wyer

For further information on Blackwell Publishing, visit our website:
http://www.blackwellpublishing.com

Contents

Dedication

I have dedicated this book to three people.

My dad was the ideal role model. He possessed incredible talent, intelligence, integrity, and humility. It has been tough to try to match up to someone who was the total package (although I will bet he never realized it). The description "he speaks softly but carries a big stick" fit him perfectly, except he didn't need a big stick since I toed the line (most of the time) simply because I did not wish to displease him.

The word "artistry" in the book title is not there by accident. My dad, my brother, and one of my sons were/are fine artists by trade, but my very rudimentary talent has been limited to drawing stick figure fetuses during counseling sessions. However, everyone in ultrasound is displaying a form of artistry—artistry in obtaining the information and artistry in putting the information into play.

Thank you, dad, for guiding me every day.

Elaine is one of the most remarkable of the thousands of patients I have had the pleasure of meeting over the past 40 years. She participated fully in her own care, and even provided me with snippets from the literature when I was struggling with her diagnosis. Her remarkable courage, determination, and impressive intellect energized me.

Elaine, this book was written for you and others like you whose fetuses have problems that might be helped by some messages contained within.

Last, I am dedicating this book to my wife, Susan. She has provided much of the inspiration for it.

After spending the first part of my career seeking new—and often invasive—ways to find out more about the fetuses, my energies then turned toward finding non-invasive substitutes. While in that mindset, Susan, a nurse midwife, helped me to further understand that in many ways we, as providers, have a tendency to interfere in what is generally a very natural and normal process. Our "ready, shoot, aim" thinking evolved to help patients, but often it can have the opposite effect. She has stimulated me to try to put the "aim" back in its proper place in the diagnostic sequence.

Susan, I deeply appreciate your support and, recently, your patience with me while I spent hours and hours sitting in front of the computer (yours)—often swearing at my inept attempts to complete the simplest tasks—when we could be playing tennis or doing something infinitely more entertaining.

Thank you for adding so much to my life.

Acknowledgments

For an academic department to be successful, it must have an excellent coordinator. Through the years I have been lucky to have had only five perinatal coordinators—all of them world-class. Jane Berg, who, as well as possessing a myriad of organizational talents, also has the ability to tweak everything possible out of the computer. In addition, she reads at least as much of the perinatal literature as our fellows, and has a "Jeopardy-like" ability to remember even obscure papers.

I know this project has not only tested her above skills, but, at times, her patience, and I am deeply indebted.

Thank you, Jane. It would have been very difficult to pull this off without you.

Wayne Persutte and I have worked together for more than 15 years, and I have thoroughly enjoyed every minute of our hundreds of discussions about ultrasound, sports, and politics. He has been responsible for many of the images in this book, which obviously are essential to the messages within it.

Thank you for everything, Wayne.

Helen MacFarlane provided most of the illustrations for this book. Since this was designed to be a "nuts-and-bolts" type of text, we decided to make the illustrations reflect this concept. Rather than "Netter-like" renditions, we resorted to the simplest of diagrams, and Helen did a remarkable job of following that pathway.

Thank you so much, Helen.

A large "thank you" goes to John Queenan, who has provided the forward to this book. Who better to write this than one of the most respected individuals in OB/GYN?

Many years ago I was an intern in a community hospital in Connecticut and John was on the staff there, as well as being a faculty member at Cornell Medical School in New York City. After watching him in action as a clinician, teacher, and leader in the therapy of Rh disease, I decided I wanted to be him. John, you are one of the 4 individuals who influenced me to do what I do, including writing this book.

Foreword

A medical pundit was once asked, "What are the three greatest advances in obstetrics and gynecology of the last decade?" His answer was swift and definitive: "Ultrasound, ultrasound, ultrasound." While all of us could add to the list, there is little doubt of the primacy of sonography in clinical medicine. This modality has made a profound improvement in the delivery of care in numerous ways: detecting congenital anomalies, early fetal life, and ectopic pregnancies; establishing gestational age; and evaluating fetal condition in Rh disease, multiple gestations or intrauterine growth restriction.

Dr. Hobbins begins this book by presenting a systematic review of the fetal physical exam. In chapter 12 he starts to define the role of sonography in many clinical problems and ends with practical uses of this technology in a changing world. He closes with vintage Hobbins, expounding on various hot topics. The appendix contains his selection of useful clinical tables.

Over the last half decade as the deputy editor of *Obstetrics and Gynecology* I have been immersed in evidence-based scientific manuscripts. While advancing medical knowledge, there is a loss of author's experience and advice in such manuscripts. Enter John C. Hobbins, MD, one of the outstanding teachers and researchers from the onset of clinical sonography, three decades ago. From the start, Dr. Hobbins' skills at scanning were artistry in practice. To me, reading this book is like following Pablo Picasso, Dr. Hobbin's favorite artist, on a personal tour of his gallery. How refreshing to read the thoughts and advice of a world-class expert. In undertaking this project Dr. Hobbins has crafted the book to serve both patients and the medical profession. I believe it fully achieves his mission.

John T. Queenan, MD
Professor of Obstetrics and Gynecology
and Chair Emeritus
Georgetown University Medical Center
Deputy Editor, *Obstetrics and Gynecology*
August 2007

Preface

During the 35 years that I have been immersed in the practice of perinatal medicine, it has been possible to chronicle intimately the evolving role of ultrasound. At first, it was used to answer a few basic questions regarding gestational age, fetal and placental position, and to rule out multiple gestations. Now the modality can unroof the innermost secrets of the fetus through two-dimensional and three-dimensional imagery and Doppler waveform analysis.

In 1977, one of the first books dedicated to ultrasound was written by Fred Winsberg and me. The second edition was coauthored with Richard Berkowitz, one of the great thinkers in the field. Both times, we had difficulty in filling up these thin books with enough information to make them worth selling. At that time, most practitioners were using a "contact scanner" that required the operator to move a small transducer attached to an articulated arm across patient's abdomen in order to create a composite image from data stored during the sweep. The first machine we used at Yale was a surprisingly small unit made by Picker that was donated by a grateful patient of the chairman at that time, C. Lee Buxton, who felt that there might a future for ultrasound in obstetrics and gynecology (after hearing a lecture by the father of obstetrical ultrasound, Ian Donald). Also, his interest was kindled further by Dr Ernest Kohorn, a British transplant in the department who had spent time with Professor Donald.

In 1975, Jim Binns, a young representative from a fledgling company, ADR, stopped by with a small real-time machine that could almost fit in a suitcase. The real-time images springing from this machine had the same wow effect on us that the four-dimensional real-time images from today's machines have on patients, and we instantly *had* to own it. This we accomplished with a check for $20,000. A few years later, this simple linear array technology morphed into the complicated, expensive, and often cumbersome units of today that, fortunately, produce exquisite images. In just a decade, the price of these machines has gone from that of a Mazda Miata to a Lamborghini, and, while during the time it took to reduce the size of a computer to something you can enclose in your hand, many of today's ultrasound machines, which ironically depend heavily on microchip technology, are so heavy that I live in fear that I might accidentally run one over my foot. In addition, because the new machines incorporate many new features to substantially improve the images, some keyboards now look like the instrument panels of a jumbo jet. Also, although companies are constantly striving to make their keyboard the most user-friendly feature ever fashioned, no keyboard is the same—something that is very frustrating to a dyslexic multiple machine-user like me.

What is the point of this stroll down memory lane (which generally produces the same gag reflex as telling a young resident that we used to work every other night)? It is to point out that, while all this was going on, ultrasound has evolved from something that would answer a few clinical questions to a now indispensable tool that plays a major role in every pregnancy. Just like the history of ultrasound technology, which has taken many tangents, the clinical pathway of ultrasound has not always followed a straight-line. However, until the next technological advance sets off a new set of challenges, most of the clinical kinks have been ironed out to a point where a book can now be written to lay out the state of contemporary knowledge in obstetrical ultrasound.

Other than a cursory mention of the past in this introduction, the only historical inserts will be used to dispel a few earlier misconceptions or to do away with some misguided rituals that have crept into ultrasound practice over the past two decades.

In contrast to our first books, the challenge now is to sift through the myriad of available clinical information and to cram selectively the most useful nuggets into this text. The format will be simple, but different than other standard textbooks. While avoiding "text book speak," I will be working backward from a topic by focusing on a specific condition or an initial finding noted during a basic examination and exploring how ultrasound can be used optimally to attain the clinician's goal of arriving upon a diagnosis and activating a plan of management. While attempting to be succinct, I have avoided including voluminous reference sections after each chapter, and have tried to be judiciously selective by citing mostly those papers whose data I have used in the text.

The goal is to inform—but with a heavy dusting of opinion.

John C. Hobbins, MD
February 2007

1 Early pregnancy loss

Most perinatologists deal more frequently with patients during the second portion of the first trimester, and I am no exception. For that reason, while drafting this chapter I needed help with the topics of early pregnancy milestones and the common problem of early first trimester embryonic/fetal loss. After a brief search, I came up with a gem in the form of syllabus material accompanying a superb lecture by Dr Steven Goldstein, given at an ultrasound course. This will be sprinkled throughout this chapter.

Early pregnancy can be divided up into three segments: the pre-embryonic period (conception to 5 menstrual weeks); the embryonic period, during which time organogenesis is the major activity (4–9 menstrual weeks); and the early developmental period, during which time the fetus simply grows while adding to the building blocks formed earlier (10–12 weeks). Not surprisingly, the third segment has been called the fetal period.

Ultrasound milestones

First, it must be stipulated that there is a major difference between when a certain finding *can* appear and when it *should* be present, the latter having more importance in early pregnancy failure. Also, one can identify structures much earlier with transvaginal ultrasound, which has a separate timetable. Frankly, up until the eleventh week, there is little reason to view a first trimester pregnancy with transabdominal ultrasound (TAU) other than as an initial quick scouting venture.

The first ultrasound sign of pregnancy is a gestational sac that is generally oblong and has a thick "rind" (Figure 1.1a). The sac should have a double ring, representing the decidua capsularis and the decidua parietalis, and should be seen when the beta human chorionic gonadotropin (hCG) is between 1000 and 2000 mIU/mL. Once seen, the sac diameter should grow by an average of 1 mm a day, and the mean sac diameter (MSD) can be used as a gauge against which to assess other findings [1]. Beware of the pseudosac, which does not have a double ring and is seen in association with ectopic pregnancy (Figure 1.1b).

The yolk sac is the second structure to be visible by ultrasound (Figure 1.2). It can be seen when the MSD is 5 mm, but it *should* be seen by the time the MSD is 8 mm [2]. It plays a crucial role in the development of the fetus—providing nourishment and producing the stem cells that develop into red blood cells, white blood cells, and platelets. In effect, the yolk sac provides the immunological potential for the fetus until about 7 menstrual weeks, when those functions are taken over by the fetal liver. From then on the functionless yolk sac becomes a circular structure without a core, after which it finally disappears by 12 menstrual weeks.

After about 8 weeks, the yolk sac has little diagnostic value and, although some studies have suggested that a macro yolk sac (more than 6 mm) is an ominous sign, our own observations have not borne this out. We have noted a "filled in" yolk sac (Figure 1.3) to be sometimes associated with fetal demise, but in these cases the embryo/fetus provides the ultimate information.

One can see an embryo by 5 menstrual weeks and a way to determine gestational age is to add 42 days to the crown–rump length (CRL) measurement in millimeters. The embryo should increase its CRL by 1 mm/d. Not seeing an embryo when the MSD has reached 6 mm is indicative of a pregnancy loss [3]. Also, the size of the embryo, relative to the MSD, is important. For example, if the MSD–CRL is <6 mm, the prognosis is very poor.

Cardiac activity should be visualized when the embryonic length is greater than or equal to 4 mm, and not seeing a beating heart at this embryonic size is an ominous sign [4]. The heart rate itself may provide insight into the fate of the pregnancy. For example, Benson and Doubilet [5] noted that if the heart rate (HR) was less than

Obstetric Ultrasound: Artistry in Practice. John C. Hobbins. Published 2008 Blackwell Publishing. ISBN 978-1-4051-5815-2.

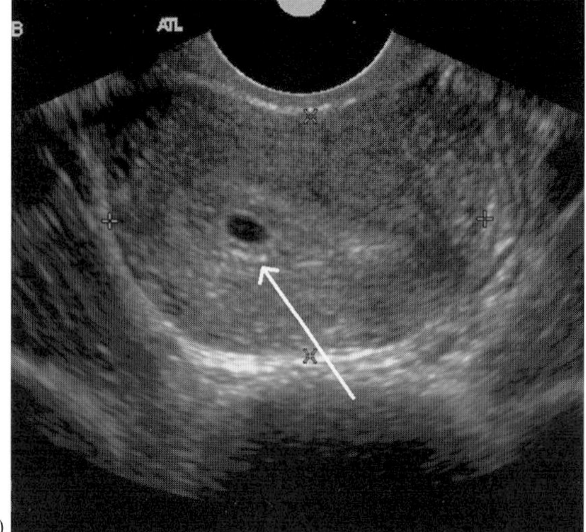

(a)

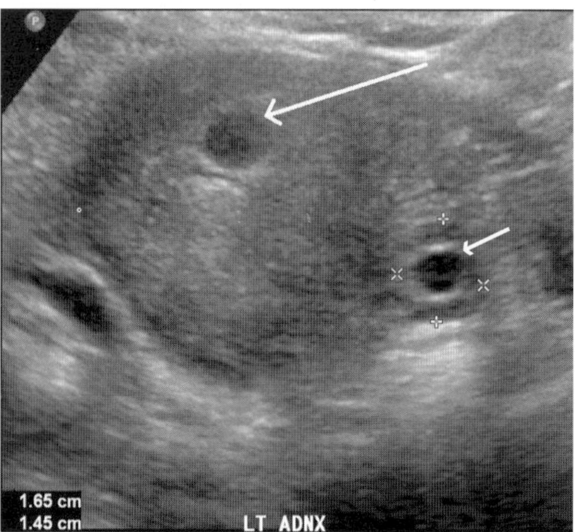

(b)

Fig 1.1 (a) Early gestational sac. (b) Ectopic. Large arrow points to pseudosac. Small arrow points to ectopic next to uterus.

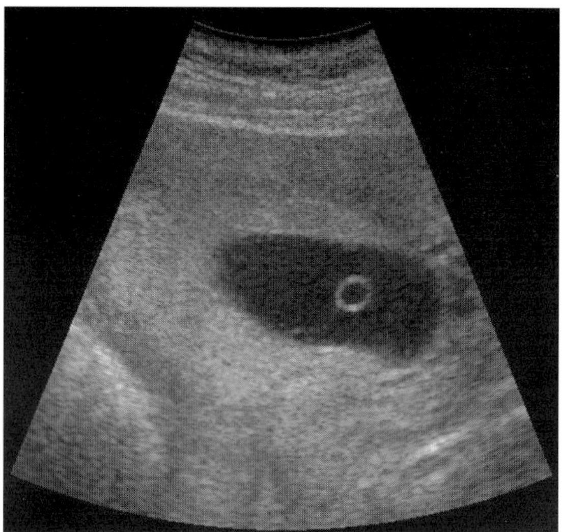

Fig 1.2 Yolk sac.

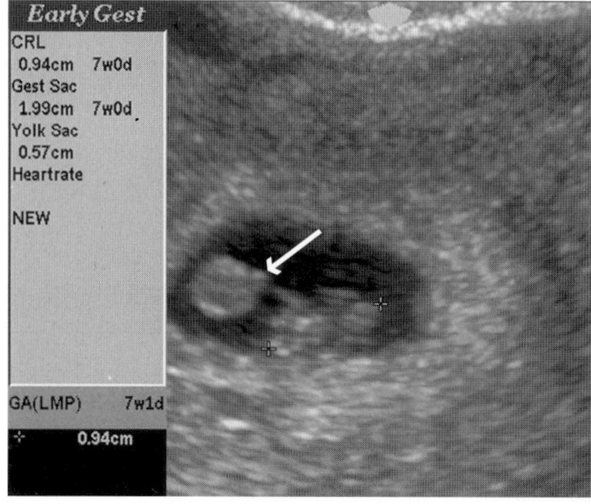

Fig 1.3 Filled-in yolk sac; calipers are on CRL and arrow points to yolk sac.

90 in pregnancies that were less than 8 weeks, there was an 80% chance of fetal death. If the HR was below 70, 100% ultimately had an intrauterine demise. Later in the first trimester, fetuses with HR above the 95th percentile have a markedly increased risk for trisomy 13 [6].

Human chorionic gonadotropin (hCG)

This is a product of the placenta that rises linearly throughout the first trimester and decreases through the second trimester. Although various investigators have explored subunits of the hCG molecule in screening for Down syndrome (beta subunit), the assays commonly used today for standard monitoring of early pregnancy measure intact hCG (not beta hCG).

Should see on TVS	Time of visualization
Gestation sac	5 menstrual weeks
Yolk sac	when MSD is >7mm
Embryonic pole	5 weeks or when hCG is >1000 mIU
Fetal heart activity	when CRL is >5 mm

Initially, Kadar et al. [7] described a "discriminatory level," above which one should see an embryo (6500 mμ/mL), to help sort out pregnancy loss from ectopic pregnancy. These initial values were based on TAU and an assay that has been replaced by another (second international standard). The hCG level, above which one should identify an embryo by transvaginal sonography, is now 1000 mIU/mL to 2000 mIU/mL, as determined by the second international standard. In a patient clinically at risk for loss or ectopic pregnancy the ideal diagnostic strategy would be to obtain serial measurements of hCG, the levels of which generally double every 48 hours, but certainly should increase by more than 66% in that time period [8].

The natural progression of early pregnancy loss

A surprising number of pregnancies are lost within days of conception. Thereafter, the loss rate diminishes steeply until the twelfth week of gestation. For example, in one study where daily hCG levels were undertaken postconception, 22% of those pregnancies with an initially positive hCG never developed to a point where ultrasound demonstrated a viable pregnancy [8]. In another study from Australia, serum hCG levels were obtained at 16 days postconception in over 1000 patients having had IVF (in vitro fertilization) [9]. The average level was 182 mIU/mL in those with later pregnancy loss (8–19 weeks), compared with 233 mIU/mL in continuing pregnancies [10]. These data again strongly suggest that the die is cast soon after conception for many pregnancy losses. Below, the chances of a continuing pregnancy are laid out according to the ultrasound findings.

Ultrasound findings

When present	Chances of loss before 12 weeks
Gestational sac only	11.5%
Yolk sac only	8.5%
Embryo <6 mm	7.2%
Embryo between 5–10 mm	3.3%
Embryo >10 mm	0.5%

If first trimester bleeding occurs, the loss rates obviously increase. It has been estimated that about 25% of all patients will have some bleeding or spotting in the first trimester, and in half of these pregnancies a viable fetus will not materialize. The most common reason for early loss is aneuploidy. Ohno [11] found that 69.4% of products of conception from 144 spontaneous abortions yielded abnormal chromosomes, the majority representing trisomies. Also, the overwhelming majority of pregnancies are nonviable many days before vaginal bleeding ensues, and the size of the embryo will provide information as to when demise has occurred.

Ectopic pregnancy

The incidence of ectopic pregnancy is about 20/1000, but those with a past history of ectopic pregnancy have a 10-fold greater risk of this complication. Other predisposing factors include pregnancy by assisted reproductive technology (ART), infertility (in general), advanced maternal age, and cigarette smoking.

Identification rates with ultrasound alone range between 20 and 85% [12]. However, using ultrasound in combination with hCG levels improves the positive predictive value to 95% [13].

Since with transvaginal sonography (TVS) it is sometimes difficult to identify an extrauterine pregnancy, the first diagnostic stop should be the uterus. A true gestation sac should be present when the hCG is >2000 mIU/mL, and, in most cases is present when an hCG is >1000 mIU/mL. In general, hCG rises sluggishly in ectopic pregnancy, rarely ever doubling in 48 hours. However, very occasionally a normal early pregnancy will not meet the criteria for an expected rise. Therefore, if no adnexal mass is seen in a patient with symptoms of an ectopic, and the initial hCG level is between 1000 and 2000, a conservative approach might be warranted. On the other hand, if the hCG level is >2000 and no intrauterine sac is identified in a patient with symptoms of ectopic pregnancy, there is a very high likelihood of an extrauterine pregnancy. Obviously, the ultrasound finding of a fetus in the tube or even an adnexal mass should trump any of the above diagnostic subtleties in a symptomatic patient with a positive pregnancy test.

As indicated above, one can be fooled by the "pseudosac" (Figure 1.1b) that masquerades as a true intrauterine sac. It does not have a double ring and is not seen in conjunction with a yolk sac. Also, seeing an intrauterine sac does not completely rule out a heterotopic pregnancy when conception has been accomplished through ART. The prevalence of heterotopic pregnancy has been cited to be about 1 in 30,000, but with ART it could be as high as 1 in 100.

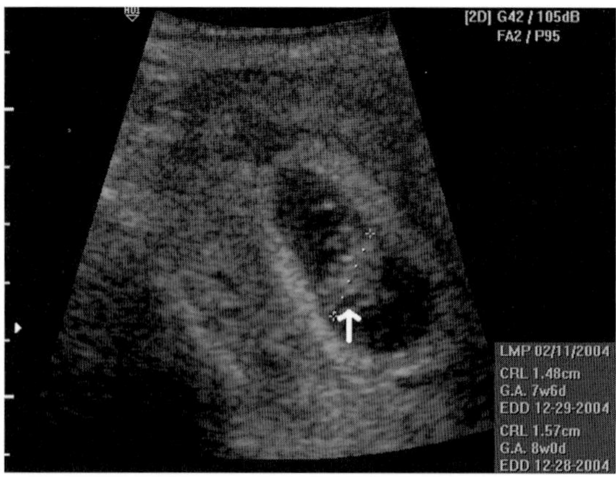

Fig 1.4 Seven-week embryo. Prominent echo-spared area is marked by an arrow.

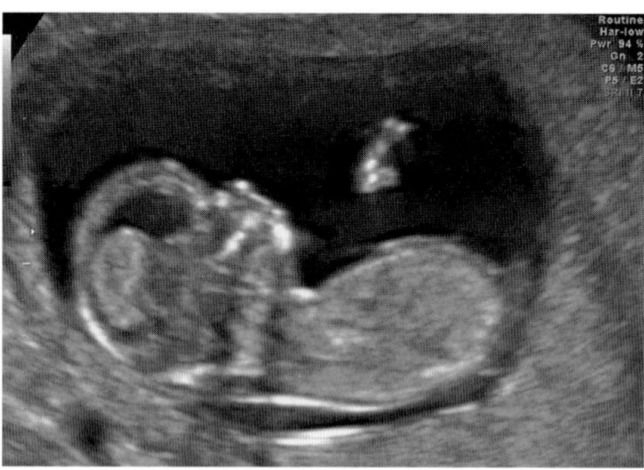

Fig 1.5 Normal first trimester fetus with frontal echo-spared area.

Identification of major fetal abnormalities in the first trimester

In the embryonic stage the organs are just forming so, in general, one must wait until organogenesis is complete and, most importantly, embryos are large enough to visualize, before making diagnostic judgments. An example of an early diagnostic misfire is thinking that an echo-spared structures in the posterior and anterior calvarium (Figures 1.4 and 1.5) before 11 menstrual weeks is an abnormality. With watchful waiting it will become clear that this finding actually represented the normal rhombencephalon that, although visually striking, should not have generated concern.

On occasion, seeing a ventral wall herniation prior to 11 1/2 weeks can raise unwarranted anxiety if one does not realize that this is a normal finding. If the herniation has a wide base, this could represent a true omphalocele, which is, fortunately, a rare finding (Figure 1.6).

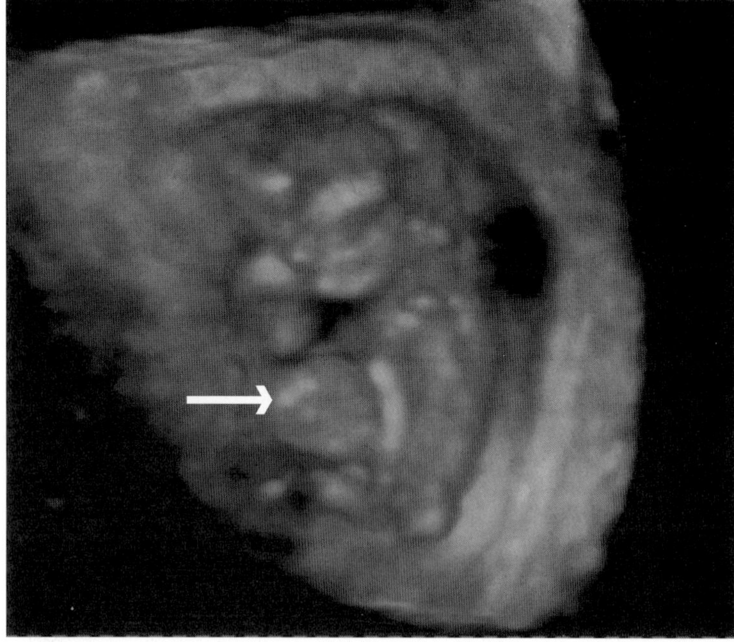

Fig 1.6 3D image of first trimester omphalocele. Arrows points to ventral wall defect.

Table 1.1 Studies in the literature dealing with the identification of anomalies with transvaginal ultrasound. (From Souka AP et al. [14], with permission from Elsevier.)

Author(s)	Population	*N*	Major anomalies (%)	First trimester sensitivity (%)	Total (%)
Hernardi and Torocsik (1997)	Low risk	3991	35 (0.9)	36	72
Economides and Braithwaite (1998)	Low risk	1632	13 (0.8)	54	77
Calvalho et al.	Low risk	2853	66 (2.3)	38	79
Taipale et al.	Low risk	4513	33 (0.7)	18	48
Chen et al.	High risk	1609	26 (1.6)	64	77
Souka et al.	Low risk	1148	14 (1.2)	50	92

Possible false negative observations can also occur. For example, the neural tube closes between 20 and 28 days postconception and a failure of closure early in that window will result in anencephaly. However, since the calvarium is not well mineralized until later in pregnancy, the rudimentary brain will herniate upward and often the fetal cranial pole will appear similar to that of an unaffected fetus. For this reason, in the past a few anencephalic fetuses have evaded diagnosis until after 11 weeks.

In the fetal period, there are now many reports of various fetal abnormalities being identified with 2D and 3D ultrasound, and the nonspecific finding of an increased nuchal translucency (NT) has allowed investigators to search more thoroughly with TVS for anomalies that might ordinarily have been missed.

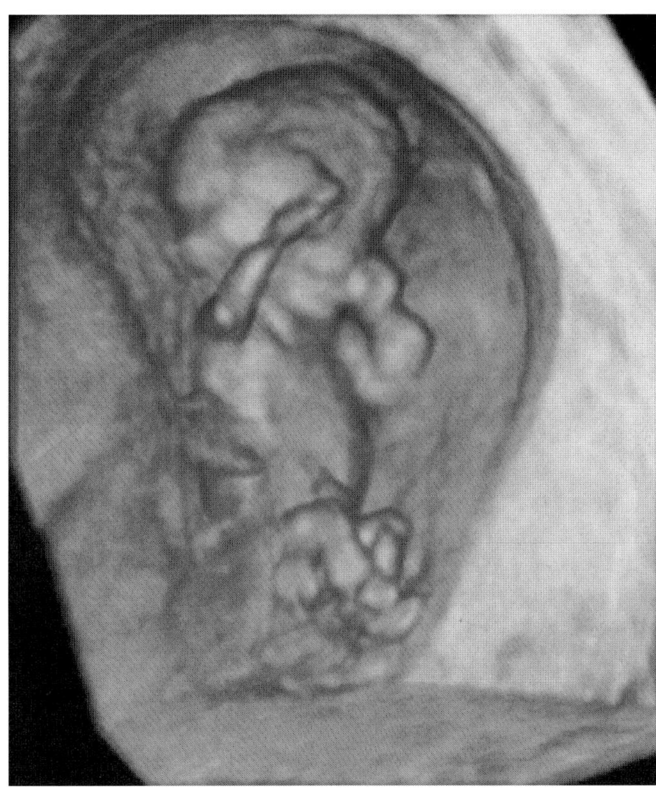

Fig 1.7 First trimester 3D.

Souka et al. [14]. published the results of studies in the literature dealing with the identification of anomalies with transvaginal ultrasound (Table 1.1).

Although 3D ultrasound can provide some beautiful images of the first trimester fetus (Figure 1.7), we utilize this generally useful tool infrequently in the first trimester except to get a better view of the NT when the position of the fetus persistently keeps us from using the necessary midline sagittal approach.

References

1 Goldstein SR, Wolfson R. Endovaginal ultrasonographic measurement of early embryonic size as a means of assessing gestational age. J Ultrasound Med 1994; 13: 27–31.

2 Wilcox AJ, Weinberg CR, O'Connor JF, et al. Incidence of early loss in pregnancy. N Engl J Med 1988; 319: 189–94.

3 Benacerraf BR, Bromley B, Laboda LA, et al. Small sac in the first trimester: a predictor of poor fetal outcome. Radiology 1991; 178: 375–7.

4 Goldstein SR. Significance of cardiac activity in very early embryos. Obstet Gynecol 1992; 80: 670–2.

5 Benson CB, Doubilet PM. Embryonic heart rate in the early first trimester: what rate is normal? J Ultrasound Med 1995; 14: 431–4.

6 Papageorghiou AT, Avigdou K, Spencer K, et al. Sonographic screening for trisomy 13 at 11 to 13^6 weeks of gestation. Am J Obstet Gynecol 2006; 194: 397–401.

7 Kadar N, Caldwell BV, Romero R. A method of screening for ectopic pregnancy and its indicator. Obstet Gynecol 1981; 58: 162–6.

8 Goldstein SR, Snyder JR, Watson C, et al. Very early pregnancy detection with endovaginal ultrasound. Obstet Gynecol 1988; 72: 200–4.

9 Tong S, Wallace EM, Rombauts L. Association between low day 16 hCG and miscarriage after proven cardiac activity. Obstet Gynecol 2006; 107: 300–4.

10 Goldstein SR. Early detection of pathologic pregnancy by tran- svaginal sonography. J Clin Ultrasound 1990; 18: 262–73.

11 Ohno M, Maeda T, Matsunobu A. A cytogenetic study of spontaneous abortions with direct analysis of chorionic villi. Obstet Gynecol 1991; 77: 394–8.

12 Brown DI, Doubilet PM. Transvaginal sonography for diagnosing ectopic pregnancy: positivity criteria and performance characteristics. J Ultrasound Med 1994; 13: 259–66.

13 Ankum WM, Hajenius PF, Schrevel LS, et al. Management of a suspected ectopic pregnancy. J Reprod Med 1996; 41: 724–8.

14 Souka AP, Pilalis A, Kavalakis I, et al. Screening for major structural anomalies at the 11-to-14 week ultrasound scan. Am J Obstet Gynecol 2006; 194: 393–6.

2 Placenta and umbilical cord

Everyone performing a standard ultrasound evaluation should systematically fulfill the criteria published jointly by the American Institute of Ultrasound in Medicine (AIUM) and the American College of Radiology (ACR). In the first part of this book, dealing with the findings unveiled during this examination, I will discuss each of the eight steps included in the above guidelines. Since each of the first three steps only warrants a few words, I will lump them together in this chapter on the placenta, a topic that deserves substantial attention.

Fetal presentation

The presentation of the fetus has little clinical meaning until the third trimester, when a breech presentation or a transverse lie should alert the clinician to the need for a cesarean section, the option of an external version, or the possibility of a placenta previa.

Very few obstetricians today will attempt to deliver a breech vaginally after a study emerged by Hannah et al. [1] suggesting a higher rate of perinatal mortality and morbidity when infants, presenting as breeches in late gestation, were delivered vaginally, rather than by cesarean section. Seemingly, this has put a permanent nail in the coffin for vaginal delivery in this setting, even though another paper later revealed the flaws in the above study, as well as later prospective studies showing no difference in outcomes between routes of delivery for breeches [2,3].

In the first and second trimester, fetal presentation has little bearing on whether a malpresentation will be found at term.

Fetal number

Looking for more than one fetus is an important 3-second task that has clinical impact, as well as providing insurance against the later embarrassment of someone else finding a missed twin or triplet. The identification of multiple gestations should single out a patient for a specific plan of management that could impact the outcome of pregnancy—as will be discussed in the section on twins.

Fetal life (viability)

I am mystified as to why the common practice today is to document scrupulously with M-mode the presence of a fetal heart rate. If you can see a heartbeat and there is clearly fetal movement, should that not be enough? I guess not, because the current paranoia is that there is always someone lurking in the shadows waiting for a sonographer/sonologist to make a diagnosis of intrauterine demise when there is no demise, or vice versa.

Examination of the placenta

This is a fetal organ, and many, if not most, of the problems fetuses can get into are linked in some way to the placenta. In fact, since early maternal complications, such as preeclampsia, can be directly traced to the placenta, it is surprising that the placenta garners so little attention in most obstetrical textbooks.

Placental position

Determining placental location is a requirement of every set of guidelines for a basic ultrasound examination. Frankly, however, the only real point of interest should be its relationship to the lower uterine segment and cervix. In other words, whether it is anterior, posterior, or fundal has little clinical bearing, as long as it is not within the immediate neighborhood of the cervix.

Let's look at the data in the literature. The incidence of placenta previa at the end of pregnancy is about 2.8/1000. However, it rises with increased parity, approaching 5%

Obstetric Ultrasound: Artistry in Practice. John C. Hobbins. Published 2008 Blackwell Publishing. ISBN 978-1-4051-5815-2.

in patients with five or more pregnancies. The rate of placenta previa is higher in AMA women, in those with twin pregnancies, and in those having had previous cesarean sections. With a cesarean section rate that has risen to 29% in the USA today, we can now expect to see an increase in the prevalence of placenta previa, and with it, an increase in associated complications, such as preterm birth and placenta accreta.

First, a low-lying placenta that is within 2 cm of the cervix (a Williams' textbook definition) should get one's attention, but the likelihood of this placenta remaining in this position is small. For example, about 5% will have a "placenta previa" diagnosed between 10 and 20 weeks, but only 10% of these will remain over, or close to, the endocervix at term [4]. However, if the diagnosis is made at 28 to 31 weeks, 62% will persist, and if found between 32 and 35 weeks, about 75% will remain at delivery.

In placenta previa, the extent to which the placenta overlaps the cervix appears to be extremely important. Studies show that if the placenta extends past the cervix by 1.5 cm in the second trimester, the likelihood of placenta previa at term is about 20% [5]. If the overlap is more than 2.4 cm, then 40% of these will remain [6]. The point is that the glass is more than half full even when the tip of the placenta is clearly over the cervix earlier in pregnancy (Figure 2.1).

Why does the placenta seem to migrate upward as pregnancy progresses? In the first trimester, the lower uterine segment makes up the lower 10% of the uterus. However, into the third trimester about 30% of the uterine volume is occupied by the lower uterine segment. The idea is that the placenta gets passively moved away from the cervix as the segment stretches out.

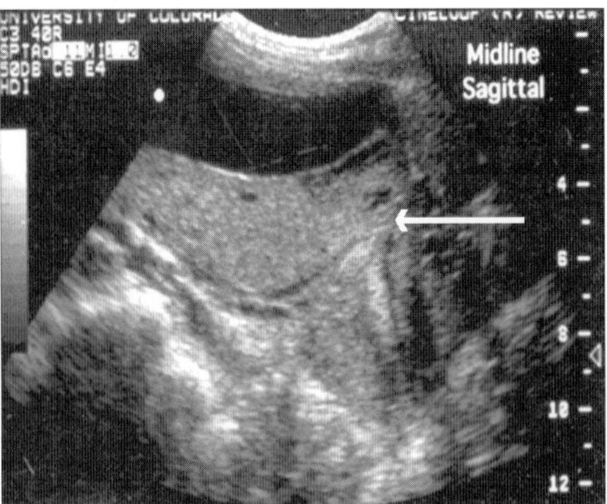

Fig 2.1 Placenta previa-transabdominal scan. Arrow points to endocervix.

Trophotropism [7] is an intriguing concept that also may explain this relative placental migration, and can also explain ectopic or velamentous insertions of the umbilical cord. The theory is that there are some areas within the uterine cavity where the placenta has chosen to alight that may not represent an ideal environment for it to flourish. So the placenta compensates by atrophying in the less hospitable area near or over the cervix, while, at the same time, proliferating northward to a territory that is more accepting. We documented this phenomenon by serial ultrasound examinations on at least two occasions where, with time, the umbilical cord insertion appeared to stay in the same relative position with regard to the cervix, while passively gravitating toward or, actually, onto the placental edge.

The message here is that, whatever the etiology, a majority of placentas initially noted to be in the neighborhood of the cervix will not remain there. If a second trimester patient has no symptoms, and the placenta does not overlap the cervix by more than 1.5 cm, there is no need to alter these patients' lifestyles by instituting "pelvic precautions," or by interdicting travel or exercise. In fact, in these patients we often avoid the use of the word "previa" and simply suggest that they return after 30 weeks for another examination unless there is intervening vaginal bleeding.

In the evaluation of a possible previa in patients with vaginal bleeding, the examination usually starts with a standard transabdominal approach. After identifying its relative location, one can then tell how high in the uterus the placenta starts. If there is any placenta in the vicinity of the fundus, it is unlikely that the placenta will be over the cervix by the end of pregnancy. However, this does not rule out an accessory lobe as a reason for the vaginal bleeding.

The next step is to evaluate the lower uterine segment. If there is truly a placenta previa, then the presenting part of the fetus will always be floating and one can easily move it out of the way so that the area of the endocervix can be examined (Figure 2.2). This should be done with a bladder that is not full because one can artificially create the impression of a low-lying placenta by the bladder compressing the lower uterine segment. The same confusion can also be created by lower uterine segment contractions that are often concentric (Figure 2.3).

The transvaginal examination with the bladder empty represents the best way ultimately to make the diagnosis of placenta previa (Figure 2.4), although the combination of transabdominal ultrasound (TAU) and transvaginal ultrasound (TVS) may be needed to identify an accessory lobe. The crux of this endeavor is to make sure

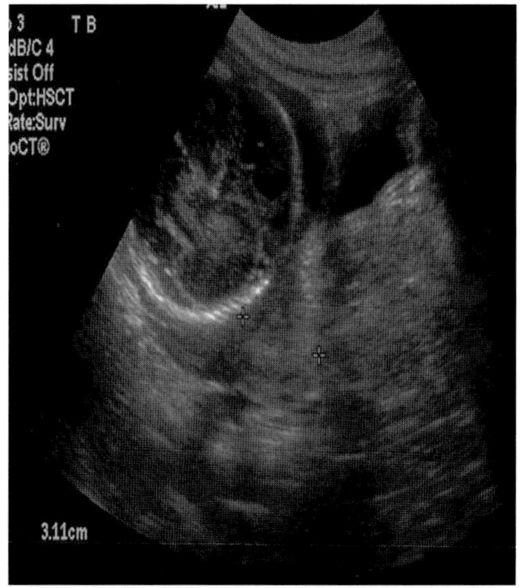

(a)

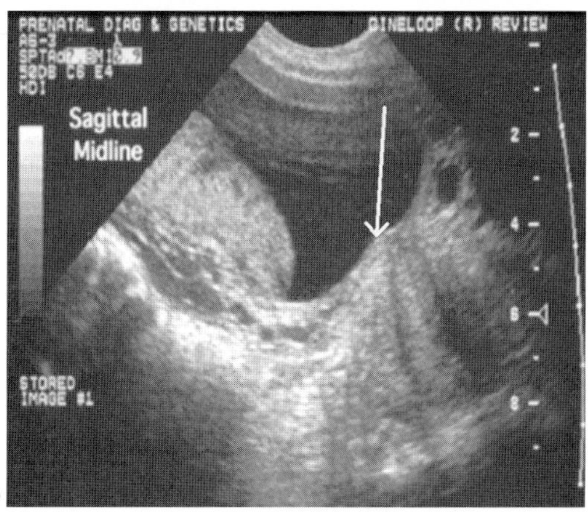

(b)

Fig 2.2 (a) Head obscuring view of cervix and placenta. (b) Previa excluded after head removed. Arrow points to endocervix.

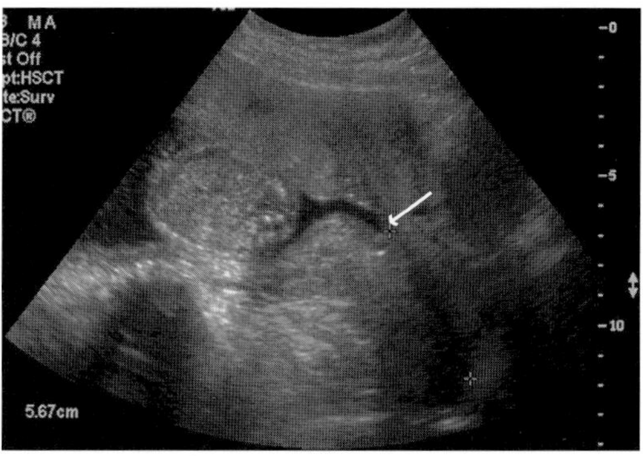

Fig 2.3 Concentric contraction obscuring endocervix. Arrow marks the probable location of the endocervix.

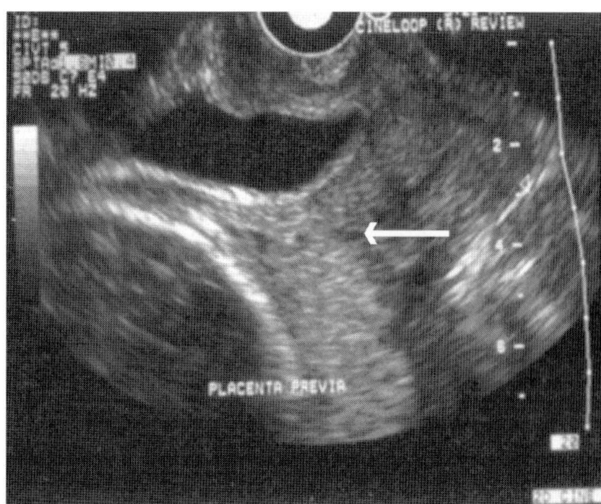

Fig 2.4 Placenta just covering cervix in late gestation by transvaginal scan. Arrow marks endocervix.

nothing—placenta, umbilical cord, or interconnecting vessels to an accessory lobe—is in the vicinity of the cervix.

Some have advocated the use of transperineal ultrasound (TPU) to evaluate the endocervix. Perhaps TPU evolved when clinicians were reluctant to enter the vagina with an ultrasound probe in someone who was bleeding from a possible placenta previa. However, the TVS probe goes in the vagina and not in the cervix and, although TPU can often produce reasonable views of the cervix, it is inferior to TVS in locating the placenta.

A case in point regarding placental position

Patient was sent in for consultation because she was noted to have "placenta previa" at 21 weeks. She reported no bleeding but had been on reduced activity and pelvic precautions, since the diagnosis was made. We found a low-lying posterior placenta that was just touching the endocervix. The cervical length measured at 3.5 cm. We indicated that the chances of her having a placenta previa at term were very small, and that she could return to normal daily activities. However, she should report any vaginal bleeding or spotting.

Our reward was a big box of candy from her husband. The couple had grown tired of their routine daily regimen of abstinence.

Vasa previa

This potentially lethal problem complicates approximately 1 in 2500 pregnancies. One recent study [8] indicates that

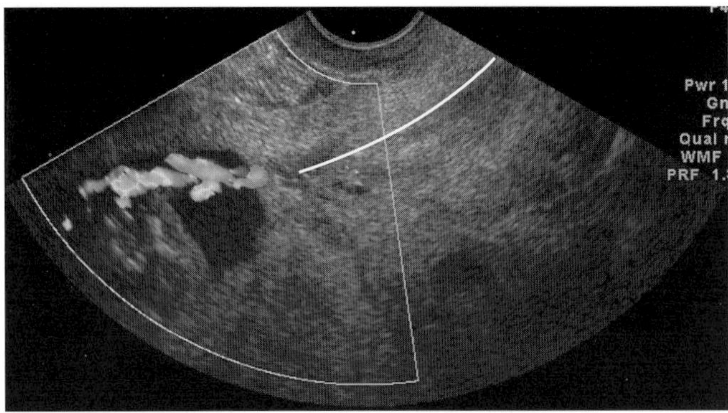

Fig 2.5 Vasa previa. Line marks cervical canal.

if the diagnosis is known prior to delivery, the perinatal survival improves from 44 to 96%.

As suggested above, there are two ways that vasa previa can occur. First, when the connecting vessels from a primary placenta to an accessory lobe course directly over the cervix. Secondly, where a velamentous insertion of the cord resides in the membranes immediately over the cervix. In the latter case, the trophotropism theory of Bernischke fits the clinical picture. Since the vascular environment of the lower uterine segment is poorly suited to support placental development, the placenta preferentially grows superiorly while atrophying inferiorly, leaving the umbilical cord in the same place—over the cervix—but with no cushion of intervening placental tissue (Figures 2.5 and 2.6).

Although standard guidelines for the performance of a basic ultrasound examination do not include a search for the cord insertion, from the above statistics it is clear that this simple task can occasionally be lifesaving by alerting the clinician to perform a timely cesarean section. Cord insertion assessment certainly should be accomplished in those in whom there is a question of placenta previa.

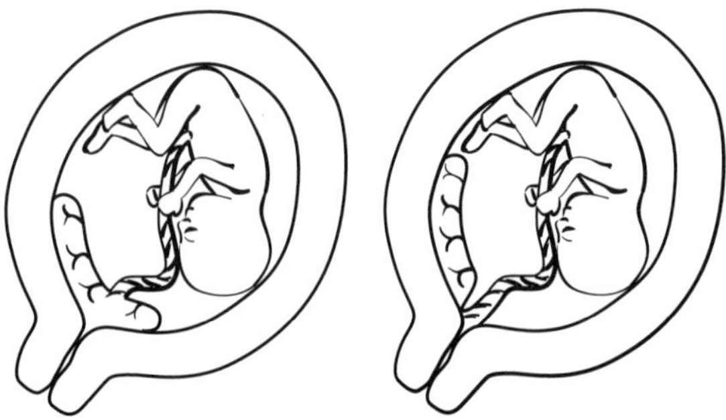

Fig 2.6 Trophotropism: evolution of vasa previa.

The diagnosis of vasa previa itself can be made with color Doppler demonstration of vessels or a cord immediately over the endocervix. This is best done with TVS, and with pulse Doppler the artery in question can be seen to be beating at a fetal rate.

Patients in whom a search for the cord insertion should always be undertaken are those conceived through IVF. One study shows that their risk of vasa previa is about 1 in 293 [9].

Placenta accreta

This complication occurs in about 1 in 10 patients with placenta previa, compared with 4 per 10,000 in others [10]. The risk for this condition is elevated in patients over 35 with previa who have had a previous cesarean section. They have a 40% chance of placenta accreta.

Finberg [11] initially laid out some diagnostic suggestions that have continued to hold true. However, the individual most recently cited in the literature is Comstock [12], who has shown that the strongest clues to its presence are placental lakes, often in the area just underneath an old cesarean scar, that possess a typical slow lacunar flow. Although, by definition, the placenta invades into the myometrium, focusing on the uterine wall can be unrewarding since, at times, it is difficult to outline an uninterrupted myometrial margin (clear space), even when there is no accreta (Plate 2.1).

The diagnosis is easier to make when there is invasion through the serosa (increta), or into the bladder (percreta), conditions which unfortunately have serious maternal consequences (Figure 2.7).

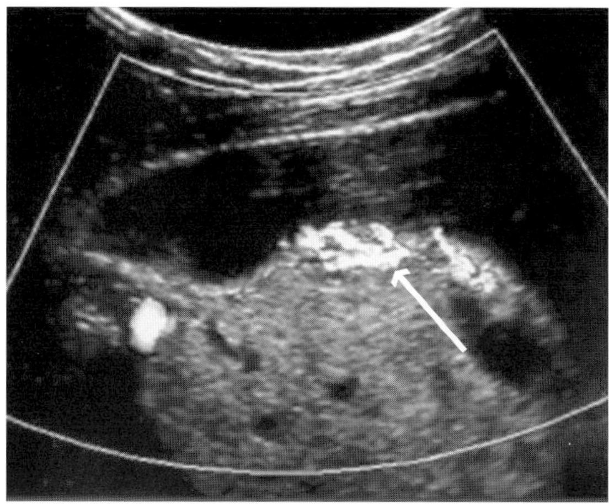

Fig 2.7 Percreta. Arrow points to bladder-uterine wall interface.

One must be careful when using color Doppler not to mistake dilated basal veins (Figure 2.8) for the tornado-shaped lacunar areas synonymous with accreta. The former will have a clear rim of myometrium under them.

Since one-half of patients with placenta accreta will have elevations of maternal serum alpha-fetoprotein (MSAFP) generally well above 2.5 multiples of the median (MoM), this finding should raise one's diagnostic antennas in a patient either at risk for placenta accreta or in someone in whom there are suspicious ultrasound signs for this condition [13,14]. Also, a normal MSAFP will provide added reassurance that imaging studies are correct in excluding accreta in those clinically at risk for this serious complication.

As opposed to some authors, we have found MRI to be useful adjunctively when the evidence for placenta accreta is equivocal. Frankly, it is often the only way to get at a posterior placenta. However, be prepared when reading the report for the hedge—the official plant of the radiologist.

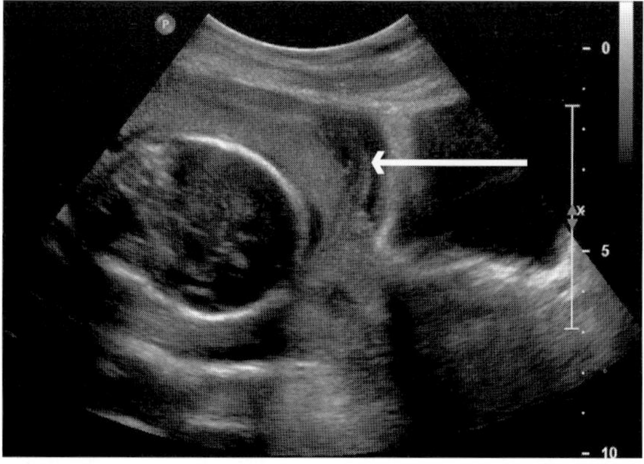

Fig 2.8 Pseudoaccreta at 19 weeks. Arrow marks normal dilated basal veins.

The umbilical cord insertion

In the vast majority of cases, it matters little where the umbilical cord inserts on the placenta. However, there are some exceptions. As noted above, if a marginal insertion is directly over the cervix, this can have disastrous consequences. Also velamentous (Plate 2.2) or marginal insertions (Plate 2.3) have been associated with a higher rate of intrauterine growth restriction (IUGR), especially in twins, and can be associated with an unusual configuration to an umbilical artery waveform (a "notch" in the systolic downslope) [15].

A very interesting paper from Japan [16] just surfaced, which should get our attention. The authors compulsively evaluated the cord insertion sites in 3446 patients and found 40 with velamentous insertions (VIs). Two important observations emerged from their data. The closer to the cervix the VI was, the longer were the exposed vessels (10 cm in the lower segment vs 4 cm in the upper or middle uterine segments). Also, the incidences of variable decelerations and "nonreassuring fetal status" were 80% when the VI was in the lower segment versus 60 and 13%, respectively, when VI was above this location, and the cesarean section rate was 80% with lower segment VIs versus 10% when the insertions were elsewhere. The idea here is that the absence of Wharton's jelly in the exposed cord makes it extremely vulnerable to compression.

Circulation of the placenta

Although the placenta functions as a well-oiled instrument that depends upon a highly integrated relationship between maternal and fetal compartments, I will deal with the two compartments separately.

The maternal side

The blood enters the intervillous space via the spiral arteries, which are the final tributaries of the uterine artery. Along the way, the uterine artery becomes the arcuate artery, which runs parallel to the uterine cavity, sending off small vascular branches (radial arteries) that are earmarked to perfuse the placenta. These ultimately become the spiral arteries that dump maternal blood into the intervillous space. Through the years, there have been

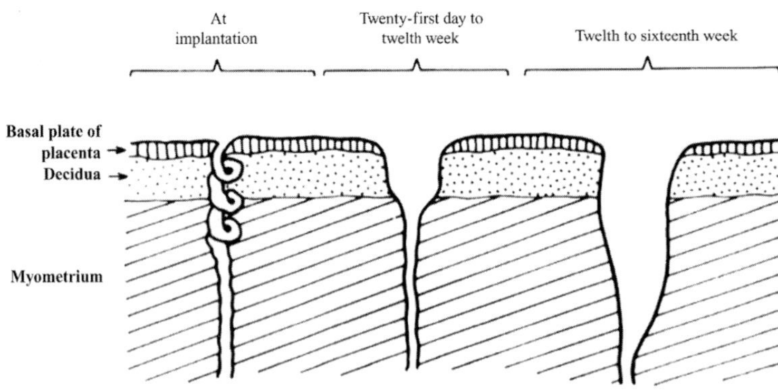

Fig 2.9 Maternal spiral artery conversion (from Reece EA, Hobbins JC (eds), Medicine of the Fetus and Mother, 2nd edition. Philadelphia: Lippincott Williams & Wilkins, 1999, with permission).

conflicting theories as to whether the blood is deposited into the middle of a fetal tissue unit where the oxygen and nutrients are transferred to the fetal side of the placenta from inside out, or whether the blood shoots up into the ubiquitous intervillous space where its bathes the fetal cotyledons from the outside in. We will let others fight that out and simply assume the blood enters the space through these tiny spiral arteries, which undergo two important transformations.

In the first trimester, the spiral arteries are rather stiff, narrow, spiral-like vessels, but by about 12 weeks, they are invaded by the trophoblast in the decidual plate, which opens the ends of these arteries, creating a decrease in resistance to flow into the intervillous space. Gradually, by 18 weeks the myometrial portions of the spiral arteries are similarly invaded, creating even lesser impedance to flow (Figure 2.9). Occasionally this trophoblastic invasion is delayed until about 24 weeks, but rarely should it occur after this time.

The fetal side of the placenta is very much dependent upon the above maternal changes evolving smoothly because during this same time a steady flow of blood into the space is required for proper development of branching angiogenesis. Also, as initially noted by Bronsens many years ago, failure of trophoblastic invasion has been associated with preeclampsia and has been linked to other conditions such as IUGR, thrombophilia, and premature rupture of the membranes. As indicated later, the way to tell whether this transformation has occurred is through Doppler waveform analysis of the upstream uterine arteries.

The fetal side

The fetal side of the placenta develops in three stages. In the first trimester primary villi, composed mostly of mesenchymal tissue, move downward toward the basal plate to provide stability during a time when the placenta plays a somewhat passive role. Toward the end of the first trimester, when the framework is more complete, the primary villi and secondary villi, along with their vessels, branch into 10 to 15 subbranches and sub-subbranches (Figure 2.10). Not surprisingly, this is called branching angiogenesis, and this process continues until the twenty-fourth week of gestation, when it gives way to a stage of nonbranching angiogenesis. Here the capillaries in the villus tissue grow faster than the underlying venules and arterioles, doubling over onto themselves while forming the terminal villi which are responsible for the transfer of oxygen and nutrient to the fetus.

Basically, the more terminal villi and the more branches there are in the placenta, the greater is the available surface area in contact with the intravillus space and the more efficient is the nutrient delivery system. Obviously, the converse situation of fewer branches and a paucity of terminal villi will result not only in a smaller fetus, but one prone to all of the morbidities of fetal growth restriction.

There are two ways to assess the lushness of the fetal circulation: Doppler waveform analysis of the umbilical

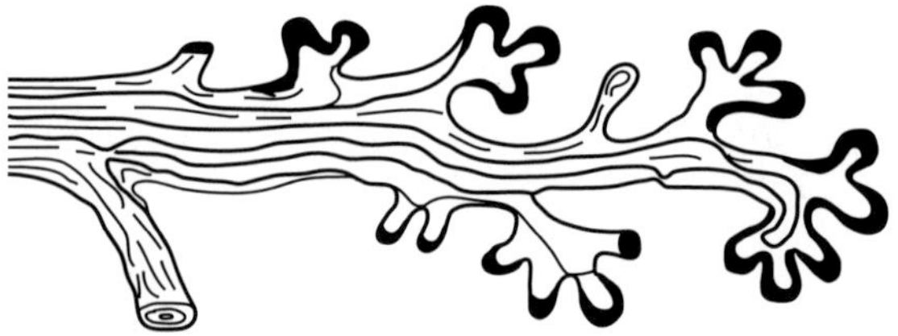

Fig 2.10 Villous tree.

arteries, and, now, 3D color Doppler mapping of the placental circulation.

Placental size

Through the years, investigators have attempted to assess placental size through three diameter calculations or, recently, by 3D volume algorithms. Anterior placentas are more accessible. They also have a fairly consistent planoconvex configuration. However, fundal placentas do not, and, in the third trimester, posterior placentas are inaccessible because they are mostly shadowed by the fetus.

Years ago we pursued the concept of measuring placental size and, after some frustration, we defaulted to simply assessing placental thickness. Although we never published these data, I will pass them on.

The thickness of the placenta (when measured at right angles to the long axis) increases linearly throughout pregnancy until about 33 weeks (when the normal process of hyperplasia stops and hypertrophy alone takes over). At that time the average thickness is 3.5 cm, and after that point, many placentas actually thin out to about 3 cm. These observations are not useful as predictors of early growth curtailment, but they were helpful in defining a true macrosomic placenta, when the measurement is over 5 cm.

Macroplacentas

In most cases, a macroplacenta is suspected by "eyeballing" how much intrauterine space it seems to be occupying (Figure 2.11). However, it is best to use the placental thickness concept mentioned above. Most often a large placenta is a normal variant. However, there are some diagnostic possibilities to explore before writing off this finding. Is the placenta uniformly echogenic poor? If so, undiagnosed diabetes is a possibility. Also, simple nondiabetic macrosomia is another explanation (big fetuses come with big placentas). Rare causes include unsuspected anemia, hydrops, or infectious agents such as cytomegalovirus. Often placentas will have large lakes that tend to expand the placenta. Other very rare causes of large placentas include "fascinomas" such as diffuse chorioangiomas, partial moles, or a rare complication of chronic abruption, a Breus mole (Figure 2.12).

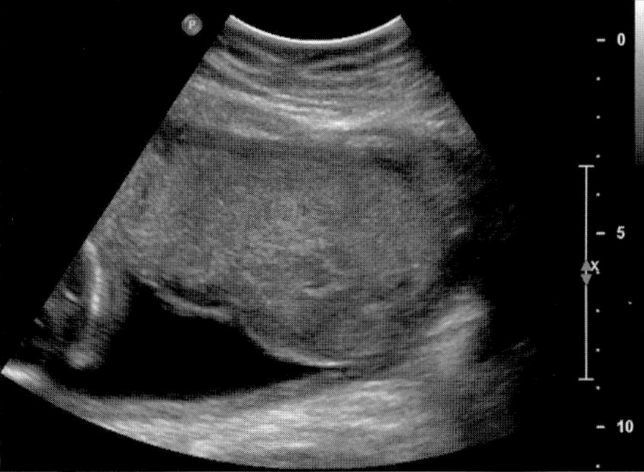

Fig 2.11 Macroplacenta.

Another case in point

This patient was referred for an ultrasound evaluation because she had had intermittent, but significant, vaginal bleeding since the first trimester. The fetus was small-for-gestational age at 21 weeks and there was very little amniotic fluid. The placenta was very large and mottled in appearance, while seemingly pinning the fetus against the back wall of the small cavity (Figure 2.12). The differential diagnosis included, in addition to the abruption, a partial mole, a bizarre form of infection, or placental mosaicism.

Since the amniotic cavity was not easily approachable and the full thickness of the placenta would have to be traversed to get there, we chose to do a placental biopsy. The sample had sparse amounts of villi and an abundance of rose-colored fluid. This came back with a normal karyotype (ruling out a partial mole accompanied by the usual triploid fetus). When on serial ultrasound evaluations the fetal growth further sputtered and the fetal lung volume plateaued to a point where the situation was unsalvageable, we and the patient jointly decided not to postpone the inevitable, and she was induced. After the delivery, she had an opportunity to hold her baby.

The placenta showed evidence of a Breus mole, a rare condition secondary to chronic abruption where blood dissects upward from the basal plate into the placental mass.

Although the possibility of this mechanism for the macroplacenta crossed our minds at the first visit, I led myself down another pathway as the clinical plot thickened. Now, for a time, I will probably think of this rare condition first every time I see a macroplacenta and will be reminded of this remarkable patient and her husband who refused to give up throughout weeks of increasingly worsening news.

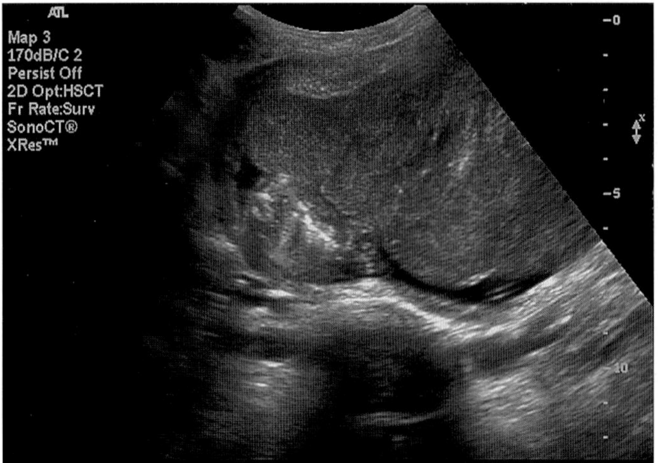

Fig 2.12 Breus mole.

Placental lakes

In the vast majority of cases placental lakes are innocuous findings, even though some of the vacant areas in placental architecture can be dramatic (Figure 2.13). They can be found anywhere in the placenta—in the margin, in the subchorionic space, or hugging the basal plate. They simply represent areas not filled in with villus tissue, which can provide a window into the fascinating dynamics of flow in the intervillous space. Do not expect to pick up this flow with color Doppler or even power Doppler, because the flow is too slow to create much of a frequency change. The way to distinguish the lake from an infarction, cystic degeneration, or clot in the placental margin is to magnify the lake and simply watch the swirling, Brownian-like movement within the echo-spared area. As indicated below, the only finding of concern is when multiple small lakes are noted in the basal portion of the placenta, especially in the neighborhood of a cesarean section scar, as seen in placenta accreta. Variations on the placental lake theme contribute the vast majority of cases to the category having the initials FLP (funny-looking placentas). They are occasionally associated with an elevation in MSAFP, which is of fetal origin and traverses the placenta more easily when lakes are present.

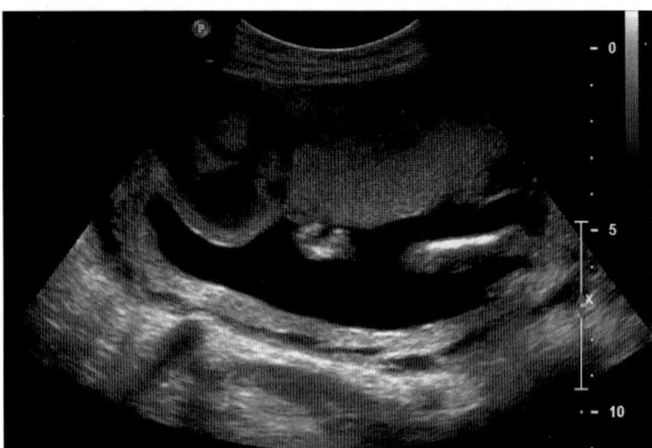

Fig 2.13 Impressive placental lakes.

Abruption

Placental separations most frequently occur in the placental periphery. The blood then tracks extramembranously to and through the cervix. If it stops along the way as a clot (Figures 2.14 and 2.15), the diagnosis can be confirmed, but about half of the time it does not, thereby leaving behind no traces. In these cases, the diagnosis is made by excluding a placenta previa and documenting clinically that the bleeding is coming from inside the cervix and not from the cervix itself.

The most common misconception is that the diagnosis can be made by identifying with ultrasound a separation between the placenta and the uterine wall. This is rarely the case, and if there is truly a large enough separation to be that obvious, the patient is usually in the operating room and not the ultrasound suite.

The easiest way to find a clot is to scout the lower uterine segment adjacent to the inferior margin of the placenta, and a tenting of the membranes will alert the operator to the presence of a clot. Later, often the clot will have been passed, leaving a potential space into which maternal blood will flow, creating a marginal lake.

Since abruption can be associated with disseminated intravascular coagulation and, very occasionally, intrauterine demise, the management of abruption used to be more

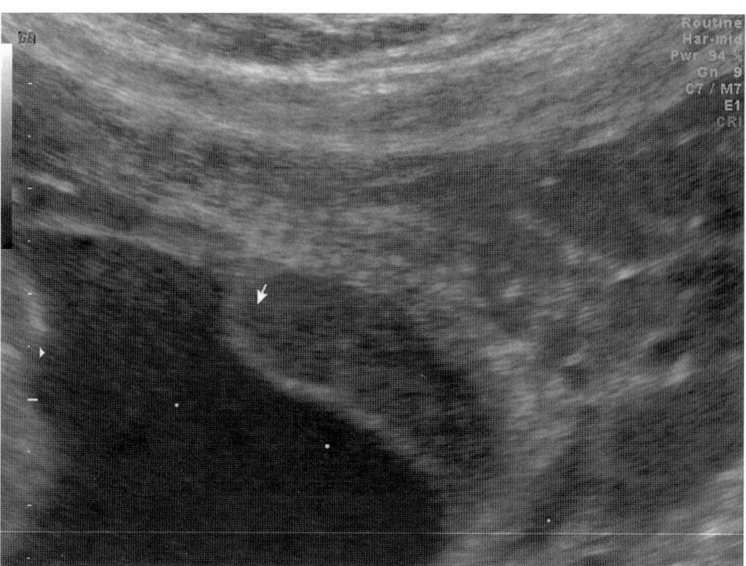

Fig 2.14 Extra membranous clot with tenting of membranes.

aggressive, resulting in a very hawk-like movement toward delivery once the diagnosis of abruption was contemplated. However, the vast majority of abruptions are minor, self-limited, and nonrecurrent, and we now have ways of safely monitoring the condition with serial ultrasound examinations and blood tests.

My feeling is, clot or no clot, the management is the same prior to term—to watch and wait if the patient is clinically stable and not contracting. Many clinicians prescribe bed rest, which, while making empiric sense, probably has little benefit, and the outcome is usually excellent after only one vaginal bleed.

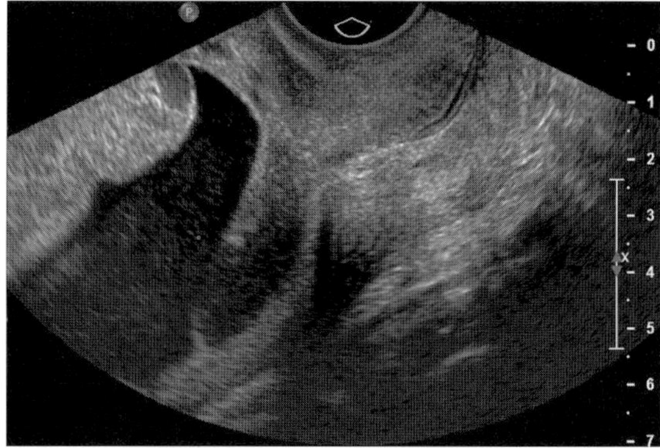

Fig 2.15 Extra membranous clot over cervix.

I have been very skeptical about the concept of "silent abruption." We have encountered patients who, although experiencing no vaginal bleeding, were referred with a diagnosis of a "clot" or an "area of placental separation." In virtually all these cases, the clot winds up being a marginal lake (Figure 2.16), or the separation being echo-spared dilated basal veins.

The overwhelming majority of patients with one vaginal bleed will not have a recurrence. However, they do have a higher rate of preterm birth, and premature rupture of the membranes. In the latter case, Lockwood has postulated that the presence of the components of the clot itself will have a direct effect on the integrity of the membranes. Also, with abruption the membranes are separated from their source of nutrition for some time, making them more susceptible to rupture.

Placental grading

In 1979, Grannum [17] published a placental grading classification that was originally designed to replace amniocentesis for fetal pulmonary maturity. Although the most mature grade [3] placenta was a very reasonable predictor of pulmonic maturity, it was only found in about 15% of term pregnancies. For a while placental grading was in vogue, and it was even incorporated by some into the standard biophysical profile (to be discussed later), but, of late, the grading system has largely fallen by the wayside.

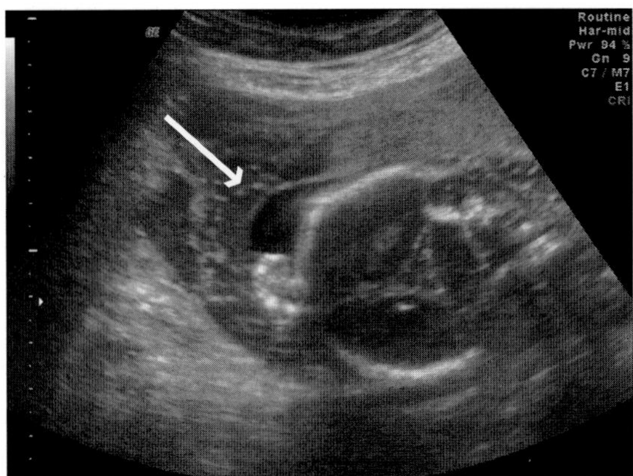

Fig 2.16 Dilated marginal veins causing pseudoabruption. Arrow points to dilated veins adjacent to placenta, mimicking a clot.

There are two observations from the initial placental grading investigation that have stood the test of time.

One study [18] showed a reduction of stillbirth when added to a standard ultrasound regimen used after 24 weeks, suggesting indirectly that a grade 3 placenta prior to 36 weeks speaks for a higher rate of perinatal mortality.

We have found that the finding of a grade 3 placenta prior to 36 weeks (premature placenta senescence) occurs quite frequently in IUGR and maternal hypertension, and often precedes the emergence of clinical signs. A good percentage of placentas demonstrating premature senescence are seen in smokers.

For the above reasons, I will present a rephrased version (Table 2.1) and schematic (Figure 2.17) of Grannum's original description of the grading system. Although, in general, the placenta always is flecked with echogenic material in later pregnancy, the feature that labels a placenta as being grade 3 is the presence of at least two echo dense septa that run all the way through the placenta, creating two separate compartments, probably representing individual cotyledons (Figure 2.17).

That said, even Grannum would want us today to move on to more specific information provided by contemporary ultrasound.

Abnormalities of the cord

Long cords can get into trouble. The mean length of an umbilical cord at term is 50 cm and, theoretically, according to some authors, the longer the cord, the more active the fetus (a good sign). In general, the longer the cord, the

Table 2.1 Placental grading system.

	Grade 0	Grade 1
Chorionic plate	Straight and well defined	Subtle undulations
Placental substance	Homogeneous	Few scattered echogenic areas
Basal layer	No densities	No densities
	Grade 2	**Grade 3**
Chorionic plate	Indentations extending into but not to the basal layer	Indentations communicating with the basal layer
Placental substance	Linear echogenic densities (comma-like densities)	Circular densities with echo-spared areas in center; large irregular densities that case acoustic shadowing
Basal layer	Linear arrangement of small echogenic areas (basal stippling)	Large and somewhat confluent basal echogenic areas; can create acoustic shadows

greater the chance for it to get tangled or to find its way around the fetus's neck, or on very rare occasions, to get tangled.

One interesting concept that has emerged is that a "sick" fetus will have a straighter cord (Plate 2.4). This has blossomed into an assessment of cord "coiling."

The idea is that a vigorous fetus will be attached to a well-coiled cord. This has stimulated some investigators to study the degree of coiling, the coiling index (CI). An umbilical cord coils on average 11 times throughout its length. There does seem to be an association between the absence of coiling and very adverse outcomes, such as fetal death, IUGR, anomalies, fetal distress (currently known by the euphemism "nonreassuring heart rate"). Now the concept is being pushed further to quantify the degree of "hypocoiling," reflected in coils per centimeter of cord. Strong [19] found that when there were less than 0.10 coils per centimeter, 40% had nuchal cords compared with only 4.8% when 0.3 coils were seen per centimeter. However, as will be discussed later, nuchal cords are common and are mainly innocuous.

I feel that a noncoiled cord should get everyone's attention, but to attempt to quantify how many coils there are per centimeter is not worth the effort and is, at best, a very weak reflector of fetal condition that can be far better appreciated by other means such as Doppler's or biophysical testing.

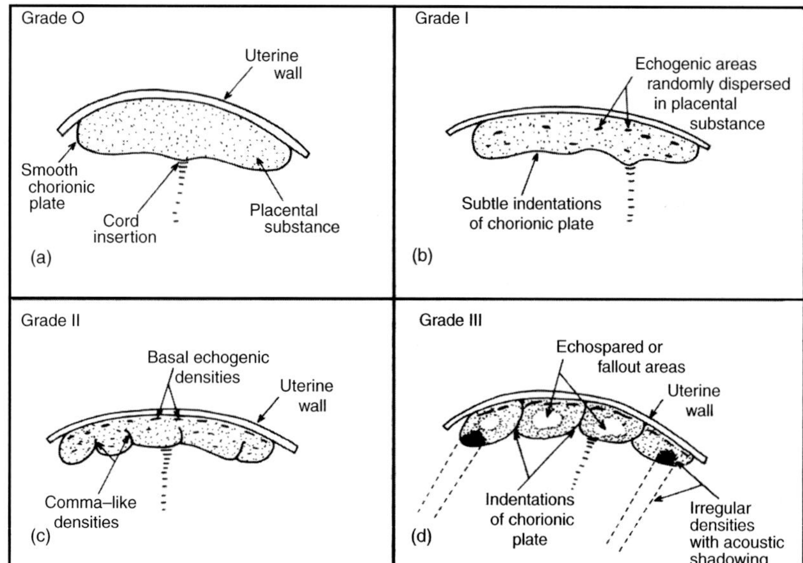

Fig 2.17 Placental grading by Grannum. Diagram showing the ultrasonic appearance of (a) grade 0 placenta, (b) grade 1 placenta, (c) grade 2 placenta, (d) grade 3 placenta. (From Grannum PA et al. [17] with permission from Elsevier.)

Single umbilical artery

A single umbilical artery is found in 0.2 to 1% of pregnancies, but it seems more common to us. Since it has been associated with a higher rate of fetal anomalies, it is important to make sure that there really is only one artery before assigning this stigma to a pregnancy. In the late second and third trimester a typical cross-section of the umbilical cord will yield an image of the larger umbilical vein alongside the paired umbilical arteries (Figure 2.18). However, the best way to confirm the diagnosis is to approach the fetal ventral wall with color Doppler to track the umbilical arteries as they split to enclose the fetal bladder (Plate 2.5). Although the angle of insonation may make one artery seem smaller than the other in the fetal pelvis, these vessels can truly be discordant in size and have different waveforms. However, it is difficult to tell if the higher resistance in the smaller vessel is due to the size of the vessel or to a difference in downstream resistance. For example, as indicated in the sections on twins and IUGR, the umbilical vessels supposedly anastomose briefly at their insertion site on the placenta before again splitting apart. According to the one and only paper describing this finding, only about 5% do not come together. However, our Doppler investigation challenges that assertion. Nevertheless, whether or not the umbilical arteries join may be a moot point since, with directional streaming, one umbilical artery could logically be assigned to one side of the placenta that might have decreased perfusion and increased resistance (fewer terminal villi or branches, or even, infarction), compared with its arterial companion, which is involved more with the more lush side.

A variant of the single umbilical artery theme is a segmental fusion occurring anywhere along the length of the umbilical cord, and this may be the reason for an erroneous diagnosis of a single umbilical artery being made with cross-sectional views alone. It is unclear if this fusion is associated with the same risk of anomalies as a true single umbilical artery. However, increased rates of velamentous and marginal insertions have been reported with this finding.

Back to a true single umbilical artery, since it is doing the work of two it often has a larger diameter (vein-to-artery ratio of less than 2) and, even in the face of IUGR, it may not show a typical decrease in end diastolic flow.

Many studies have documented the association between single umbilical artery and congenital anomalies. These rates varied in the literature between 33 and 74%. The major anomalies most commonly associated with single umbilical artery involve the fetal heart, central nervous system, and renal system [20]. The only chromosome abnormalities linked with single umbilical artery are trisomy 18 and 13. Unfortunately, this has stimulated some authors to recommend karyotyping for this finding. I disagree. In the second trimester trisomy 18 and trisomy 13 are not likely to be missed, and if a thorough search for ultrasound markers for trisomies is unproductive, the likelihood of the

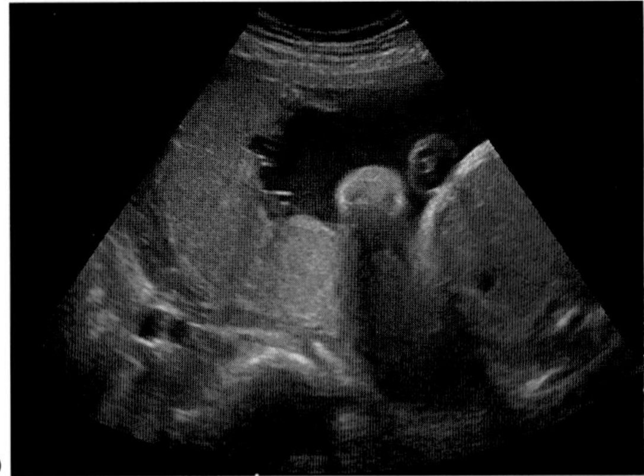

(a)

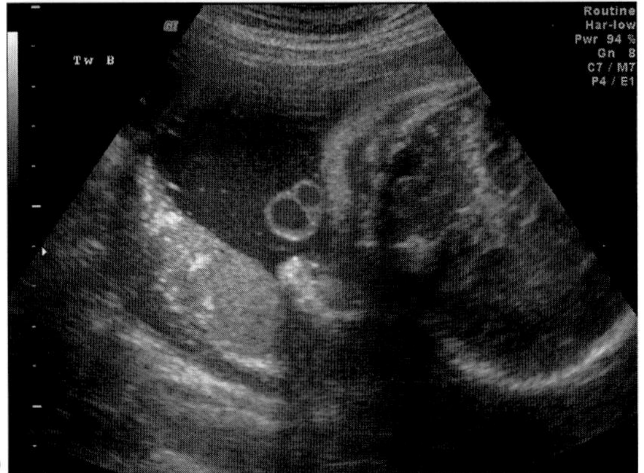

(b)

Fig 2.18 (a) A cross-section through three-vessel cord. (b) Single umbilical artery.

fetus having either chromosome abnormality is less than the risk of amniocentesis.

Regarding the risk of a nonchromosome abnormality, the above-mentioned organ systems must be thoroughly evaluated when a single umbilical artery is found. If any fetal anomaly is found, then the risk of any aneuploidy also increases appreciably and would warrant amniocentesis and a fetal echocardiogram.

Cord around the neck (CAN)

The inadvertent finding of an umbilical CAN (Plate 2.6) creates angst that in virtually every case is unnecessary [16]. Nevertheless, once this is found, the management becomes a conundrum. The major reason for the extra attention that it generates is that stillbirth occurs in approximately 6/1000 pregnancies in the USA, and a good proportion of these are unexplained. Since about 1 in 5 fetuses have at least one loop of CAN at delivery, the "unexplained" has a tendency to become the "explained." Obviously, there are rare cases where a true knot is seen in the cord or where there is pathological evidence of clot or obstruction to the umbilical vein that can explain the fetal demise. Occasionally, these cases wind up in the courts and, therefore, it is no wonder that this ultrasound finding strikes fear in the hearts of not only the patient, but also her provider.

Let's put this finding in perspective. In one observational study [21] involving 11,200 deliveries, 19% of infants were born with one loop of CAN, 5.3% had two loops, and 1.2% had three. From an ultrasound perspective, in a recent study follow-up information was obtained from 118 consecutive fetuses diagnosed with ultrasound to have cords around the neck between 17 and 36 weeks [22]. These data were compared with 233 matched controls. There was no difference in time of birth, cesarean section rate, abnormal fetal heartrate patterns, meconium-stained amniotic fluid, low Apgar scores, or admissions to the newborn special care unit. In another study [23] in which 18% of infants had a nuchal cord at delivery, there were no differences in outcomes, but, interestingly, only 37.5% of those with nuchal cords were detected by ultrasound prior to induction or cesarean section. Perhaps this is good news from a clinical standpoint, based on the unnecessary anxiety this inadvertent finding creates.

Based on all of the available data, here is what I feel should be done with the chance finding of a CAN. If a single loop is noted and the patient does not complain of decreased fetal movement, then there is every indication that this is a normal variant. If the provider feels that it is necessary to apprise the patient of the finding, then it should be couched in a very reassuring manner. If more than one loop of cord is seen, then a simple nonstress test can be accomplished, looking for any sign of repetitive bradycardia or decreased beat-to-beat variability.

There have been a few isolated and conflicting reports of changes in Doppler waveform that have been seen in conjunction with CAN, and Abuhamad has described a small notch in the downslope of the umbilical artery waveform in association with VIs of the cord, tangled cords

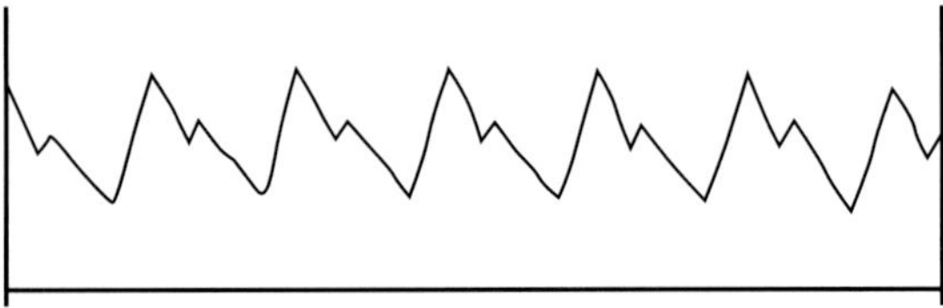

Fig 2.19 Schematic of circulation of CSF in aqueductal stenosis. Notch in downslop when cord is impinged.

in monoamniotic twins, and, although not yet published, rare cases of CAN [15] (Figure 2.19).

On the basis of the rarity of a CAN being associated with, or certainly responsible for, intrauterine demise, the clinician would be most wise to interrupt the pregnancy only if there is a sign of impending trouble, such as decreased fetal movement and/or fetal heartrate abnormalities suggestive of cord impingement. Also, this should only be considered if the fetus is, or is close to being, mature.

References

1 Hannah ME, Hannah WJ, Hewson SA, et al. Planned caesarean section versus planned vaginal birth at breech presentation at term: a randomized multicentre trial. Term Breech Trial Collaborative Group. Lancet 2000; 356: 1375–83.

2 Goffinet F, Carayol M, Foidart JM, et al. Is planned vaginal delivery for breech presentation at term still an option? Results of an observational prospective study in France and Belgium. Am J Obstet Gynecol 2006; 194: 1002–11.

3 Alarab M, Regan C, O'Connell MP, et al. Singleton vaginal breech delivery at term: still a safe option. Obstet Gynecol 2004; 103: 407–12.

4 Dashe JS, McIntire DD, Ramus RM, et al. Persistence of placenta previa according to gestational age at ultrasound detection. Obstet Gynecol 2002; 99: 692–7.

5 Becker RH, Vonk R, Mende BC, et al. The relevance of placental location at 20–23 gestational weeks for prediction of placenta previa at delivery evaluation of 8650 cases. Ultrasound Obstet Gynecol 2001; 17: 496–501.

6 Taipale P, Hiilesmaa B, Ylostalo P. Transvaginal ultrasound at 18–23 weeks in predicting placenta previa at delivery. Ultrasound Obstet Gynecol 1998; 12: 422–5.

7 Benirschke K, Kaufmann P, Baergen, R. Pathology of the Human Placenta, 5th ed. New York: Springer, 2006.

8 Oyelese Y, Catanzarite V, Prefumo F, et al. Vasa previa: the impact of prenatal diagnosis of outcomes. Obstet Gynecol 2004; 103: 937–42.

9 Schachter M, Tovbin Y, Arieli S, et al. In vitro fertilization is a risk factor for vasa previa. Fertil Steril 2002; 78: 642–3.

10 Clark SL, Koonings PP, Phelan JP. Placenta previa/accreta and poor cesarean section. Obstet Gynecol 1985; 66: 89–92.

11 Finberg HJ, Williams JW. Placenta accreta: perspective Sonographic diagnosis in patients with placenta previa and prior cesarean section. J Ultrasound Med 1992; 11: 333–43.

12 Comstock CH. Antenatal diagnosis of placenta accreta: a review. Ultrasound Obstet Gynecol 2005; 26: 89–96.

13 Kupferminc MJ, Tamura RK, Wigton TR, et al. Placenta accreta is associated with elevated maternal serum alphafetoprotein. Obstet Gynecol 1993; 82: 266–9.

14 Zelop C, Nadel A, Figoletto FD, et al. Placenta accreta/percreta/increta: a cause of elevated maternal serum alphafetoprotein. Obstet Gynecol 1992; 80: 693–5.

15 Abuhamad A, Sclater AJ, Carlson EJ, et al. Umbilical artery Doppler waveform notching: is it a marker for cord and placental abnormalities? J Ultrasound Med 2002; 21: 857–960.

16 Hasegawa J, Matsuoka R, Ichizuka K, et al. Velamentous cord insertion into the lower third of the uterus is associated with intrapartum fetal heart rate abnormalities. Ultrasound Obstet Gynecol 2006; 27: 425–9.

17 Grannum PA, Berkowitz RL, Hobbins JC. The ultrasonic changes in the maturing placenta and their relation to fetal pulmonic maturity. Am J Obstet Gynecol 1979: 133: 915–22.

18 Bricker L, Nielson JP. Routine ultrasound in late pregnancy. Cochrane Database Syst Rev 2000; CD001451.

19 Strong TH, Jarles VL, Vega JS, et al. The umbilical coiling index. Am J Obstet Gynecol 1994; 170: 29–32.

20 Persutte WH, Hobbins JC. Single umbilical artery: a clinical enigma in modern prenatal diagnosis. Ultrasound Obstet Gynecol 1995; 6: 216–29.

21 Sornes T. Umbilical cord encirclement and fetal growth restriction. Obstet Gynecol 1995; 86: 725–8.

22 Gonzalez-Quintero VH, Tolaymat L, Muller AC, et al. Outcomes of pregnancies with sonographically detected nuchal cords remote from delivery. J Ultrasound Med 2004; 23: 43–7.

23 Peregrine E, O'Brien P, Jauniaux E. Ultrasound detection of nuchal cord prior to labor induction and the risk of cesarian section. Ultrasound Obstet Gynecol 2005; 25:160–4.

3 Assessment of amniotic fluid

It is quite clear that the fetus is afforded protective benefits from his/her aquatic environment, and if deprived of it, especially early in pregnancy, he/she can suffer severe consequences. An overabundance of fluid does not directly affect the fetus but can have a major indirect effect if the overfilling of the uterus triggers preterm birth labor. In contrast, oligohydramnios can have a negative impact on fetal lung and limb development, both of which need adequate amniotic fluid to develop.

In many cases of polyhydramnios or oligohydramnios, the fetus is already affected by something that is directly causing the fluid abnormality. To sort out the cause of polyhydramnios or oligohydramnios, it is worth reviewing the dynamics of amniotic fluid.

Amniotic fluid comes from many sources. After the first trimester the greatest contribution is from the fetal kidneys, producing 800 to 1200 cc per day. Also, there is a positive flow across the membranes of about 200 to 500 cc per day. Interestingly, although the fetal lungs contribute about 360 cc to the amniotic cavity per day, about half of this moves back into the lungs.

Fluid is removed mostly through fetal swallowing (500 to 1000 cc per day). Inconsequential amounts leave the cavity through the membranes.

The amniotic fluid volume rises linearly to about 33 to 34 weeks, when the average is about 1000 cc, after which it generally drops slowly to about 800 cc at 40 weeks of gestation and to 600 cc at 42 weeks.

Basically, there are three methods commonly used to assess the adequacy of amniotic fluid: (1) the vertical pocket technique, (2) the amniotic fluid index (AFI) and (3) the subjective ("eyeball") assessment.

The largest vertical pocket concept came into being when it was first described by Manning and Platt [1] in 1981 as part of the biophysical profile (BPP). Initially, the lower cut-off of a vertical pocket of 1 cm was found to be too stringent because this represented the most severe end of the oligohydramnios spectrum. The upper limit evolved later, with most investigators using a pocket exceeding 8 cm to connote polyhydramnios (Figure 3.1).

The AFI was devised by Phelan [2] in 1987, and was based on the idea that four pockets were better than one. The technique depends upon the uterus being divided up into four quadrants and the largest vertical pockets in each quadrant being totaled. An AFI of equal to, or greater than, 20 cm constitutes polyhydramnios.

Some authors have pitted the single vertical pocket technique (now with a mostly excepted minimum threshold of 2 cm) against the AFI, often using dye dilution calculations at the time of amniocentesis as an accurate indicator of amniotic fluid volume. Three studies [3–5] showed that AFI had a poor correlation with amniotic fluid volume (R^2 of 0.55, 0.30, and 0. 24) and two of these three studies demonstrated a slightly better performance with a cut-off of either a single vertical diameter of 2 cm or two pockets of 2 cm. For some reason, it has been generally assumed that the interobserver variation with AFI is minimal. However, a contemporary study [6] showed a 10.8% coefficient of variation within examiners and a 15.4% variation between examiners. Also, there appears to be no uniformity as to what AFI threshold to use to define oligohydramnios. For example, the 5th percentile at 37 weeks in Moore's publication is 8.8 cm [7], compared with Magann's [8] 5th percentile of 6.9 cm.

The umbilical cord poses a problem of quantification. For example, it is unclear as to whether one should pick a pocket without umbilical cord in the image, or to subtract out the diameter of the cord, or to push on as if the cord were not there, and simply measure the vertical distance between the inner walls (as the forefathers did when color Doppler was unavailable). Although one might surmise that subtracting out a cord defined by color Doppler would improve the accuracy of the assessment of the true amniotic fluid volume, one author [9] demonstrated, paradoxically, that using color gave a false diagnosis of

Obstetric Ultrasound: Artistry in Practice. John C. Hobbins. Published 2008 Blackwell Publishing. ISBN 978-1-4051-5815-2.

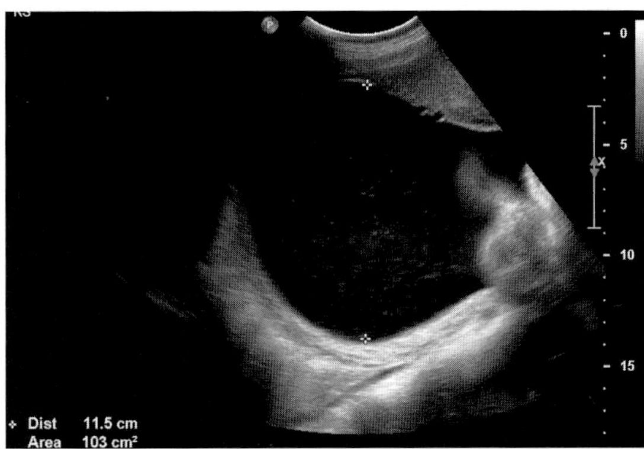

Fig 3.1 Polyhydramnios.

oligohydramnios in 21% of patients, compared with 3% when color Doppler was not used (amniotic fluid volume was determined with a dye dilution method). It seems that the way around this confusing issue is to find a vertical pocket that does not seem to contain cord on standard 2D ultrasound, and, although it may seem counterintuitive, to "bag" the use of color Doppler in amniotic fluid assessment.

My take on this is not to obsess about a subjective technique that is clearly inexact. There is little clinical difference after 30 weeks between an 11 cm and a 17 cm AFI, or even, for that matter, a 3 cm and a 5 cm AFI. In the former case, there is a reassuringly adequate amount of amniotic fluid, and in the latter case there is oligohydramnios, which, as indicated below, should warrant further evaluation.

One must be impressed, however, with the study by Magann [10] in which he found that high-risk patients, randomized to having AFI as part of their BPP, had twice the rate of ultrasound-diagnosed oligohydramnios (38% vs 16%), inductions (30% vs 15%), and cesarean sections for fetal distress (13% vs 7%) as their counterparts randomized to having a vertical pocket method. Since every perinatal outcome endpoint was identical, they concluded that the vertical pocket method avoided unnecessary intervention. We are now moving back to this technique, especially in twins where attempts at an AFI can actually be counterproductive.

Last, I think that the subjective assessment of amniotic fluid volume by an experienced operator is at least as good as any of the above attempts at overquantification, since the aim of the exercise simply is to determine if there is too much, too little, or an adequate amount of amniotic fluid present.

Abnormalities of amniotic fluid volume

Oligohydramnios

If one decides by any method that there is oligohydramnios, then further diagnostic testing is in order. The big three possible problematic causes of oligohydramnios are a fetal renal abnormality, IUGR, or ruptured membranes, and these should be ruled out before contemplating the fourth possibility—a normal variant.

The first place to start would be the fetal kidneys, and for any degree of oligohydramnios both kidneys would have to be affected. It is important to assess the size and texture of the kidneys. The average kidneys' circumference (of the two together) should be about one-third of the abdominal circumference through pregnancy (0.30) and the texture should be mildly heterogeneously echogenic (see Appendix). Most often the individual pyramids can be appreciated.

The two most common dysplasias associated with oligohydramnios are multicystic dysplastic kidney disease (MDKD) and infantile polycystic kidney disease (IPKD). The former appears as large kidneys replete with cysts of varying size throughout the renal parenchyma (Figure 3.2) and the latter emerges in the later portion of the second trimester as bilaterally enlarged, uniformly hyperechogenic kidneys (Figure 3.3). The cysts in these kidneys are not grossly visible. Unfortunately, the prognosis for these conditions is dismal although, obviously, if MDKD is unilateral, the prognosis is excellent. However, oligohydramnios is not generally a feature of unilateral disease, since the unaffected kidney easily takes over the urine production for two.

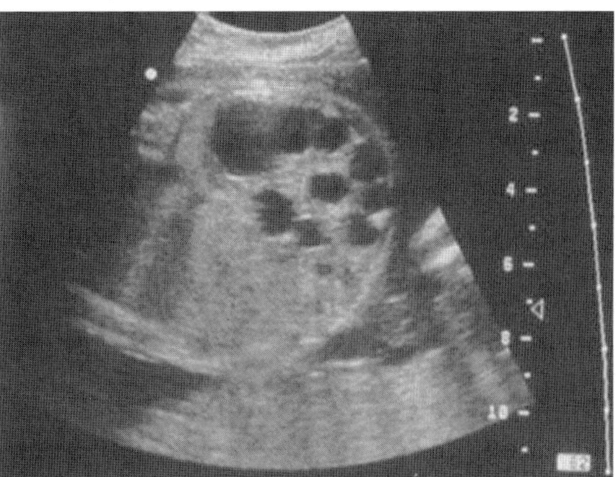

Fig 3.2 Multicystic dysplastic kidney.

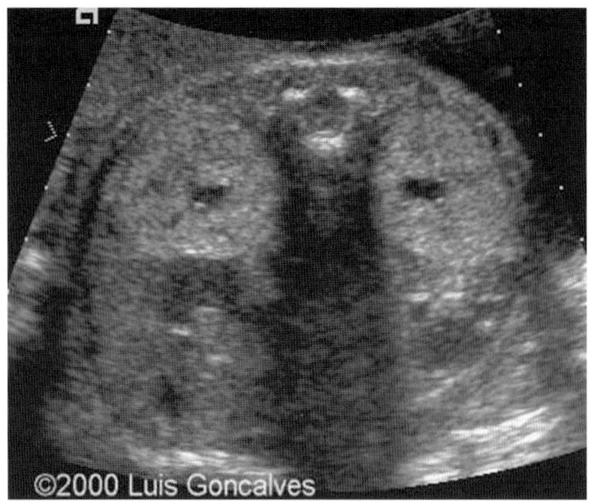

Fig 3.3 Infantile polycystic kidney disease. (Copyright 2000 Luis Goncalves.)

Another possibility in severe oligohydramnios is renal agenesis. This is a difficult diagnosis to make because kidneys are not easy to image when there is no acoustic window. However, the diagnosis can be suspected by an inability to identify renal arteries on color Doppler, which can be imaged on every fetus (Plate 3.1).

A lower urinary tract obstruction, such as posterior urethral valves, is an uncommon yet problematic cause of oligohydramnios and in these cases everything above the urethra is dilated (Figure 3.4). In the case of incomplete urethral obstruction, the prognosis is not hopeless, especially if the kidneys are not hyperechogenic and if there is no evidence of subcortical cysts, suggesting irreversible type 4 cystic dysplasia. In these cases intervention through shunting can be contemplated.

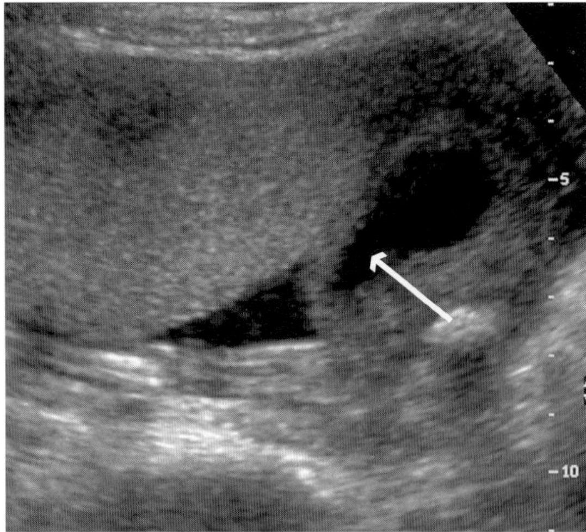

Fig 3.4 Keyhole bladder.

Bilateral upper tract obstructions such as ureteropelvic junction (UPJ) obstruction or ureterovesical junction (UVJ) obstruction are very rare causes of oligohydramnios, and, interestingly, the fetal renal cortex seems to fare better when obstructions are above the bladder. So, in essence, the size and configuration of the kidneys, ureters, and bladder should all be investigated carefully in the face of oligohydramnios.

A case in point of oligohydramnios

A 28-year-old woman presented at 18 weeks with a history of having delivered an infant in Mexico with a severe renal abnormality that resulted in his death a few minutes after birth. She remembers her doctors feeling that the infant had a "cystic kidney problem" but the actual autopsy information was not available.

On examination, the amount of amniotic fluid was diminished, with the largest vertical pocket being 1 cm, a small bladder was seen, but the kidneys were slightly enlarged (0.40 KC/AC ratio) and had a fluffy appearance.

We invited her back 2 weeks later and there was more pronounced oligohydramnios. The kidneys were more enlarged and were uniformly bright. The fetal bladder did not fill during the 40-minute examination.

We told her that the findings and her history were compatible with the diagnosis of infantile polycystic kidney disease and we painted a very bleak picture regarding the prognosis.

She continued her pregnancy and she temporarily was lost to follow-up, but later was admitted to the hospital in active labor at 35 weeks. Two hours later she delivered a fetus with Potter facies who died after a few minutes of pulmonary failure. An autopsy confirmed the diagnosis of infantile polycystic kidney disease and she was counseled about a 25% chance of recurrence.

Another avenue to pursue would be placentally mediated growth restriction. This will be covered later, but in IUGR, the fetus will spare his/her brain by shunting blood to the cerebral cortex at the expense of what would ordinarily be going to the kidneys. With less renal plasma flow, less urine is produced and oligohydramnios occurs. Although there are exceptions to this rule, the oligohydramnios generally occurs in concert with increased end diastolic flow in the middle cerebral artery. However, even

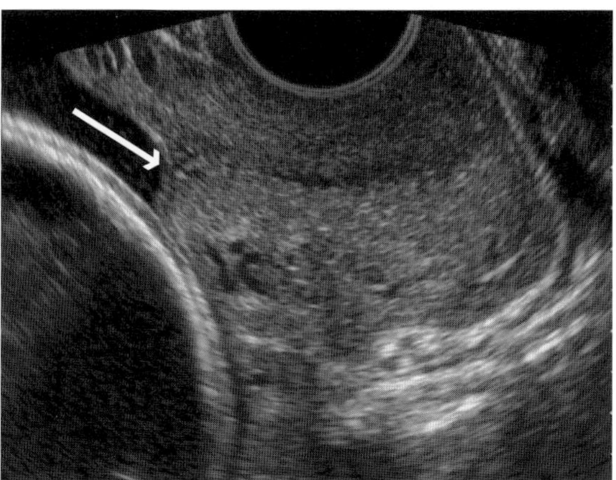

Fig 3.5 Arrow points to intact membranes running across the endocervix.

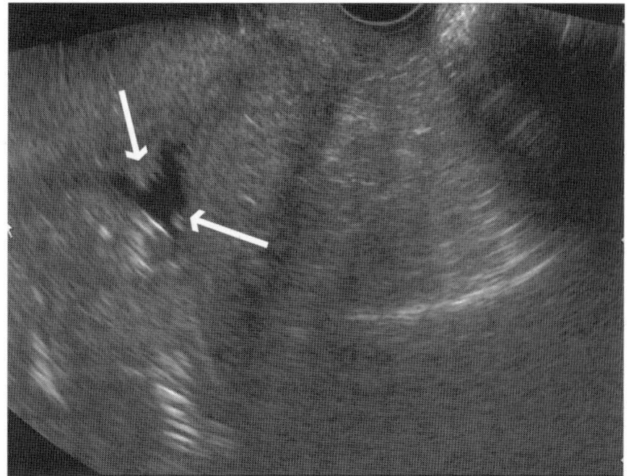

Fig 3.6 Rent in membranes. Arrows point to remnants of membranes.

before turning one's attention to Dopplers, the presence of a small-for-dates fetus should alert the clinician to a supply line cause for the oligohydramnios. Here the oligohydramnios must be considered as a sign of IUGR, or really as an example of an adaptive mechanism in IUGR, and not necessarily as an indicator of fetal jeopardy.

It has been difficult to prove, but the same mechanism for oligohydramnios could be occasionally occurring in fetuses that may not be, by definition, growth restricted, but rather are genetically destined to be much larger. Here, the fetal demand outstrips the placenta's ability to keep up, and a circulatory cascade enfolds that is similar to that seen in IUGR. We have noted increased end diastolic flow in the middle cerebral arteries in appropriate-for-gestational age (AGA) fetuses toward term with modestly diminished amniotic fluid. These mothers often go into labor soon after the Doppler changes occur.

In later gestation, the other possibility for oligohydramnios has little to do with the fetus and is more about the integrity of the membranes. Most often, the patient will complain of leakage of fluid per vagina and the diagnosis is evident. However, on occasion, the history is equivocal or, frankly, not helpful. In these cases, once a renal anomaly or obstruction has been ruled out and a normal-sized fetal bladder is seen, a transvaginal ultrasound examination can be extremely helpful. If the transducer is gently angled in such a way as to optimize its axial resolution, the membranes can be seen coursing over the cervix (Figure 3.5) if they are intact. In contrast, the integrity of the membranes cannot be demonstrated when oligohydramnios is secondary to ruptured membranes (Figure 3.6). Unfortunately, the method is a better excluder of ruptured membranes than an includer, since sometimes because of oligohydramnios the ability to visualize the membranes is hampered.

Also, one can get a rough estimate of the length of the latent period (from the time of rupture of membranes to the time of spontaneous initiation of labor). For example, in one study [11] the average latency period, when the cervical length was greater than 2 cm, was 10 days versus 50 hours if the cervical length was less than 2 cm. This information can provide the clinician with an idea of whether expectant management has a real chance of extending the pregnancy. Also, there may be a rebirth of an option to manage some patients with ruptured membranes at home with careful surveillance, and only patients with long cervices might be considered for this approach.

In severe oligohydramnios or anhydramnios, irrespective of the cause, the major threat to the fetus is pulmonary hypoplasia; especially if the fetus is deprived of amniotic fluid during the second trimester, when bronchiolar branching is in progress. Management decisions often depend upon direct 3D or indirect 2D measurements of fetal lung volume and the prognosis is very poor for fetuses in pregnancies with oligohydramnios and small lungs, whatever the etiology.

Unfortunately, based on the above potential problems being linked to oligohydramnios, many clinicians have concluded that every fetus with an AFI of less than 5 cm is at substantial risk for hypoxia, pulmonary hypoplasia, or cord impingement. For that reason, attempts have been made to noninvasively and invasively increase amniotic fluid volume.

Kilpatrick [12] found that loading women with oligohydramnios and intact membranes with isotonic saline increased the AFI by an average of 2 cm. However, in a more recent study, Malhotra [13] found that, although fluid loading significantly increased the AFI after 3 hours, it was not appreciably different by 24 hours.

Unfortunately, the tendency today is to overreact when oligohydramnios is found. However, the operative word here is "isolated," and when it is truly isolated there is a place for watchful waiting. A typical example of unnecessary meddling is the common practice of inducing labor toward the end of pregnancy when oligohydramnios is found. In one study of 147 high-risk patients [14], presenting at 34 weeks or greater with AFIs of less than 5 cm, induction doubled the number of cesarean sections, yet had no effect on perinatal outcome, when compared with matched high-risk pregnancies with AFIs above 5 cm. In another very similar study [15] involving 183 patients induced between 37 and 42 weeks for isolated oligohydramnios, the cesarean section rate was 15.8%, compared with 6.6% in a control group entering spontaneous labor at the same gestational age with normal amniotic fluid. Yet there was no difference in any perinatal outcome, including fetal distress in labor.

Other studies have shown a higher rate of cesarean section when inductions are undertaken for any reason; a practice that occurs now in about 1 in 5 pregnancies in the United States.

The case in point

A hard charging 36-year-old real estate broker was referred in from Vail, Colorado. This was her first pregnancy and she was sent in for an ultrasound evaluation because her AFI measured 5 cm. We obtained an estimated fetal weight that was in the 20th percentile, and no obvious fetal abnormalities were noted. The bladder was of normal size and there were no signs of rupture of membranes.

The Dopplers were instructive. Both umbilical arteries had normal waveforms, suggesting an adequate villus circulation. However, there was increased end diastolic flow in the middle cerebral artery.

We put the picture together this way. Since both parents were large people, this fetus probably was genetically programmed to be in the 80th percentile. However, this high-intensity mother, operating at 7500 feet above sea level had a placenta that could not keep up with what was asked of it. The fetus adapted by brain sparing and the kidney flow became a lower priority.

We suggested that she curtail her activity, sprinkling her day with periods of rest, and to increase her fluid intake. Two weeks later the AFI was 12 cm and there was more than expected interval growth.

Often patients are put on strict bed rest so that they won't compete with the blood supply to the fetus. Unfortunately, in high-energy individuals, bed rest can generate enough frustration-stimulated adrenaline to be counterproductive.

Polyhydramnios

An AFI of greater than 20 cm or a single pocket of greater than 8 cm defines polyhydramnios, which theoretically means an amniotic fluid volume exceeding 2000 cc. This happens in 0.25–3% of pregnancies. When present, a variety of causes need to be explored. It is estimated that about 20% of the time the reason lies with the fetus. The typical fetal problems associated with polyhydramnios involve gastrointestinal (GI) obstruction above the ileum, a central nervous system (CNS) abnormality, or a condition that would interfere with fetal swallowing. Occasionally, a mass causing compression of the mediastinum can result in interference with absorption of fluid. Some studies have shown the incidence of aneuploidy to be as high as 20% in polyhydramnios. However, Carlson and Platt [16] noted the increase in fetal anomalies to be mostly in those with AFIs of greater than 24 cm.

Diabetes can be associated with polyhydramnios, and the mechanism appears to be simply an increased urine production secondary to fetal hyperglycemia. Actually, fetal macrosomia, with or without diabetes, can result in a generous amniotic fluid volume, apparently secondary to a substantial, but proportional, production of urine. Nevertheless, any patient with polyhydramnios, a large fetus with body-to-head disproportion, and a large fetal bladder should be investigated for diabetes. If this is found late in pregnancy, it would be worth repeating the glucose screen even if the 26-week test was normal.

To recap

The diagnostic workup for oligohydramnios should include an evaluation of fetal biometry, kidneys, and bladder, and, if normal, an attempt should be made to document the integrity of the membranes. If there is still no obvious cause, and one is dealing with oligohydramnios and not anhydramnios, another examination should be scheduled in 2 weeks with the hope that the clinical picture will be clearer then. If the oligohydramnios seems to be of long duration, then an attempt should be made to assess directly or indirectly the size of the fetal lungs through the abdominal circumference to thoracic circumference ratio, the lung length, or 3D algorithms to calculate lung volume.

If the patient is more than 32 weeks, some authors, simply citing an association between oligohydramnios and adverse outcome, have advocated delivery. However, today we have reasonably precise ways to evaluate fetal condition and, as indicated above, it seems unreasonable to decide that fetuses with isolated oligohydramnios and no evidence of compromise be delivered, only to spend many unnecessary days or weeks in the nursery.

In polyhydramnios, it is essential to obtain fetal biometry. If macrosomia is found, diabetes should be contemplated. Attention should also be directed to the fetal GI tract. A small or seemingly absent stomach should cue the clinician to the distinct possibility of a tracheal esophageal fistula, either the blind pouch variety or the more common communicating variant (with the trachea). Also, a careful evaluation of the fetal heart, CNS, and limbs is in order. If an abnormality is found, karyotyping should be undertaken.

A conundrum arises over whether or not to do a chromosome analysis when a full genetic sonogram is negative. Those suggesting this tack cite earlier studies where it was unclear whether the polyhydramnios was truly isolated. I feel that this exercise would be unrewarding if the AFI is between 20 and 24 cm or the vertical pocket is between 7 and 9 cm, but in any case, it should depend upon the comfort level of the clinician with the ultrasound evaluation.

In severe polyhydramnios, therapeutic amniocentesis may well be required for patient comfort or to discourage the development of preterm labor. Obviously, karyotyping would be worthwhile once the fluid has been obtained.

Another case in point

The patient was referred at 22 weeks because the AFI was 22 cm. The finding appeared to be isolated. Our examination revealed the largest vertical pocket to be 9 cm. The fetus was AGA and, as indicated above, no anomalies were noted. The stomach was visualized but was consistently small on serial examinations. We alerted the neonatologist to the possibility of a tracheal esophageal fistula and we looked like champs when the infant was later diagnosed to have this condition.

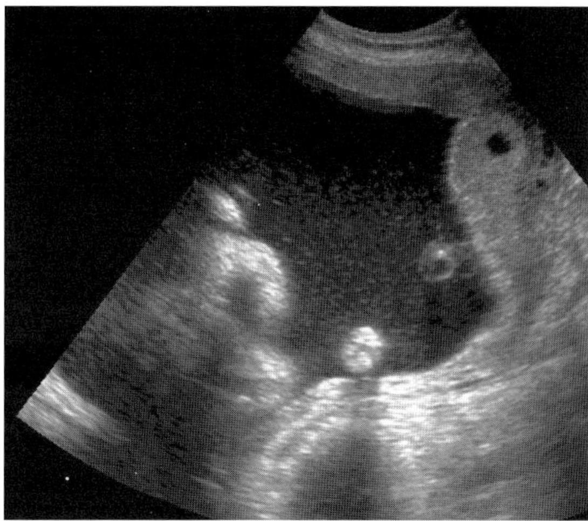

Fig 3.7 Light flecking in fluid.

The idea here is not necessarily to share with you our triumphs (which on some days are matched with our less-than-stellar calls), but to alert the reader to a possible diagnosis that, when recognized, can trigger a neonatal plan that will avoid significant morbidity secondary to aspiration.

In polyhydramnios, the fetal stomach should generally be larger than usual, since the fetuses seem to swallow more fluid in an effort to control the size of their aquatic environment. A consistently small stomach, or nonvisualized stomach, in the face of polyhydramnios, should get everyone's attention.

Unusual findings in the amniotic cavity

"Flecking" of amniotic fluid

In very late pregnancy, vernix can be responsible for the echogenic particles (Figure 3.7) frequently seen in amniotic fluid [7]. However, prior to about 34 weeks, these flecks cannot be attributed to vernix. We have noticed that heme pigments, seen after placental abruption or a bloody amniocentesis, become specular reflectors and, through fetal swallowing, are often responsible for echogenic bowel. In the majority of cases the flecking is of no great concern. However, there is one variation of the echogenic particle theme that does have some worrisome connotations. Espinoza [17] has described "sludge" of echogenic material, usually settling, by gravity, into the area of the cervix (Figure 3.8). This has been linked to fetal

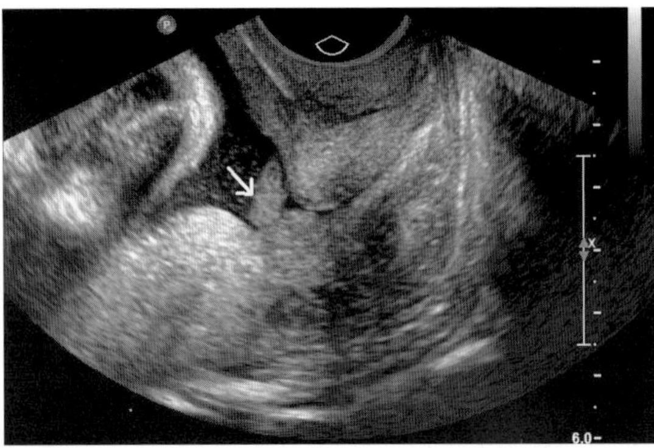

Fig 3.8 Cervical sludge.

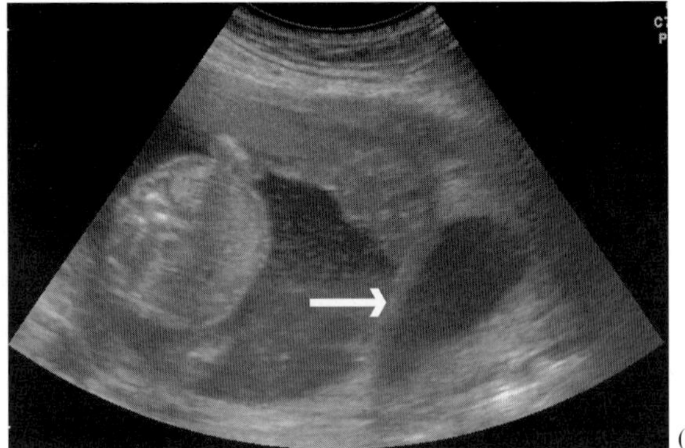

(a)

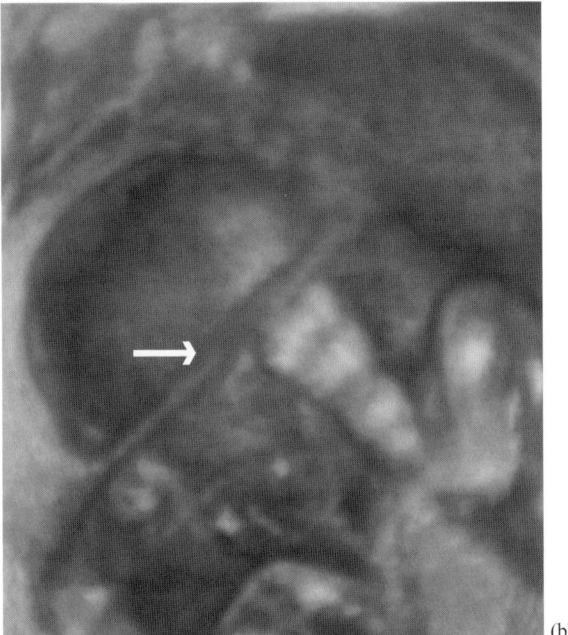

(b)

Fig 3.9 Uterine sheet: 2D (a) and 3D (b) depiction.

infection. When seen in about 1% of pregnancies there is a strong relationship with preterm birth, histological chorioamnionitis, and neonatal morbidity.

Meconium will often produce a snowflake pattern, and in late pregnancy, when amniotic fluid volume diminishes, the particles are more concentrated, producing a gravel-like appearance. Since meconium passage is not unusual in pregnancies with normal outcomes, when specular reflectors are noted in light amounts, one wonders what to do with this information in a seemingly uncomplicated pregnancy. However, when the fluid around the cord is more uniformly echogenic than the umbilical vein, this should get our attention.

Uterine sheets

A uterine sheet is a shelf-like structure that runs from north to south within the uterine cavity and probably represents in most cases a uterine adhesion (Figure 3.9). This finding is observed in 0.4–0.6% of pregnancies. Although some authors have noted a somewhat higher cesarean section rate in those with uterine sheets, these studies have not demonstrated an adverse effect on the fetus, and certainly should be distinguished from a true amniotic band, which has a different clinical connotation. Only one recent series of uterine sheets from Asia [18] contained two intrauterine fetal demises, presumably due to a cord accident. The authors described two variants of uterine sheets: complete, where there are no loose ends, and incomplete, where the shelf appears to be waving in the breeze. Fetal demise occurred in the two cases of "complete" sheets while the remaining 36 "incomplete" sheets were not associated with adverse outcome. They postulated that a complete sheet was not necessarily innocuous.

In contrast, my experience is that most of our sheets fall into the complete variety, and none has ever been associated with intrauterine demise or any other adverse outcome. The only complication we have encountered has been the anxiety created by patients being told that they have an amniotic "band." After a quick search on the Internet, these patients are so wired by the time they arrive at our office, their feet are barely touching the ground. Amniotic band syndrome is a rare condition that, unfortunately, *is* associated with severe fetal abnormalities and is, much of the time, lethal. This will be described in more detail in the section on limb abnormalities.

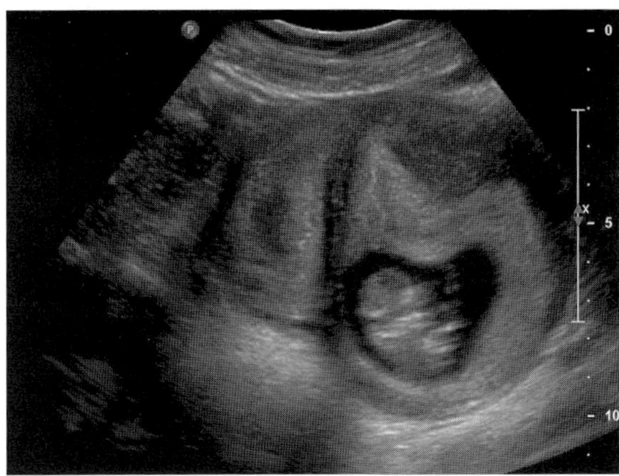

Fig 3.10 Bicornuate uterus with pregnancy in the left horn.

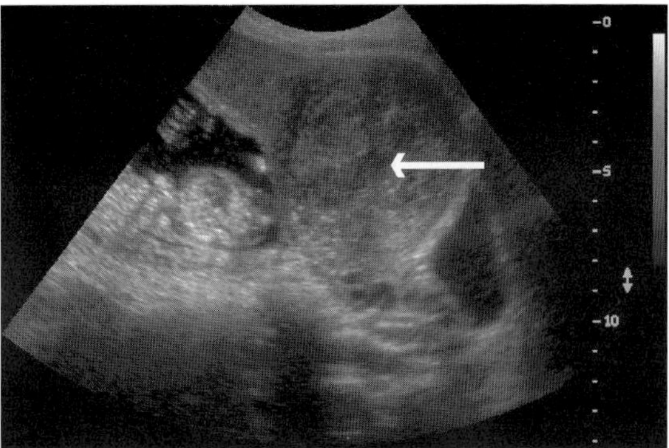

Fig 3.11 Lower uterine segment fibroid.

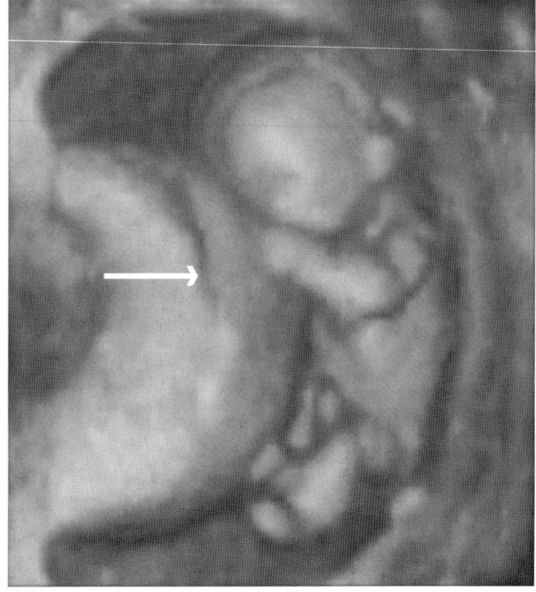

Fig 3.12 Contraction compressing cavity in first trimester. Arrow points to placenta/uterine wall interface.

Uterine abnormalities

Bicornuate uterus

Most commonly the sonologist or sonographer is forewarned that the patient has two uterine horns, but sometimes not. The typical picture when two separate horns are encountered is a seemingly normal-sized uterus containing all of the pregnancy and a much smaller, laterally rotated, opposite horn, often containing a lush decidual reaction (Figure 3.10).

The mildest variant is a heart-shaped uterus in which a small septum can be visualized with cross-sections through the uterine fundus. Most pregnancies with bicornuate uteri fare well, but the more separated the horns, the greater is the chance of preterm birth. For that reason, we generally follow these patients with serial cervical length measurements measured transvaginally.

Fibroids

Fibroids are overrated. They grow in early pregnancy under the influence of various hormones. The greatest acceleration in growth occurs in the first trimester of pregnancy, after which there is a slowing until about 20 weeks, when the growth generally stops. Usually, when they have outstripped their blood supply they take on a mottled appearance that often is related temporally to the patient's complaints of pain in the area of the fibroid.

One problem with large fibroids (Figure 3.11) is that they sometimes situate themselves in the lower uterine segment and can later impede the passage of the fetus through the birth canal. Nevertheless, even when located in the area above the cervix, they soften and can gravitate away from the lower uterine segment.

Some studies suggest a higher rate of abruption when the placenta implants over a fibroid, but this has not been my experience. Also, there has been some concern about IUGR secondary to competition for the uterine blood supply. This is a myth, because when the fetus's requirements are the greatest, the fibroid's demands are long gone.

Although a recent study [19] has suggested a correlation statistically with seemingly everything bad that can

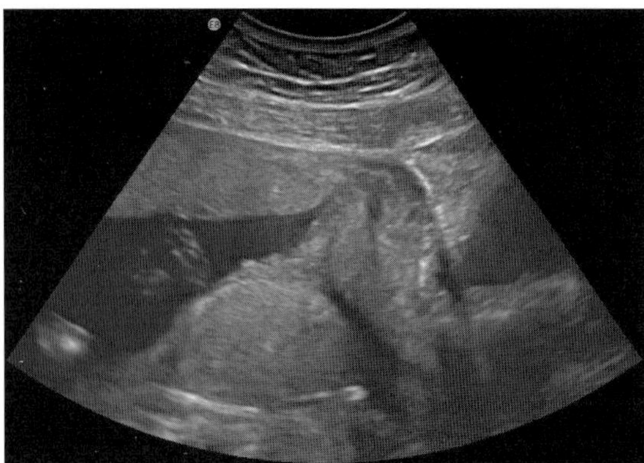

Fig 3.13 Concentric contraction confusing the ability to locate the endocervix.

happen to a pregnancy, the actual incidence of these complications in this population is still quite low, and I wonder if the problem may be more with the host (the mother) rather than with the fibroid itself, since, for example, fibroids are more prevalent in older women.

In any case, it is not necessary to monitor fibroid size after 20 weeks, and clinically one should simply be alert to the possibility of preterm labor, perhaps abruption, and postpartum hemorrhage (because the uterus may not contract as well after the placenta has been delivered, especially if the fibroid is in the lower segment). Nevertheless, the overwhelming majority of women with fibroids will sail through pregnancy without any problems, and these women need not be constantly reminded of their greater risk for the above complications (which I would rate as modestly increased).

Uterine contractions

Localized uterine contractions often masquerade as fibroids, and can occur at any time in pregnancy. If a contraction is located in the fundus or mid-portion of the uterus, it will appear as a uterine wall thickening, which most often juts downward into the uterine cavity (Figure 3.12). A contraction rarely pushes upward, breaking the smooth contour of the serosa of the uterus. If it occurs in the lower uterine segment, it can appear as a localized wall thickening or as a circumferential contraction compressing both walls of the lower uterine segment and making it difficult to visualize the true endocervix (Figure 3.13).

Contractions can last for many minutes but will eventually disappear and the diagnosis will become clear.

References

1 Manning FA, Platt LP, Sipos L. Antepartum fetal evaluation: development of a fetal biophysical profile. Am J Obstet Gynecol 1980: 136: 787–95.

2 Phelan JM, Smith CV, Broussard P, et al. Amniotic fluid volume assessment with the four-quadrant technique at 36–42 weeks' gestation. J Reprod Med 1987; 32: 540–2.

3 Chauhan SP, Magann EF, Morrison JC, et al. Ultrasonic assessment of amniotic fluid does not reflect actual amniotic fluid volume. Am J Obstet Gynecol 1997; 177: 291–5.

4 Croom SC, Bonias BB, Ramos Santos E, et al. Do quantitative amniotic fluid indices reflect actual volume? Am J Obstet Gynecol 1992; 167: 995–9.

5 Dildy GA III, Lira N, Moise KJ Jr, et al. Amniotic fluid volume assessment: comparison of ultrasonographic estimates versus direct measurements with dye-dilution technique in human pregnancy. Am J Obstet Gynecol 1992; 167: 986–94.

6 Bruner JP, Reed GW, Sarno AP, et al. Inter-observer variability and amniotic fluid index. Am J Obstet Gynecol 1993; 168: 1309–13.

7 Moore TR, Cayle JE. The amniotic fluid index in normal human pregnancy. Am J Obstet Gynecol 1990; 162: 1168–73.

8 Magann EF, Sanderson M, Martin JM, et al. The amniotic fluid index, single deepest pocket, and two-diameter pocket in normal human pregnancy. Am J Obstet Gynecol 2000; 182: 1581–8.

9 Magann SF, Chauhan SP, Barrilleaux PS, et al. Ultrasound estimate of amniotic fluid volume: color Doppler overdiagnosis of oligohydramnios. Obstet Gynecol 2001; 98: 71–4.

10 Magann EF, Doherty DA, Field K, et al. Biophysical profile with amniotic fluid volume assessments. Obstet Gynecol 2004; 104: 5–10.

11 Gire C, Faggianelli P, Nicaise C, et al. Ultrasonographic evaluation of cervical length in pregnancies complicated by preterm premature rupture of membranes. Ultrasound Obstet Gynecol 2001; 19: 565–9.

12 Kilpatrick SJ, Safford KL, et al. Maternal hydration increases AFI in women with normal amniotic fluid. Obstet Gynecol 1993; 81: 49–52.

13 Malhotra B, Deka P. Duration of the increase in amniotic fluid index (AFI) after acute maternal hydration. Arch Gynecol Obstet 2004; 269: 173–5.

14 Casey BM, McIntire DD, Bloom SL, et al. Pregnancy outcomes after antepartum diagnosis of oligohydramnios at or beyond 34 weeks' gestation. Am J Obstet Gynecol 2000; 182: 909–12.

15 Conway DL, Adkins WB, Schroeder B, et al. Isolated oligohydramnios in the term pregnancy: is it a clinical entity? J Matern Fetal Med 1998; 7: 197–200.

16 Carlson DE, Platt LD, Medearis AL. The ultrasound triad of fetal hydramnios, abnormal hand posturing, and any other

anomaly predicts autosomal trisomy. Obstet Gynecol 1992; 79: 731–4.

17 Espinoza J, Goncalves LF, Romero R, et al. The prevalence and clinical significance of amniotic fluid 'sludge' in patients with preterm labor and intact membranes. Ultrasound Obstet Gynecol 2005; 25: 346–52.

18 Tan KBL, Tan TYT, Tan JVK, et al. The amniotic sheet: a truly benign condition? Ultrasound Obstet Gynecol 2005; 26: 639–43.

19 Qidwai GI, Caughey AB, Jacoby AF. Obstetric outcomes in women with sonographically identified uterine leiomyomata. Obstet Gynecol 2006; 107: 376–82.

4 Fetal biometry

Before launching into the following chapters on biometry and fetal anatomy, a few imaging ground rules need to be addressed. The common tomograms (slices) used to assess a portion of the fetal anatomy are the axial slice (Figure 4.1a), the coronal slice (Figure 4.1b), and the sagittal slice, most often midline (Figure 4.1c). Although the above figures only pertain to the head, these views will be referred to throughout the text, and obviously pertain to every portion of the fetal anatomy to be discussed.

In this chapter, I will deal with the standard fetal biometry and how to deal with biometric discrepancies.

Biparietal diameter (BPD)

This was the first fetal measurement attempted, first by A-mode and then later by 2D contact scanning. The measurement is made axially at a level just above the ear and, although others have obsessed over standardization, it is very difficult to mess up this measurement. Hopefully, everyone reading this book knows that the BPD is measured at the level of the thalami (Figure 4.2) and is made from the outer margin of the calvarium to the inner surface of the downside of the skull. Since the degree of tucking has little to do with the measurement, as it does with the head circumference, the interobserver variability is small, and one can rely on this measurement as one of the best indicators of gestational age.

As with all biometry, there are multiple formulas correlating a given BPD with gestational age, but most clinicians and sonographers simply use the formula that is already in the software of their ultrasound machines. Unlike estimated fetal weight, there are only modest differences in BPDs across different populations, so using a built-in formula is acceptable.

Head circumference

This measurement puts into play a diameter made east to west across the skull, which depends upon the inferior lateral resolution of the transducer, and is also dependent upon the degree of fetal tucking. Perhaps its greatest benefit is when, because of either oligohydramnios or a breech presentation, there is dolichocephaly, rendering the BPD less accurate.

Most clinicians will use both measurements to evaluate fetal head size.

Abdominal circumference (AC)

Of all the usually performed biometric measurements, this is the best one to assess the size of the fetus and, indirectly, the status of fetal nutrition. This concept will be dealt with in the section on IUGR. However, AC is the worst way, by itself, to determine gestational age, because of its wide biological variation. The reason why the AC was originally chosen as a standard part of the biometric profile is because the measurement is made at the level of the bifurcation of the right and left portal veins, e.g., smack in the middle of the liver, an organ that is quite large in macrosomia and very small in small-for-gestational age (SGA) fetuses (Figure 4.3).

The measurement must be precisely performed because it is, unfortunately, easy to get a tangential cut through the abdomen, which will cause an overestimation of the abdomen size; especially when a large portion of the umbilical vein is incorporated in the image.

Femur and humerus

The femur has always been part of the AIUM/ACR guidelines for basic ultrasound examination (Figure 4.4), but

Obstetric Ultrasound: Artistry in Practice. John C. Hobbins. Published 2008 Blackwell Publishing. ISBN 978-1-4051-5815-2.

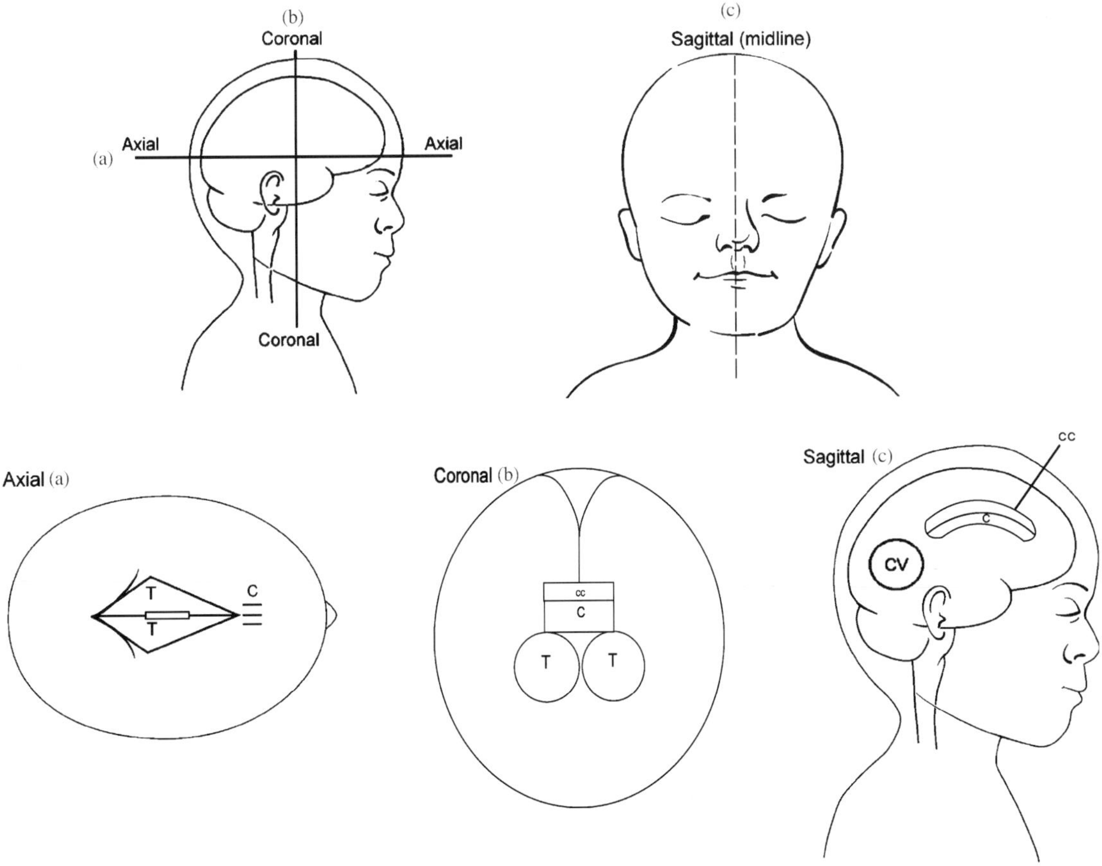

Fig 4.1 Schematic of the essential planes for ultrasound scanning: axial (a) and coronal planes (b), sagittal (midline) (c) incorporating T, thalami; C, cavum; CC, corpus callosum; CV, cerebellar vermis. For example, (a) is plane of the biparietal diameter.

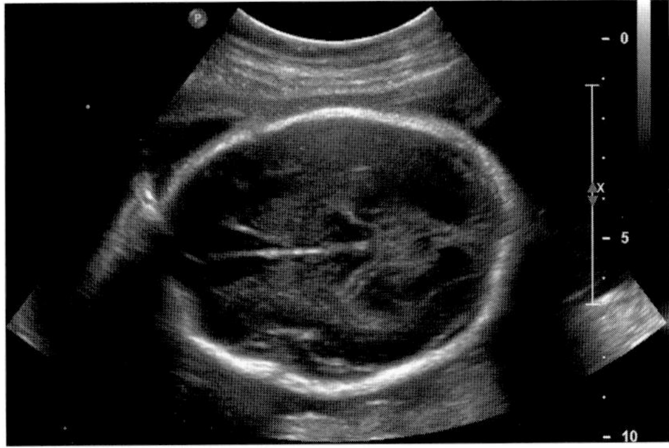

Fig 4.2 Plane of the biparietal diameter.

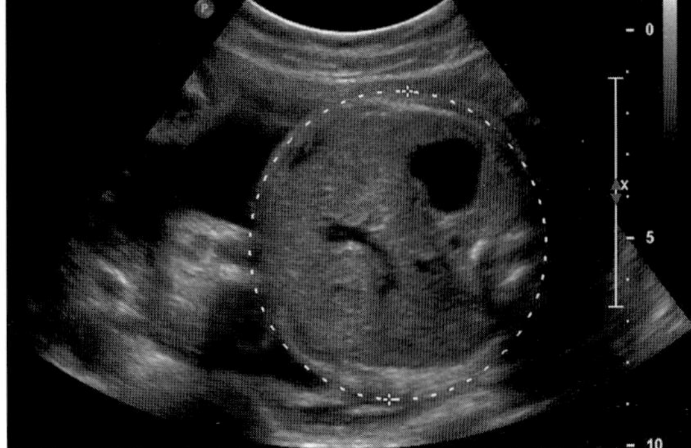

Fig 4.3 The abdominal circumference.

not many laboratories will add the humerus to the mix. The femur is indirectly reflective of the crown heel length of the fetus (length in cm times 6.9) and is subject to familial tendencies toward shortness or tallness. The humerus simply adds more to the biometric mix, but is not included in formulas to estimate fetal weight, as is the femur.

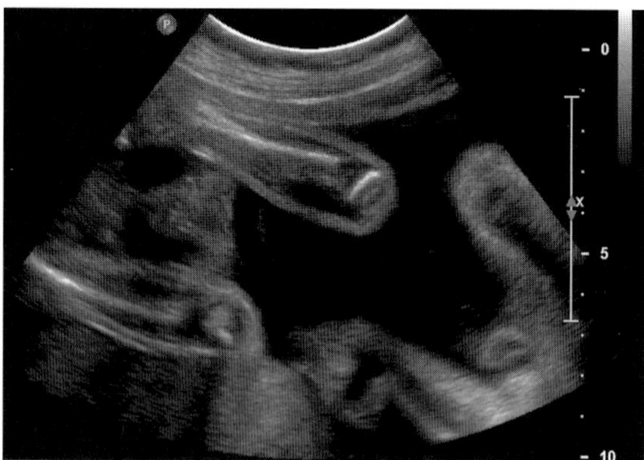

Fig 4.4 Femur.

One word of caution when measuring the femur: today's equipment will light up the thin upper edge of the cartilaginous end of the long bone. Since the authors of the nomograms included in the software packages of contemporary machines were using vintage equipment not capable of outlining the cartilage, the measurement of the femur and humerus should only include the ossified shaft.

Transcerebellar diameter (TCD)

I cannot understand why this measurement is utilized so infrequently. First, it is the best dater of pregnancy, and second, it is not difficult to obtain, at least in the second trimester (Figure 4.5). The TCD in millimeters roughly equals gestational age in weeks until about 22 weeks, after which a nomogram is needed. In later gestation, it is more difficult to obtain the measurement because of shadowing from the skull, but with some fine-tuning and perseverance this difficulty can be overcome. We have found the TCD to be very useful in late care patients to sort out an SGA fetus from an off-on-dates fetus.

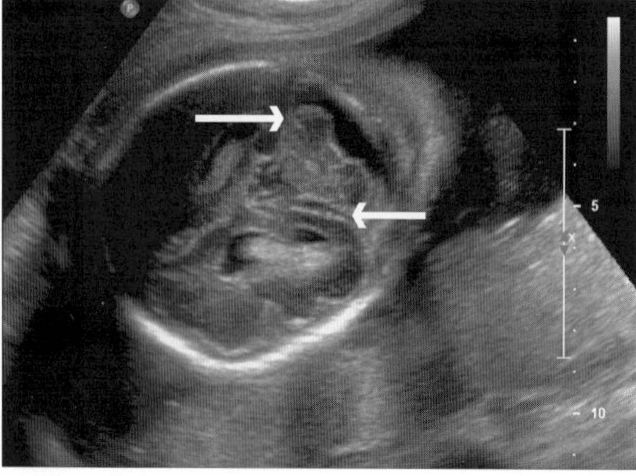

Fig 4.5 Plane for measuring the transcerebellar diameter, marked by arrows.

The bonus with the TCD is that it forces the operator to image the entire posterior fossa, which is a rich source of information regarding the cerebellar vermis itself and, indirectly, is a reflector of the integrity of the neural tube. In addition, in the same plane the nuchal skin fold thickness, our best marker of Down syndrome, can be measured.

Estimated fetal weight (EFW)

There are more than 40 formulas in the literature for EFW. The Hadlock formula that is incorporated into most North American ultrasound machine software packages utilizes four variables: the BPD, HC, AC, and femur. The Shepard formula uses only the BPD and AC, and another Hadlock formula, called upon when head measurements are difficult to obtain, involves the AC and the femur.

Anyone trying to compare the accuracy of each formula by scrutinizing the literature would be totally confused because the results are not laid out in consistent terms. Years ago we found that, using the Shepard formula, 80% of the time we were within 10% of the true fetal weight and 50% of the time we were within 5% of the actual fetal weight. That would mean that if the formula indicated an EFW of 2000 g, 4 out of 5 times the fetus would not weigh more than 2200 g or less than 1800 g. In effect, for small fetuses the EFW is reasonably precise. However, if the EFW is 4000 g, there is a possible splay of 800 g (plus or minus 400 g), and 1 out of 5 times the EFW is even less accurate than that. This has caused some authors to gang up on the concept of the EFW, and one author [1] even indicated in a nonblinded study that his "hands-on" clinical estimates outperformed his ultrasound estimates of fetal weight. This must mean that he is far better than I am at clinical estimation (where I am accurate to within plus or minus 2 lb), or he is far worse than I am in obtaining basic ultrasound biometry.

I feel that the EFW should be put in a better light. Its general purpose is to tell whether the fetus is too big or too small. On the small end, the formulas work reasonably well. However, for large fetuses in late pregnancy, estimates of size probably should be done by AC alone, since the EFW incorporates head measurements into the calculation, which are often difficult to obtain toward term.

Perhaps the greatest problem with EFW is not the accuracy of the formula but the growth curves into which the EFWs are plotted. Most North American machines have Hadlock's growth curve, which was constructed from a mixed population at sea level in Houston, Texas. Other growth curves available are from the East Coast, West Coast of the United States, and from countries in Europe and Asia. We have found that in Denver, Colorado, where we are 5000 feet above sea level, our EFWs are about 5% lower than the EFWs from Houston, translating into our 15th percentile being analogous to Houston's 10th percentile.

To compound the confusion, growth curves in the literature are not only from different populations, but also are based on a variety of EFW formulas.

Lest we dwell too much on the downside of the EFW, the advantage of the concept is that it does allow the clinician to quantify a deficit and to see if there has been adequate growth in grams over a time interval. Also, it enables us to consult with neonatologists in terms they and we can use to counsel patients regarding the prognosis for a premature fetus.

Last, and perhaps this is a rationalization, the EFW is based on diameters and circumferences that are simply reflecting the volume of the fetus. However, in order to convert this volume to mass (in grams), one has to multiply the volume by density, which is about 1.0 at 20 weeks, but is quite variable later in pregnancy. In other words, 1 cc of fetal tissue in late gestation does not necessarily equal 1 g of fetal tissue. In fact, the volume may well be the better estimator of true fetal size than fetal weight.

Deter [3] was one of the first to use 2D fetal thigh measurement as a reasonable reflector of fetal "beefiness" or "scrawniness." New techniques for the EFW have now emerged using a 3D ultrasound to multislice through the fetus. Initially, investigation has shown that these 3D attempts are superior to standard 2D formulas [4]. However, at the moment, these methods are cumbersome and time-consuming, and prospective investigation will have to show them to be clearly superior to existing methods, which depend only upon standard biometry and a 2D machine.

Estimating gestational age

The common practice is to take an average of the biometry (BPD, HC, AC, femur) that is displayed on the ultrasound report page as an average ultrasound age (AUA). This can then be compared with the patient's menstrual dates. The dating precision varies according to the gestational age of the patient. For example, it used to be thought that the CRL was the most accurate way to date pregnancy, but Chervenak [2] has found that the BPD in the second trimester has very reasonable accuracy. Although I have found that the TCD is a very good indicator of gestational age in the second trimester, it is, by far, the best dater of pregnancy in the third trimester, because it rarely is affected appreciably by aberrations in fetal growth.

In the second trimester, I use the AUA to date the pregnancy, and if the result is discrepant by more than 1 week from the patient's clinical dates, I will look at the individual values to see if there is a "maverick value" that is pulling the AUA up or down. If all measurements are in sync, including the TCD, then, unless there is a compelling historical reason to stay with the clinical dates, I will change the patient's dates to reflect the AUA. However, although many studies, including the RADIUS trial, suggest that relying upon clinical dating is a dubious practice, these studies included patients who were only sure of one thing—their last menstrual period. Unfortunately, there is always more to a story, and the sonographer/sonologist must delve into the history more deeply when there is a major discordance between AUA and dates. Does the length of her cycles suggest that she is an early or late ovulater? Did she get pregnant through assisted reproductive technology? Does she have information regarding the timing of intercourse? (Occasionally, this line of questioning can open a can of worms regarding paternity that requires some creative dancing when a large, menacing husband/partner is present.) Did she have a very early pregnancy test or ultrasound examination? A majority of the time these questions will sort out dating discrepancies.

It drives me crazy when a patient indicates that she has had her due date changed four times based on each ultrasound examination she has had. The way to handle this is to give priority to the earliest scan, and if the AUA is within a week of the patient's clinical dates, to keep the clinical dates, no matter what later examinations show.

Discordant measurements

BPD and HC

For practical purposes, a discrepancy between the fetal head measurements and the patient's dates of greater than 2 weeks should get the attention of the ultrasound examiner. If the head is bigger, then a quick evaluation of the intracranial anatomy should assure the examiner that this relative macrocephaly is simply a normal variant and, most often, a familial feature. I ask the patient her baseball cap size (everyone has a baseball cap). Also, if the father looks like Mr. Potato Head, you have the answer.

If the head circumference is smaller by about 2 weeks, this most often is a normal variation, especially in the third trimester. However, the larger the discrepancy, the more one will have to explore the rare condition of pathologic microcephaly, which will be covered later.

AC

By far the most common reason for a small AC is IUGR, and if it is out of sync with the rest of the biometry, it represents early asymmetric growth restriction. Gastroschisis is associated with a small AC, but, fortunately, in the scheme of things, this is an uncommon condition and is easily diagnosed.

Long bones

Long limbs generally signify tall genes, and there are only a few rare circumstances where a very long femur or humerus is concerning, such as in Marfan syndrome.

Almost every day on a busy ultrasound service a fetus shows up with a femur that is smaller than expected. When the discordance is in the 2- to 3-week range, this virtually always represents a genetic predisposition toward shortness; especially when found well into the third trimester, and, without fail, the patient, her partner, or someone in the immediate family is vertically challenged. Unfortunately, since a short femur may be a marker for Down syndrome, other markers, including the humerus (which generally is even smaller in Down syndrome than the femur) need to be assessed, as well as the results of the patient's quad screen. If this investigation is unremarkable, then the patient actually can be reassured. If the fetus is very short (greater than a 3-week discrepancy), then two other clinical avenues need to be explored. Very early primary placental growth failure will sometimes emerge with a short femur representing the first biometric measurement to fall off the growth curve. Most often this occurs together with abnormal uterine artery waveforms. Also, a very short femur should trigger a short-limb dysplasia investigation, which, as indicated later, is quite extensive.

A case in point

This patient arrived at our office billed as having a uterus that was large for dates. She seemed to have regular periods prior to her well-recalled last menstrual period, which suggested her to be 32 weeks. The BPD and HC were appropriate for 33 weeks, as well as the femur. The AC was in sync for 34 weeks and the EFW was in the 90th percentile.

The patient had a previous delivery of an 8.5 lb baby. Her 1-hour glucose screen was "positive," but her full glucose tolerance test at 27 weeks was "negative." Also, the above scan was productive of a single vertical pocket of 7.5 cm, the stomach was large, and the bladder was generous in size.

The combination of a large baby, body-to-head disproportion, a large bladder and generous amniotic fluid (suggesting polyuria) made this patient seem like a genuine grade A gestational diabetic—despite her negative glucose tolerance test. The 1-hour glucose screen was repeated, which was 150 mg%.

Some gestational diabetics are late bloomers, and all they need is a larger dose of anti-insulin factors springing from the placenta (like human placental lactogen) to kick them into bona fide glucose intolerance. What is perhaps debatable is whether knowing this will make a major difference in outcome. Nevertheless, altering one's diet for the better cannot be a badthing.

References

1 Chauhan SP, Lutton PM, Bailey KH, et al. Intrapartum clinical, sonographic, and parous patients' estimates of newborn birth weight. Obstet Gynecol 1992; 79: 956–8.

2 Chervenak FA, Skupski DW, Romero R, et al. How accurate is fetal biometry in the assessment of fetal age? Am J Obstet Gynecol 1998; 178: 678–87.

3 Warda A, Deter RL, Duncan G, et al. Evaluation of fetal thigh circumference measurements: a comparative ultrasound and anatomical study. J Clin Ultrasound 1986; 14:99–103.

4 Lee W, Deter R, Ebersole JD, et al. Birth weight prediction by three-dimensional ultrasonography: fractional limb volume. J Ultrasound Med 2001; 20:1283–92.

5 Intrauterine growth restriction

In this segment, we will be concentrating on fetuses that are small-for-gestational age (SGA). Following the lead from our neonatal colleagues, in North America we have been inclined to define SGA as being in or below the 10th percentile of mean weight for gestation. However, clinicians in some other areas of the world have used an abdominal circumference (AC) of greater than 2SDs below the mean for gestation as a threshold to identify the SGA fetus. Although this may seem to further confuse an already muddy identification process (see above), the AC alone makes more sense as a definer of fetal smallness for many reasons. First, it involves only one measurement that always can be imaged. Secondly, it incorporates two portions of the anatomy that are always compromised in a nutritionally deprived fetus: the liver and the rim of subcutaneous fat surrounding the abdominal cavity. Last, factors having little to do with nutrient supply can influence the size of the head and limbs, which are incorporated into most EFW formulas.

Actually there is no way an SGA fetus will have an AC that is within 2SDs of the mean (in the absence of a second problem such as ascites or organomegaly).

The reason the SGA fetuses get our attention is that they have higher rates of perinatal mortality and morbidity than AGA fetuses, depending upon the degree of the deficit. When lumped together, they have higher rates of cesarean section, fetal distress, low Apgar scores, and low pH, compared with AGA fetuses. Their immediate neonatal course is often complicated by prematurity (with all of its own problems), hypoglycemia (they have depleted glycogen stores), and hypothermia (diminished subcutaneous fat means thermal instability). A little later in their nursery stay they are vulnerable to necrotizing enterocolitis, probably because of in utero shunting away from the mesenteric arteries. Also, they have higher rates of neurological disability. Last, after becoming adults, they are prone to high rates of diabetes and cardiovascular disease.

So, while we may occasionally obsess over some rare condition having a prevalence in the overall population of, let's say, 1 in 2000, SGA fetuses complicate a whopping 1 in 10 to 1 in 20 pregnancies, and early identification and proper management can have a major impact on these individuals throughout their lives.

A recent Swedish study put into proper perspective the importance of simply diagnosing a SGA fetus. Lindqvist [1] looked at data from 1990 through 1998 involving 27,000 patients and found that the neonatal morbidity and mortality rates were fourfold higher for SGA fetuses who were not diagnosed in utero, compared with those who were (with ultrasound).

Before exploring the task of diagnosing an SGA fetus, I will touch upon some confusion regarding the terms, SGA and intrauterine growth restriction (IUGR). To some they are synonymous, while to others, SGA simply represents a small fetus (by the above definitions alone), and IUGR indicates a small fetus that is deprived (usually for a placental reason). For practical purposes, I will not use them interchangeably since, for me, the term IUGR actually connotes a condition and SGA simply means that the fetus is biometrically small.

There are four basic reasons why fetuses can be smaller than expected: (1) there is a supply line problem; (2) they are genetically programmed to be small; (3) there is a condition responsible for the primary growth failure such as aneuploidy or fetal infection; and (4) the patient is off/on dates.

Once the fetus is determined to be small, the individual biometric parameters can be compared against each other to get an idea of whether the fetus is symmetrically or asymmetrically small. Campbell [2] first described the head circumference (HC)/AC ratio as a way to determine the degree of head-to-body disproportion, which, by being reflective of "brain sparing," will point toward placentally mediated IUGR. Hadlock's AC/femur ratio [3] is simply

Obstetric Ultrasound: Artistry in Practice. John C. Hobbins. Published 2008 Blackwell Publishing. ISBN 978-1-4051-5815-2.

an adaptation of the neonatal "ponderal index" to suggest how "scrawny" the fetus is.

Although these ratios are often spit out on the standard report page, one can get a feel for symmetry and asymmetry by simply looking at the individual gestational age readout for each biometric parameter, and to use a 2-week difference between measurements as an indicator of discordance.

Yes, one can suspect the placenta as being the culprit in asymmetric IUGR, but every other reason for a small fetus, including constitutional smallness and being off/on dates, tend to result in symmetrically small fetuses, and frequently there may be more than one etiology for IUGR. Therefore, the rest of the workup becomes very important, especially the Doppler investigation.

One last word about biometry: the best way to separate out an off on dates fetus from an IUGR fetus is through the transverse cerebellar diameter (TCD). All but one investigator have found that TCD is relatively unaffected in IUGR. However, even in the less common instance where the TCD is more than one week smaller than actual dates in an IUGR fetus, the TCD still remains closer to the real dates than any of the other biometric measurements, especially the AC.

Once the fetus by estimated fetal weight (EFW) or AC is determined to be smaller than expected, an attempt should be made to whittle down the diagnostic possibilities by exploring carefully the legitimacy of the patient's dates, her family tendencies (genes for smallness), history of possible infection (CMV), or whether her second trimester biochemistry gave her a higher risk for aneuploidy or IUGR.

Next, further scrutiny of the individual biometric parameters often will help to settle an off-/on-dates question. The presence or absence of oligohydramnios will also aid somewhat in narrowing down the diagnosis. Last, a very detailed fetal survey should be undertaken to rule out a major anomaly syndrome, and a search for markers for aneuploidy should be initiated to exclude the more common trisomies.

Many authors have advocated the liberal use of amniocentesis in patients with IUGR and I disagree. The more common aneuploidies associated with curtailed fetal growth are trisomy 18, 13, and triploidy, all of which can be ruled out with a reassuring genetic sonogram. Although fetuses with trisomy 21 do tend to be smaller than expected, this is mostly because of slightly small limbs (1 1/2 to 2 weeks less than dates). The AC and biparietal diameter (BPD) are relatively unaffected. Therefore, the EFW generally does not fall below the 10th percentile in Down syndrome. The chance for a chromosome abnormality further drops with a reassuring quad screen. Therefore, if the genetic sonogram and the quad screen check out as normal, the likelihood of the growth-restricted fetus having aneuploidy is less than the risk of the amniocentesis. On the other hand, if there is a marker for trisomy 18 in a patient with IUGR and polyhydramnios, that patient rarely would leave our center without a Band-Aid® on her abdomen.

The next step is to assess the condition of the fetus through Doppler analysis of the fetal circulation and, often the maternal circulation. At the first visit, if no obvious reason for the growth curtailment is found and the Dopplers are reassuring, the patient can then be scheduled for a fetal growth check in 2 weeks (since the standard error of the method precludes any meaningful information to come from measurements made at a lesser interval). However, the Doppler examinations should be scheduled for weekly intervals.

Doppler in the management of IUGR

Umbilical artery

The umbilical artery waveform reflects the degree of impedance downstream and, indirectly, the amount of "lushness" of the fetal placental circulation. Since in IUGR investigators have shown less villus branching, fewer terminal villi, smaller lumens in the fetal arterioles and, even recently, evidence of dynamic vasoconstriction, it is not surprising that one of the earliest signs of IUGR is a decrease in umbilical artery end diastolic flow.

The common method used to evaluate umbilical artery waveform is to pick any free-floating loop of cord, usually with color Doppler, and to obtain the waveform from it with pulsed Doppler (Figures 5.1a and 5.1b). Although the amplitude of the signal is greater if one has a small angle of insonation, it is not essential, since the technique involves measuring a ratio between the systolic peak and the diastolic trough. However, if the aim is to measure peak velocity, as in assessing the middle cerebral artery waveform in fetal anemia, then the angle of insonation should be as close as possible to 0°. Any result at an angle of greater than 30° is suspect.

A breathing fetus can frustrate one's ability to get a consistent measurement of a waveform (Figure 5.2), so I suggest waiting for a period of quiescence before attempting this. Since breathing and moving are good signs, the examiner is usually rewarded eventually with a reassuring result.

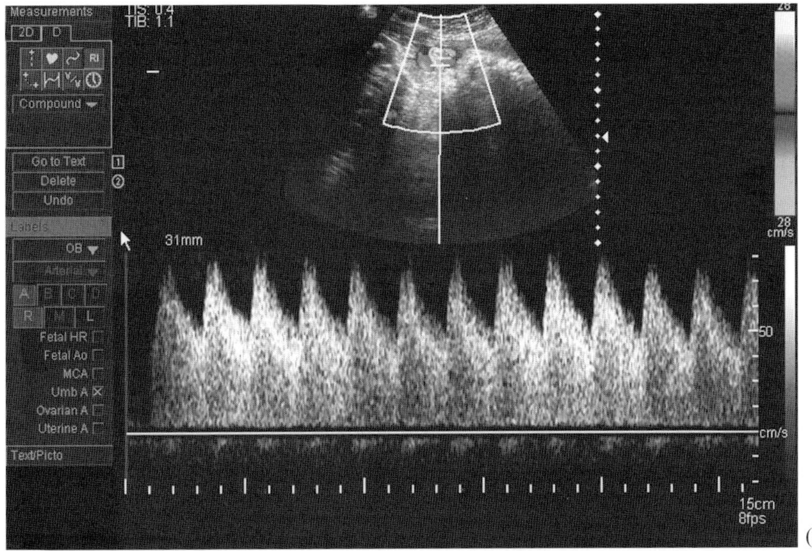

(a)

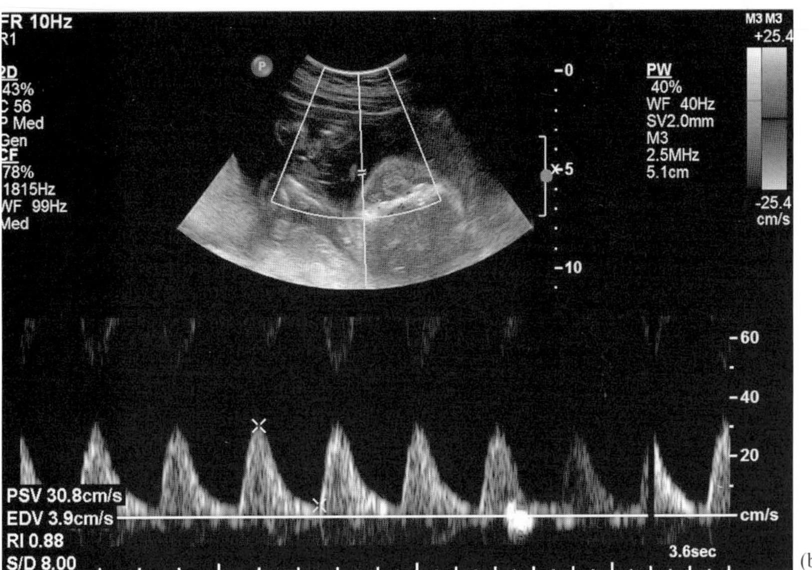

(b)

Fig 5.1 (a) Normal umbilical artery waveform. (b) Umbilical artery with low end diastolic flow.

The most common ways of quantifying the relationship between systole and diastole are as follows: (1) the S/D ratio; (2) the pulsatility index (PI); and (3) the resistance index (RI). For no particular reason, we have been consistently using the S/D ratio, but some authors have preferred the other indices, especially if the end diastolic flow is close to, or at, zero. However, all we are interested in is whether there is less end diastolic flow, absent end diastolic flow, or reversed flow, and compulsing over a number may be unproductive since the decision to deliver will not be based exclusively on whether the S/D ratio is, let's say, 4 instead of 3.5.

I have included nomograms for S/D ratios and RIs (see Appendix), which are obviously dependent upon gestational age, but, in general, the S/D ratio should not be much above 3 (RI of 0.60) after 30 weeks. In IUGR, especially the variety that emerges early, the first sign of fetal compromise is a decrease in end diastolic flow. This will often worsen as pregnancy progresses.

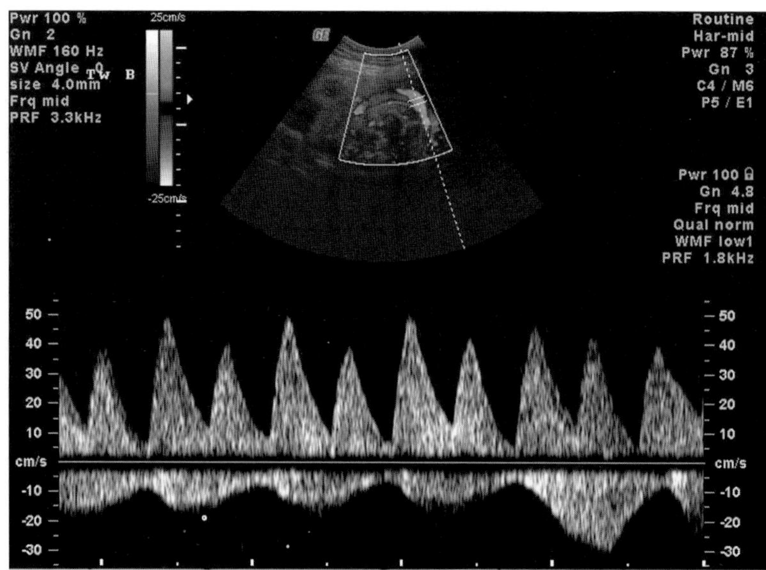

Fig 5.2 Umbilical artery waveform during fetal breathing.

Absent end diastolic flow at any time signifies trouble, and reverse flow is an ominous sign. The latter is a very late finding, correlating strongly with fetal death or neonatal morbidity.

For years, since Giles and Trudinger, pioneers in Doppler ultrasound, in 1989 showed that there were fewer terminal villi in the placentas of pregnancies in which umbilical artery end diastolic flow was diminished [4], investigators have realized that the die is cast early in pregnancy, and if the vascular bed is not overly arborized, the umbilical artery waveform will reflect this. However, this explanation would not explain the day-to-day dynamic changes often seen in umbilical artery waveforms. Now there is a suggestion that the placenta has a built-in mechanism to shunt blood away from poorly perfused areas, secondary to selective vasoconstriction and vasodilation of primary villi through a paracrine mechanism (similar to that seen in the adult lung).

Reams of information are now available in the literature to validate the use of umbilical artery waveform in the management of IUGR. For example, three meta-analyses [5–7] have shown that simply adding umbilical artery waveform to a surveillance plan will halve the perinatal mortality rate, and perhaps the most compelling case for using this approach comes from Karsdorp [8], who correlated various adverse outcomes with the level of end diastolic flow (Table 5.1).

Middle cerebral artery

These arteries come off the circle of Willis and head straight toward the cortex, generally in a direction that

Table 5.1 Doppler flow studies and outcome. (From Karsdorp VHM et al. [9], with permission from Elsevier.)

	Present end diastolic (%)	Absent end diastolic (%)	Reverse end diastolic (%)
Intrauterine death	6/214 (3)	25/178 (14)	16/67 (24)
Severe RDS	4/124 (3)	21/122 (17)	19/46 (41)
Admitted to NICU	126/208 (60)	147/153 (96)	50/51 (98)
Cerebral hemorrhage	1/124 (1)	11/122 (9)	16/46 (9)
Severe NEC	3/124 (3)	6/122 (5)	4/46 (9)

NEC, necrotizing enterocolitis; NICU, neonatal intensive care unit; RDS, respiratory distress syndrome.

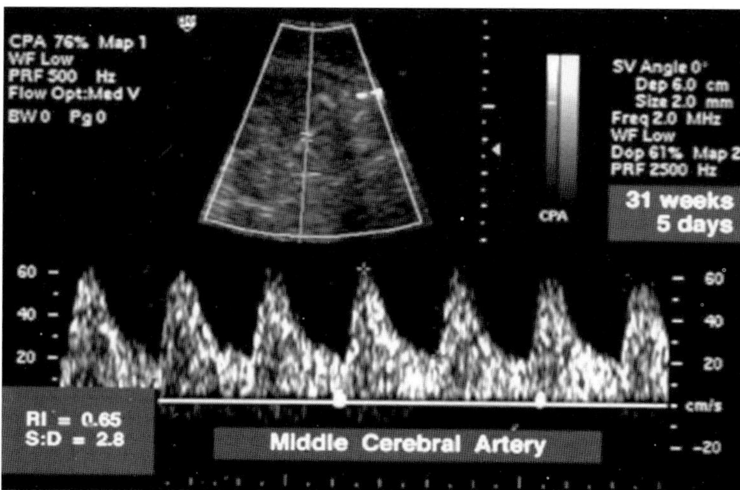

Fig 5.3 MCA: increased end diastolic flow.

lends itself to Doppler investigation (Plate 5.1). However, the waveform must be performed precisely. For example, the vessel should be sampled almost immediately after it leaves the circle of Willis (Plate 5.2). As opposed to the placental circulation, the cerebral vessels have a higher resistance with usual S/D ratios of 6 and RIs of greater than 0.80. However, in IUGR the fetus will spare his/her brain, heart, and adrenals, when hypoxic, which will result in a drop in resistance in these areas. Under these circumstances the end diastolic flow rises and the S/D ratio drops below 4, looking like a waveform from the umbilical artery (Figure 5.3). The good news is that when this is found in early IUGR, the fetus has activated his/her adaptive mechanism that generally accomplishes the mission—to protect the brain. The bad news is that the fetus has reached a point in the deprivation process to feel the need to trigger this maneuver, which has an off/on switch that is linked to the partial pressure of oxygen (PO_2) of the fetus.

It is clear that every truly deprived IUGR fetus will have increased end diastolic flow in middle cerebral artery (MCA) before delivery, but the timing is variable. In general, in early growth curtailment, the umbilical artery usually is abnormal many days before the MCA shows an increase in end diastolic flow. However, if there is a late plateauing of fetal growth after 30 weeks of gestation, then the MCA findings often precede umbilical artery changes. Most importantly, both umbilical artery and MCA waveform abnormalities are early changes in IUGR, and, in isolation, are not necessarily reasons to interrupt a preterm pregnancy.

The oligohydramnios seen in IUGR is due to autoregulation and is virtually always found in association with increased end diastolic flow in the MCA.

The fetal venous circulation

Oxygenated blood enters the umbilical vein and about 60% of this blood will continue upward through the ductus venosus (DV) to the heart. The remaining blood splits off at the bifurcation of the right and left portal vein to perfuse the right lobe of the liver. In IUGR about 80% of the umbilical vein flow gets shuttled through the DV to the right heart where, because of preferential directional streaming, the blood shoots across the foramen ovale to the left atrium and, ultimately, up the aorta to the brain. This is Mother Nature's way of assuring adequate brain oxygenation, while oxygen-poor blood entering the right atrium from the inferior vena cava, superior vena cava, and hepatic veins winds up in the right ventricle and then out the pulmonary arteries (Figure 5.4).

The point is that the system is heavily dependent on one small cone-shaped vessel that will alter its waveform according to the fetal cardiac demands and, actually, the cardiac efficiency. The ability of the fetus to move blood through the right atrium is dependent upon competition for access into this compartment, as well as on the contractility of the growth-restricted fetus's heart, which often has been laboring for many days against an after load (secondary to increased placental resistance). So, in the later stages of IUGR, there is less forward flow into the right atrium during atrial contraction, and the closer the

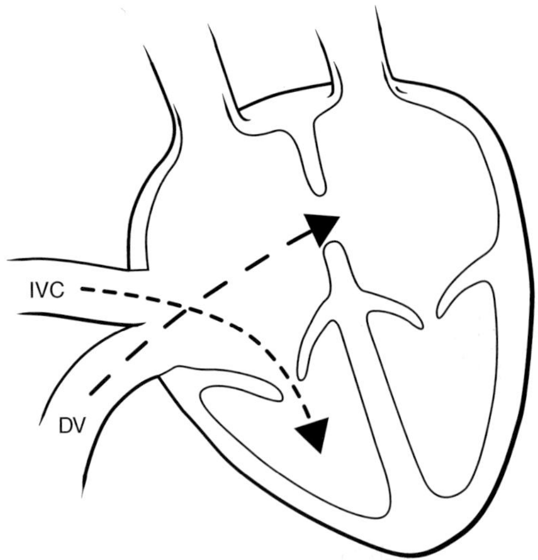

Fig 5.4 Preferential streaming of ductus venosus.

downward deflection is to the baseline, the more the fetus is in jeopardy (Figures 5.5a and 5.5b). This can be quantified by the distance (S/A) between the peak and trough of the wave form, which should not exceed 3.

Other veins that can be sampled with Doppler include the inferior vena cava, hepatic veins, umbilical part of the portal vein, and, furthest away from the heart, the umbilical vein in the cord. The latter two will show notch-like pulsations in severe IUGR.

The meaning of various waveform changes in IUGR

The umbilical arteries have been shown to be gross indicators of fetal circulatory status in general and, by representing the very earliest sign of trouble, are excellent excluders of fetal hypoxia and or metabolic acidosis when they are normal. The literature shows a distinct downturn in outcome when SGA fetuses have abnormal umbilical artery waveforms. However, many of the studies in which umbilical artery waveforms were abnormal had no other Doppler information and often the very severely compromised fetuses were lumped in with modestly affected ones. Interestingly, a few years ago investigators were able to invasively sample the fetal circulation through percutaneous umbilical blood sampling methods, and it was found that increased end diastolic flow in the MCA correlated with the PO_2 of the fetus and decreased flow during atrial contraction in the ductus venosus and inferior vena cava were correlated with the presence of fetal metabolic acidosis.

Years ago Soothill [10] followed 65 children who were admitted, as fetuses, to King's College Hospital for Doppler and percutaneous umbilical blood sampling studies because they were diagnosed to have IUGR. Neurological function was evaluated in each child with a Griffith developmental quotient test (Griffith DQ). The results were correlated against their in utero cord blood profile. There were only two variables that correlated with the Griffith DQ: the fetal pH and maternal smoking. The PO_2 had little bearing on the DQ score. This indirectly suggested that metabolic acidosis, and not hypoxia, by itself, had the greatest effect on subsequent neurological performance.

Three comprehensive Doppler studies [11–13] have shed light on the sequence of Doppler events associated with progressive worsening of fetal condition in early severe IUGR. In these studies, the fetuses were delivered only when fetal heart rate monitoring or biophysical profiles indicated fetal jeopardy (and the clinicians were interdicted from using Doppler information in their management). The umbilical artery and the MCA were affected early in the course of worsening fetal condition. The changes in these two vessels occurred up to 3 weeks before delivery and had a variable correlation with outcome. However, there was a strong correlation between abnormal ductus venosus (DV) waveforms, representing late findings, and fetal death and CNS abnormalities.

The latest study addressing Doppler's ability to predict fetal acidosis emanates from Brazil [14]. Only fetuses with absent or reversed end diastolic were included in this recent study. The authors found a strong relationship between the depth of the deflection during atrial contraction in the DV (in their words "the pulsatility index for veins") and the cord pH at birth. The correlation was so strong that they could predict the degree of acidemia from the DV alone.

Not all studies have shown the strong correlation between DV and outcome. However, until other information surfaces, I will weigh heavily the DV results in the clinical management of IUGR because (1) the results in the above studies were compelling, (2) the results make sense regarding the physiology of the process, and (3) I am biased because our group was involved in one of these studies [11].

In 1993, Pardi et al. [15] published a landmark paper in which IUGR fetuses were studied with periodic percutaneous umbilical cord blood samplings, serial umbilical artery Doppler evaluations, and fetal heart rate monitoring. The fetuses were broken down into three groups. Group 1 consisted of those with normal fetal heart rate and normal Dopplers. None of these had evidence

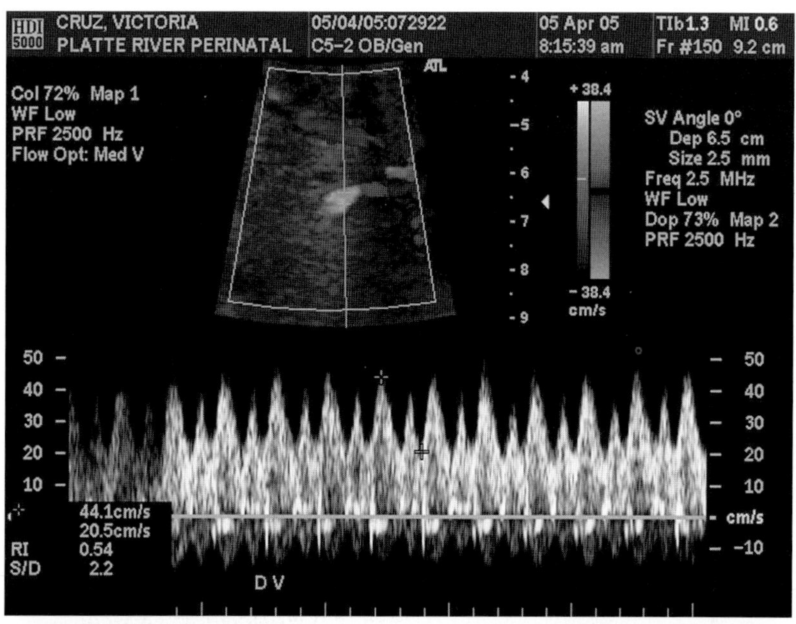

(a)

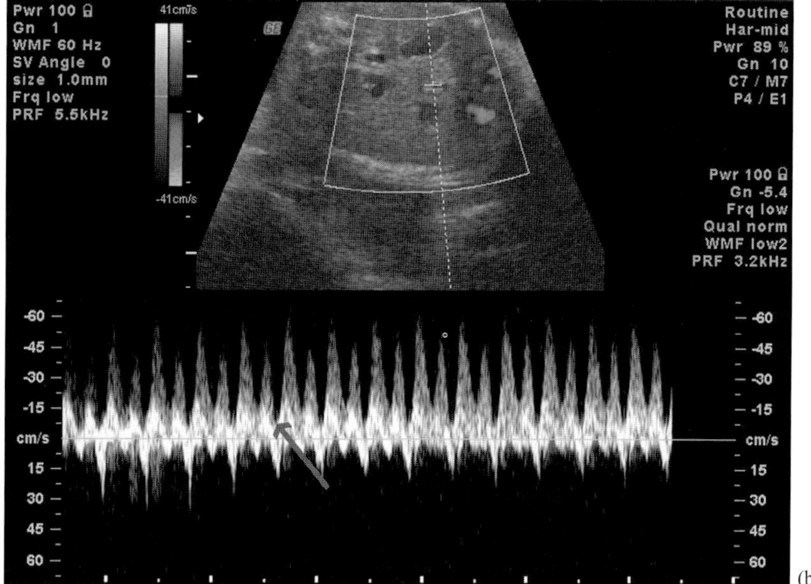

(b)

Fig 5.5 (a) Normal ductous venosus. Calipers on systolic peak and velocity during atrial contractions. Note the S/D of 2.2 is within normal limits. (b) Abnormal wave form from ductus venosus. Arrow marks decreased velocity during atrial contraction.

of hypoxia or acidosis. Group 2 consisted of those with "abnormal" Dopplers and normal fetal heart rate, and less than 5% of these fetuses had either a low PO_2 or pH. Group 3 fetuses had both abnormal fetal heart rate and abnormal Dopplers. Sixty percent of these fetuses had acidosis and/or hypoxia.

The take-home message is that umbilical artery abnormalities alone are probably not enough to warrant delivery, especially in very premature fetuses, but if we wait until the fetal heart rate becomes nonreassuring, we may have waited too long. This is why the DV information is so enlightening. However, Baschat also makes the point that the biophysical profile should not be abandoned, because it is testing independently another fetal variable, the CNS. Both can be useful adjunctively in making difficult management decisions.

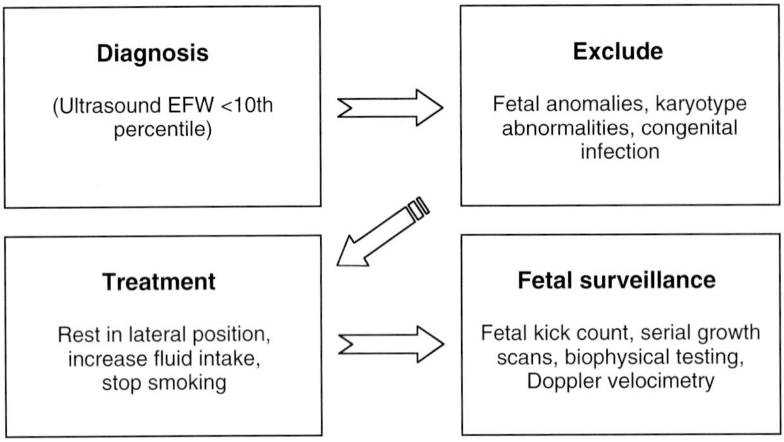

Diagnosis	→	Exclude
(Ultrasound EFW <10th percentile)		Fetal anomalies, karyotype abnormalities, congenital infection
Treatment	→	**Fetal surveillance**
Rest in lateral position, increase fluid intake, stop smoking		Fetal kick count, serial growth scans, biophysical testing, Doppler velocimetry

Fig 5.6 Algorithm for fetal surveillance and management of IUGR (courtesy of University of Colorado School of Medicine).

We use our University of Colorado algorithm (Figure 5.6) for fetal surveillance and management of IUGR once the fetus has been labeled as small-for-dates.

26–34 weeks nonstress test (NST) and Doppler studies in fetuses with EFW of <10th percentile

1 NST reactive
  a Umbilical artery Doppler reassuring
    i Repeat in 1 week
  b Umbilical artery Doppler nonreassuring
    i Venous Dopplers
      1 Reassuring: repeat in 1 week
      2 Nonreassuring: deliver
2 NST nonreactive*
  a Umbilical artery Doppler nonreassuring (absent/reverse EDF)
    i Deliver

34–36 weeks NST and Doppler studies

1 Both tests reassuring
  a Repeat in 1 week (OR)
  b Test for fetal lung maturity
    i Immature: repeat in 1 week
    ii Mature: deliver
2 Either test nonreassuring
  a Deliver

≥36 weeks: deliver

*It is realized that NSTs are often "non-reactive" in normal fetuses below 30 weeks, but in this context, absent beat-to-beat variability and *no* accelerations are ominous signs.

Case in point

This patient was referred in at 30 weeks with a diagnosis of IUGR. We found the estimated fetal weight to be 1000 g, which was well below the10th percentile.

The TCD was appropriate for 30 weeks, the HC for 19 weeks, and the AC for 28 weeks. Although morphologically normal appearing, the placenta was small. There was oligohydramnios with the largest vertical pocket being 1.5 cm. The umbilical arteries were slightly discordant with one having absent end diastolic flow and the other had a very low end diastolic component (S/D ratio of 6.8). The MCA had evidence of brain sparing (S/D ratio of 3.2). The NST was reactive and the ductus had a normal waveform.

We hospitalized her and initiated steroids to accelerate fetal lung maturity. Over the next week both umbilical arteries had absent diastolic flow but no hint of reversed flow. Although the NSTs remained reactive, the velocity of the ductus flow during atrial contraction began to stray downward toward the baseline.

We bailed out at 31 weeks 2 days, just as the patient was becoming overtly preeclamptic. The NST was weakly reactive at that time.

The fetus was born by cesarean section with a cord pH of 7.16, a base excess of 8, and Apgars of 8–9. The baby weighed 1200 g and did well enough in the nursery to enter her first spelling Bee.

References

1 Lindqvist PG, Molin J. Does antenatal identification of small-for-gestational age fetuses significantly improve their

outcome? Ultrasound Obstet Gynecol 2005; 25: 258–64.

2 Campbell S, Thoms A. Ultrasound measurement of the fetal head to abdomen circumference ration in the assessment of growth retardation. Br J Obstet Gynaecol 1977; 84: 165–74.

3 Hadlock FP, Deter RL, Harrist RB, et al. A date-independent predictor of intrauterine growth retardation: femur length/abdominal circumference. Am J Roentgenol 1983; 141: 979–84.

4 Giles WB, Trudinger BJ. Umbilical cord whole blood viscosity and the umbilical artery flow velocity time waveforms: a correlation. Br J Obstet Gynaecol 1986; 93: 466–70.

5 Divon MY. Umbilical artery Doppler velocimetry: clinical utility in high-risk pregnancies. Am J Obstet Gynecol 1996; 174: 10–14.

6 Alfirevic Z, Neilson JP. Doppler ultrasonography in high-risk pregnancies: systematic review with meta-analysis. Am J Obstet Gynecol 1995; 172: 1379–87.

7 Westergaard HB, Langhoff-Roos J, Lingman G, et al. A critical appraisal of the use of umbilical artery Doppler ultrasound high-risk pregnancies: use of metal-analysis in evidence-based obstetrics. Ultrasound Obstet Gynecol 2001; 17: 466–76.

8 Karsdorp VH, Dirks BK, van der Linden JC, et al. Placenta morphology and absent or reversed end diastolic flow velocities in the umbilical artery: a clinical and morphometrical study. Placenta 1996; 17: 393–9.

9 Karsdorp VHM, van Vugt JM, van Geijn HP, et al. Clinical significant of absent or reversed end diastolic velocity waveforms in umbilical artery. Lancet 1994; 344: 1664–8.

10 Soothill PW, Ajayi RA, Campbell S, et al. Fetal oxygenation at cordocentesis, maternal smoking and child neurodevelopment. Eur J Obstet Gynecol Reprod Biol 1995; 59: 21–4.

11 Ferrazzi E, Bozzo M, Rigano S, et al. Temporal sequence of abnormal Doppler changes in the peripheral and central circulatory systems of the severely growth-restricted fetus. Ultrasound Obstet Gynecol 2002; 19: 140–6.

12 Baschat AA, Gembruch U, Harmon CR. The sequent of changes in Doppler and biophysical parameters as several fetal growth restriction worsens. Ultrasound Obstet Gynecol 2001; 18: 571–7.

13 Hecher K, Bilardo CM, Stigter RH, et al. Monitoring of fetuses with intrauterine growth restriction: a longitudinal study. Ultrasound Obstet Gynecol 2001; 18: 564–70.

14 Francisco RPV, Miyadahira S, Zugaib M, et al. Predicting pH at birth in absent or reverse end diastolic velocity in umbilical arteries. Obstet Gynecol 2006; 107: 1042–8.

15 Pardi G, Cetin I, Marconi AM, et al. Diagnostic value of blood sampling and fetuses with growth retardation. N Engl J Med 1993; 328: 692–6.

6 Examination of the fetal cranium

During the fetal survey three areas within the cranium need to be examined (Figure 6.1). The first view is part of the standard biometry: a slice through the thalami, which would include a glimpse of the frontal horns, a view of the slit-like third ventricle, and an appreciation of the size and shape of the cavum septi pellucidi (Figure 6.2). Generous size frontal horns, a dilated third ventricle, or a poorly defined cavum should alert the operator to delve more deeply into the intracranial anatomy.

The second area to explore is a section through the lateral ventricles. This involves obtaining an axial cross-section of the fetal cranium at a level just above that used for the biparietal diameter (BPD) (Figure 6.3). Once obtained, a visual assessment of the size of the lateral ventricles is made at the level of the atrium, as well as a subjective judgment as to whether the downside choroid plexus is "dangling" (Figure 6.4). Also the ventricles should be at a slight angle with the midline and the long axis should not run parallel to the falx (as in agenesis of the corpus callosum). If the ventricles seem generous in size, then a measurement is made from the inner wall to the outer wall of the lateral ventricle at the level of the atrium. A method to indirectly quantify the amount of dangle is to measure the distance from the medial wall of the lateral ventricle to the medial margin of the choroid plexus, again at the level of the atrium (Figures 6.5 and 6.6). The upper limits of normal are 10 mm for the lateral ventricle and 4 mm for the medial gap measurement. Most investigators use a lateral ventricular range of 10–15 mm to denote "minimal or modest" enlargement and anything over 15 mm to represent "significant" or "severe" dilation.

The third stop for the operator following the standard guidelines for a basic ultrasound examination is the posterior fossa, which involves a small rotation of the transducer occipitally, while moving first through a cross-section of the superior cerebellar vermis, on the way to the inferior vermis, where the image is then frozen, as indicated in level 3 of Figure 6.1 (Figure 6.7). In this slice the size of the cisterna magna can be evaluated, as well as the integrity of the vermis itself. If a portion of the inferior cerebellar vermis is missing, then a diagnosis of partial vermal agenesis can be confirmed with mid-sagittal and coronal views, often obtained transvaginally or through 3D. If the entire vermis is missing, then the diagnosis of complete agenesis, or Dandy–Walker syndrome, can be made by noting a communication between the fourth ventricle and the cisterna magna (later). Last, the diagnosis of an open spina bifida can be excluded by the finding of a normal posterior fossa.

Filly, a leader in obstetric ultrasound, has long maintained that these three views should enable the sonographer/sonologist to rule out over 90% of the intracranial anomalies affecting the fetus. On the other hand, if any of the views produces concern about the anatomy, other techniques can be added to accomplish further investigation.

The next section will deal with the more worrisome findings that may emerge from the three basic views described above. First, a word about the normal pathway taken by cerebral spinal fluid.

Circulation of cerebral spinal fluid

The cerebral spinal fluid is produced predominantly by the choroid plexus in both lateral ventricles, with a modest amount coming from the choroid plexus forming the roof of the third ventricle. The fluid then passes bilaterally from the lateral ventricles into the third ventricle through the foramen of Monroe. From there it moves south through the aqueduct of Sylvius to the fourth ventricle, where the fluid finds its way into the subarachnoid space via the foramens of Lushka and Magendie. Finally, the fluid is absorbed in the superior sagittal sinus (Figure 6.8).

Obstetric Ultrasound: Artistry in Practice. John C. Hobbins. Published 2008 Blackwell Publishing. ISBN 978-1-4051-5815-2.

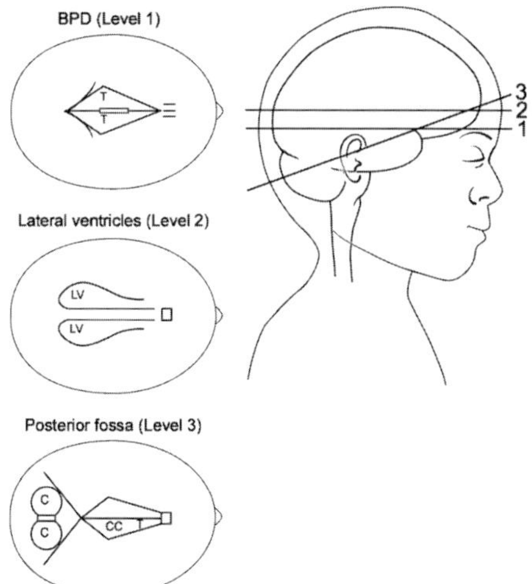

Fig 6.1 Schematic of three essential planes in screening for cranial abnormalities. (1) BPD plane, (2) Lateral ventricle plane. (3) Posterior fossa plane. T = thalami, LV = lateral ventricle, C = cavum, CC = corpus callosum, CV = cerebellar vermis.

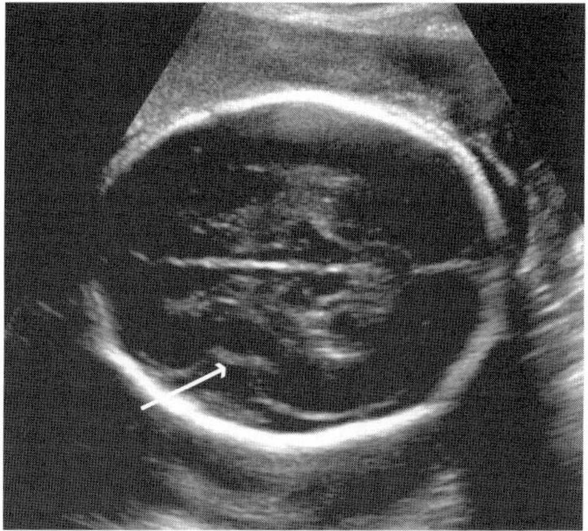

Fig 6.2 Plane of BPD, obtained at level 1 of schematic, demonstrating cavum, thalami, and Sylvian fissure as indicated by arrow.

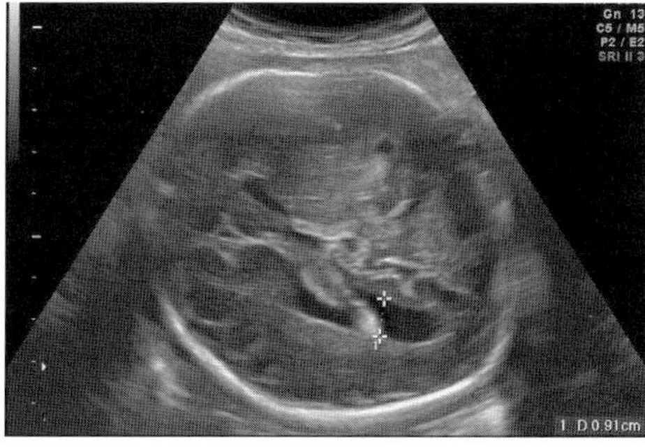

Fig 6.3 Proper plane to demonstrate lateral ventricles at level 2.

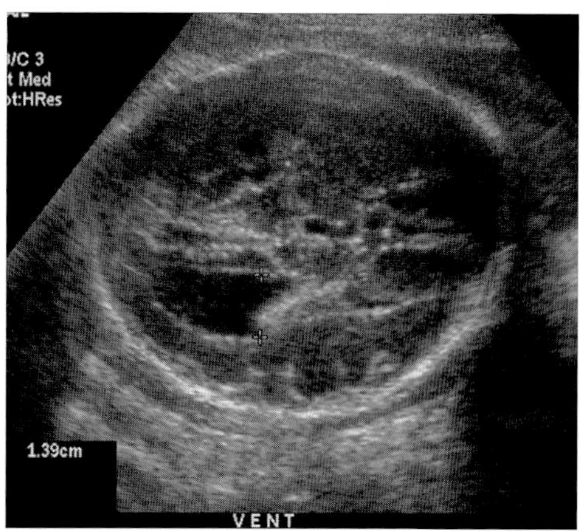

Fig 6.4 Dangling choroid plexus in fetus with modest ventriculomegaly in agenesis of the corpus callosum.

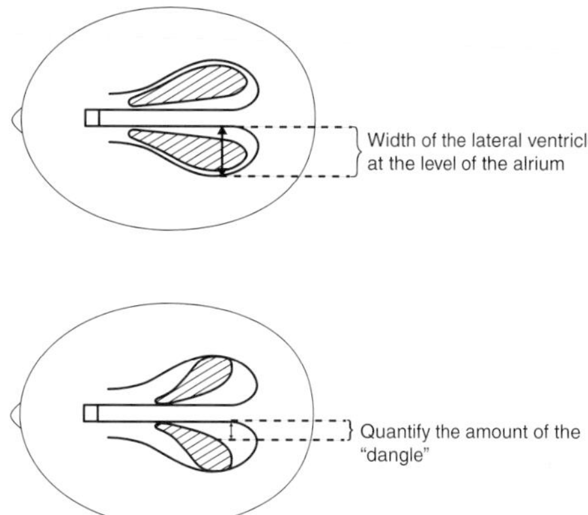

Fig 6.5 Normal alignment of choroids plexus compared with "dangling" impression in ventriculomegaly.

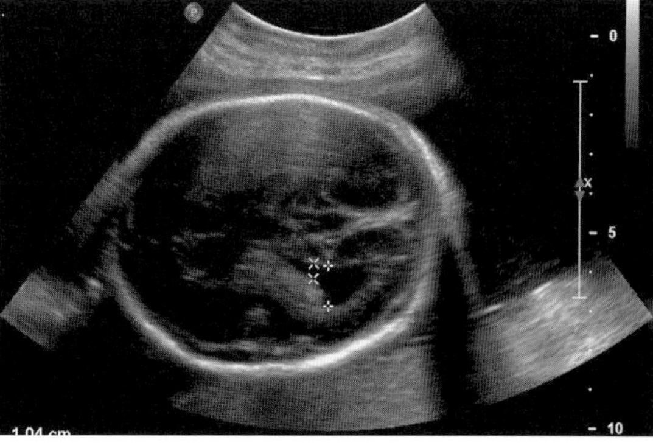

Fig 6.6 Measurements for lateral ventricle.

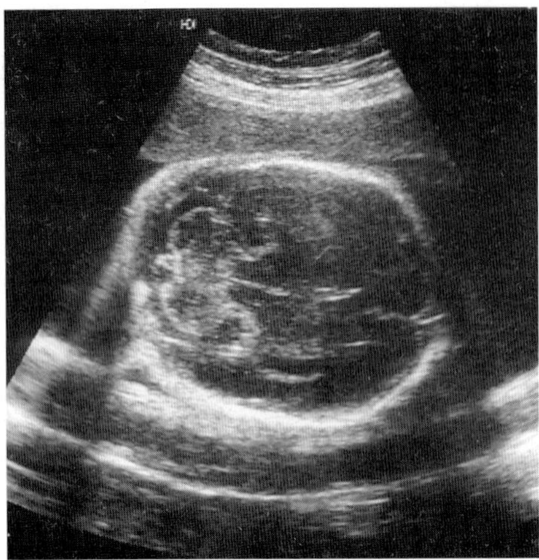

Fig 6.7 Posterior fossa, obtained at level 3 of schematic.

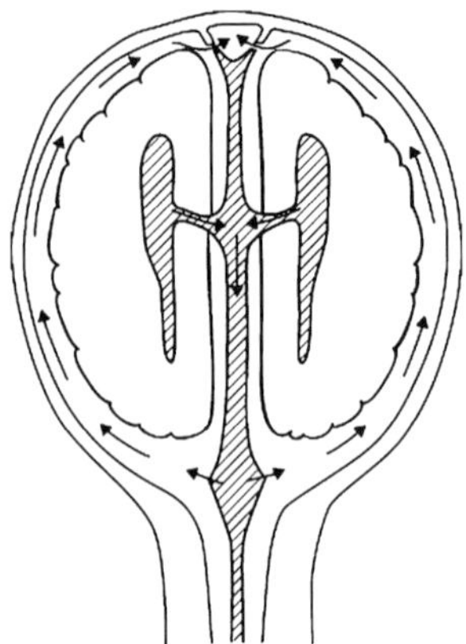

Fig 6.8 Circulation of cerebral spinal fluid; normal pathway.

Hydrocephalus generally is defined by a lateral ventricular width of greater than 1.5 cm, and can be broken down into two types: communicating or noncommunicating. The former means that the above pathways are open, but there is either an overproduction, as in choroid plexus papillomas, or an inherent problem with absorption in the superior sagittal sinus. These are uncommon findings in the fetus. The classification of obstructive hydrocephalus, which points to an impedance to the flow of cerebral spinal fluid somewhere along the pathway, can be due to aqueductal stenosis or to disruption of the posterior fossa structures, as in the Arnold–Chiari 2 anomaly noted in all fetuses with open spina bifida, or Dandy–Walker syndrome, both disallowing fluid to move out into the subarachnoid space.

The job of the clinician is to piece the diagnostic puzzle together by assessing the relative size of the intracranial compartments (Table 6.1).

Ventriculomegaly

If ventriculomegaly is present, then a very thorough search for other intracranial or extracranial abnormalities must be undertaken because a truly isolated mild ventriculomegaly has a far different prognosis than one found in conjunction with other findings. The recent literature must be explored to sort out the real prognosis for this finding in isolation, especially since older studies did not benefit from today's techniques and technology. Three recent studies have provided the greatest insight regarding the outcome of the isolated ventriculomegaly. Goldstein et al. [1] contributed 34 cases of mild ventriculomegaly

Table 6.1 Assessing intracranial compartments.

	Lat Ventricles	Third Ventricle	Cortex	Subarachnoid space	Cisterna Magna	Fourth Ventricle
Aqueductal stenosis	↑	↑	↓	↓	↔	↔
Communicating hydrocephaly	↑	↑	↔	↑	↔	↑
Dandy–Walker syndrome	↑	↑	↔	↓	↑	↑
Agenesis of the corpus callosum	↑	↑	↔	↔	↔	↔
Cortical dysgenesis	↑	↔	↓	↑	↔	↔
Open spina bifida	↑	↑	↔	↓ ↔	↓↓	↔

↑, Increased; ↓, decreased; ↔, unaffected.

and Breeze [2] another 30 cases. In the former study one-third resolved by birth and in the latter study 50% spontaneously regressed to normal. Breeze found that 21 of the 30 cases were isolated and only 4 of these had a neurological abnormality after birth.

The last study, involving 176 cases of ventriculomegaly was very enlightening. Gaglioti [3] further divided ventricular width into mild (10–12.5 mm), moderate (12.5–15 mm), or severe (greater than 15 mm).

In the mild group, 58.7% were isolated and the chances of intact survival (up to 24 months) in those with isolated mild ventriculomegaly were 97.7%, compared with 80% in the isolated moderate group and 33% in the isolated severe group. In all three studies there were 15 of 240 cases (5.9%) with abnormal karyotypes and 110 cases (45%) with major abnormalities. However, in truly isolated ventriculomegaly, especially when the measurement was between 10 and 12.5 mm, the prognosis was excellent.

Since the term "isolated" carries so much meaning with regard to prognosis, the workup for ventriculomegaly should be aggressive. First, a very thorough search for anomalies should start at the fetal head and standard 2D axial scans will not suffice. Investigation of the posterior fossa can be undertaken axially to rule out any signs of Arnold–Chiari 2 malformation by demonstrating the presence of fluid in the cisterna magna, the absence of a banana sign, and the absence of herniation downward into the foramen magnum of the cerebellar vermis. At the same time, the integrity of the cerebellar vermis can be assessed. Then there should be an attempt to obtain coronal and mid-sagittal views of the intracranial anatomy through either a transvaginal approach in a vertex presentation or a forceful fundal approach in the breech presentation. 3D has been very useful in getting these views after-the-fact through planar reconstruction. However, an axial sweep at the level of, let's say, the BPD puts into play lateral resolution, so no amount of off-site manipulation of the image can get you the same quality definition as those initially acquired coronally or sagittally.

One of the most common associated intracranial anomalies is agenesis of the corpus callosum, which can be suspected by an inability to visualize the cavum septi pellucidi, a high placement of the third ventricle, and/or, as indicated above, by noting a parallel alignment of the lateral ventricles on standard axial views (Figure 6.9). However, this diagnosis can be clinched with coronal and sagittal views, allowing the operator to trace out the entire length of the corpus callosum and to identify the elevated third ventricle, uncontained by the absent corpus callosum (Figure 6.10).

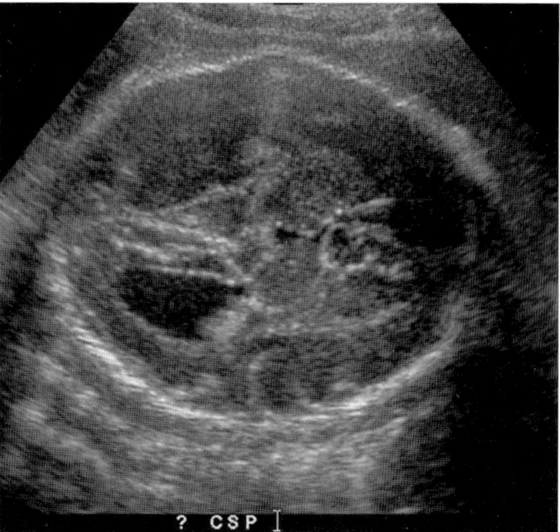

Fig 6.9 Parallel ventricles in agenesis of the corpus callosum.

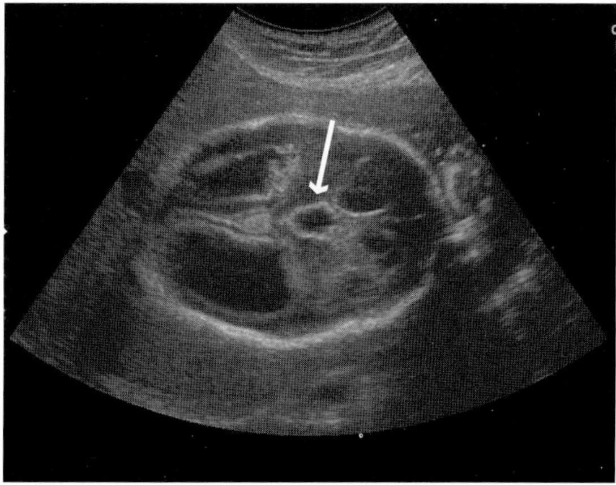

Fig 6.10 Uncontained dilated third ventricle in plane above BPD.

It is possible that modest ventriculomegaly in the second trimester could represent a clue to later full-blown hydrocephalus secondary to an aqueductal stenosis, but the ventricles generally are more than modestly dilated in this condition. The tip-off here would be a dilated third ventricle (Figure 6.11). Last, the enlarged ventricles could represent cortical dysplasia, which should be suspected by a small head circumference, a relatively enlarged subarachnoid space, a thin cortex, and a blunted or poorly defined insula.

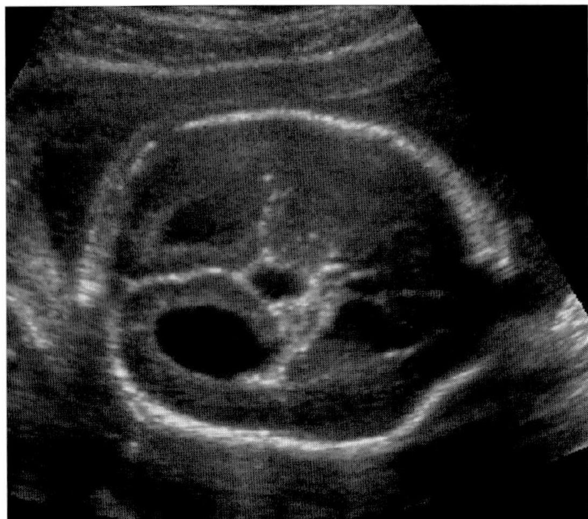

Fig 6.11 Dilated third and lateral ventricles in aqueductal stenosis.

Other areas to explore would be the fetal heart and limbs, and, since 6% of the fetuses with ventriculomegaly in the above studies had chromosomal abnormalities, an amniocentesis would be strongly recommended; especially if another abnormality is noted.

Again, most importantly, if the ventricular dilation is in the modest range, and an investigation for associated abnormalities is negative, the prognosis generally is good for these fetuses.

Aqueductal stenosis

This condition is caused by a narrowing of the aqueduct of Sylvius, resulting in dilation of the ventricular system above the obstruction (Figure 6.12). Often the lateral ventricles are markedly dilated, resulting in significant compression of the cortex and subarachnoid space (Figure 6.13).

Since shunting of the cerebral ventricles after birth can have a beneficial "bounce back" effect on the cortex, a few attempts at in utero shunting were carried out with the idea that earlier relief of the cortical compression would be of benefit. Unfortunately, when these cases were lumped together in a registry, the results were no better than if one were to wait until birth for the performance of invasive measures, and it became clear that the procedure itself had significant morbidity. At present, there is a moratorium on this type of in utero therapy.

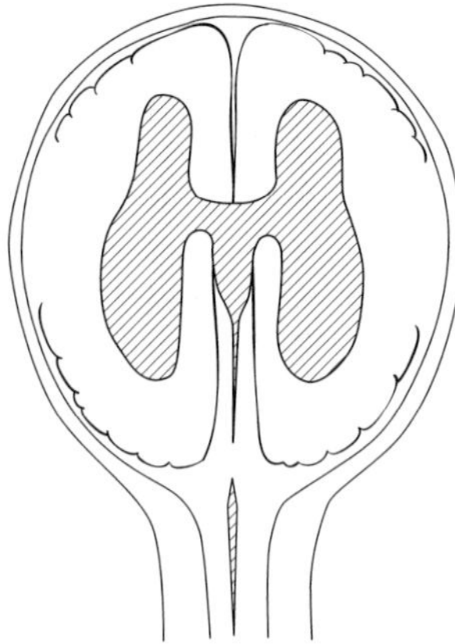

Fig 6.12 Schematic of circulation of CSF in aqueductal stenosis.

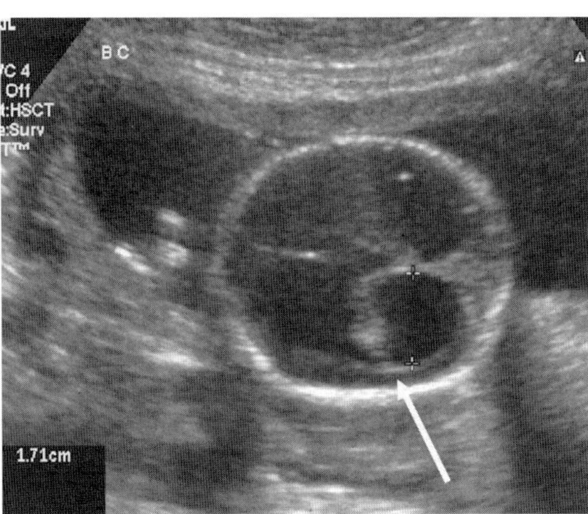

Fig 6.13 Aqueductal stenosis. Compressed cortex marked by arrow.

If an obstruction to the aqueduct is not enough of a problem alone, some fetuses with this abnormality will also have other anomalies, which are often more serious than the aqueductal stenosis. Obviously, every fetus with hydrocephalus should be carefully examined for other anomalies.

A rare variant of this condition will reappear in families as an X-linked disorder.

Agenesis of the corpus callosum

This condition is found in 0.3–0.7% of the overall population and has been noted in 2–3% of the mentally disabled.

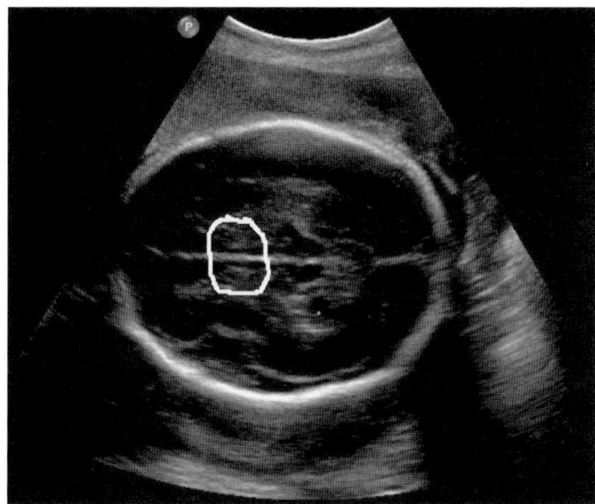

Fig 6.14 Base of the cavum represented by three lines within white circle.

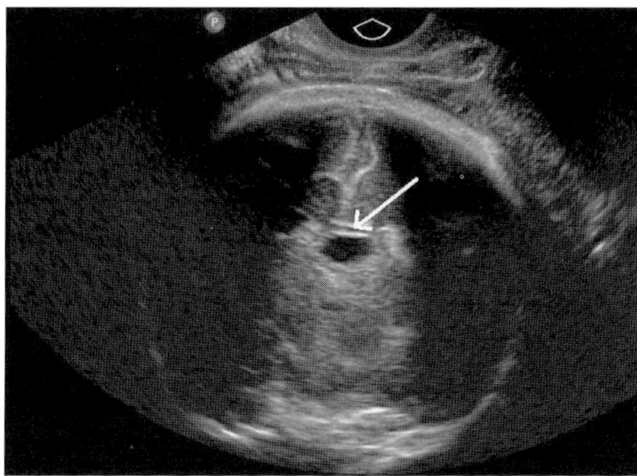

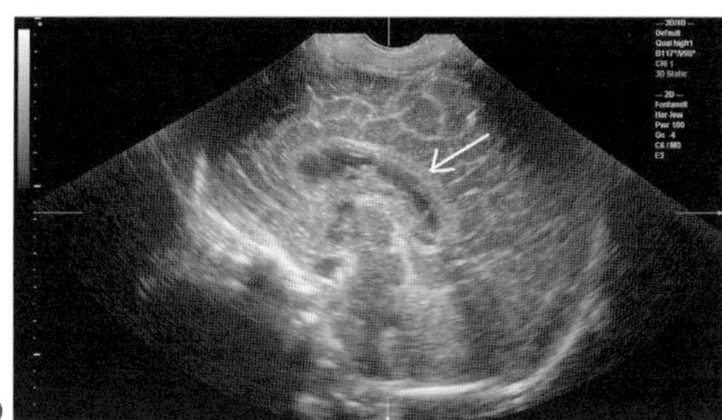

Fig 6.15 (a) Coronal view of corpus callosum, marked by arrow. (b) Mid-sagittal view, arrow points to corpus callosum.

Since the corpus callosum is not completely formed until after 18 weeks, the diagnosis in the second trimester can be challenging. The diagnosis can be suspected when, on axial scan, the lateral ventricles run parallel to the midline (Figure 6.9), instead of having the usual slightly diagonal pathway across the occipital portion of the brain. Since the cavum is never present in this condition, one might think that its presence would exclude the diagnosis. However, at times, in agenesis of the corpus callosum one can be fooled on axial scan by a midline alignment of echoes mimicking the cavum. I have found that the best way to demonstrate the integrity of the cavum is to use an image at the level of the BPD that has three lines, representing the base of the cavum (Figure 6.14).

If agenesis of the corpus callosum is suspected on standard axial views, the diagnosis can be confirmed by noting a conspicuous absence of the cavum and the accompanying superior rim of corpus callosum on coronal (Figure 6.15a) and/or mid-sagittal (Figure 6.15b) views. Also, not infrequently, the third ventricle, uncontained by the corpus callosum, will herniate upward into an unoccupied space. Midline sagittal views can also separate partial from complete agenesis (Figure 6.16) where, in the former condition, a portion of the caudal part of the corpus callosum is missing. Also mid-sagittal views will allow the sonologist/ sonographers to identify the pericallosal artery (Plate 6.1), which is absent in complete agenesis, or will veer off in partial agenesis.

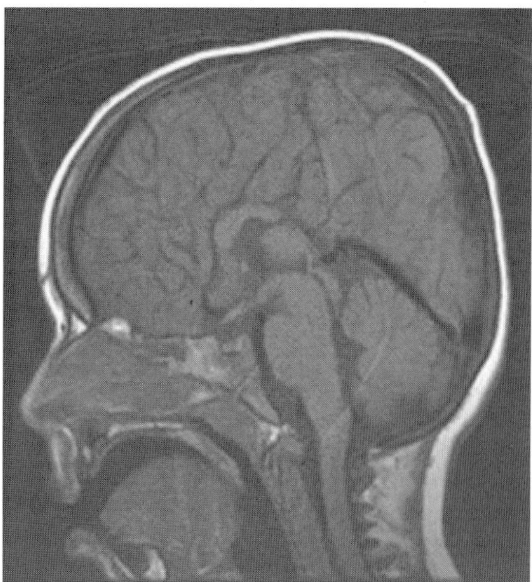

Fig 6.16 MRI of partial agenesis of the corpus callosum.

As with other cranial abnormalities, the bad news with this condition is that about half the time it is associated with other, more serious, abnormalities. The good news is that if it is truly isolated, infants/adults can often adapt well to life without it. Pilu [4] reported in 2002 on 30 infants with truly isolated agenesis of the corpus callosum who were followed from a few months after birth to 11 years of age. Twenty-six children had normal to borderline IQs (87%).

Midline defects

The holoprosencephalies are fortunately rare, and involve the absence of midline intracranial structures. The most common variation is the most severe—alobar holoprosencephaly—in which there is a single rudimentary ventricle spanning the midline. In essence, the cavum and corpus callosum are absent, but, in addition, there is central fusion of the frontal horns, which, in turn, communicate fully with the third ventricle (Figure 6.17).

This condition by itself has a bad enough prognosis, but often it is accompanied by other abnormalities of the posterior fossa and face (hypotelorism, cyclopia, proboscis formation, and midline cleft lip). The combination of holoprosencephaly with a midline cleft should alert the clinician to the strong likelihood of trisomy 13, especially if there is evidence of polydactyly.

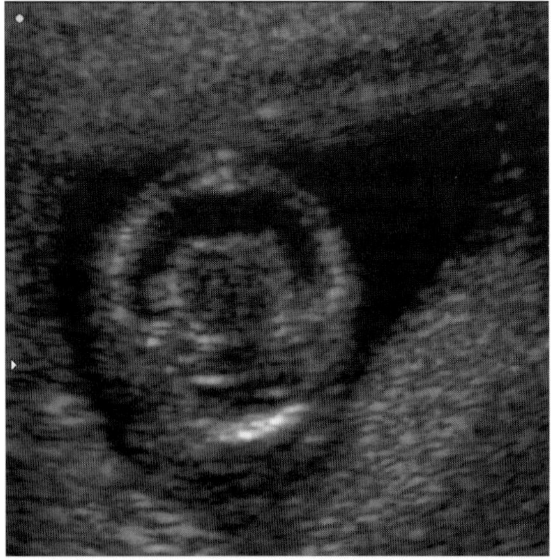

Fig 6.17 Holoprosencephaly at 14 weeks (T13).

Septal optic dysplasia

This is a very rare condition that can be difficult to distinguish from lobar holoprosencephaly. It can best be diagnosed by midline sagittal views showing a thin rim of corpus callosum without an underlying cavum. On coronal views, the channel across the space vacated by the cavum can often be appreciated (Figure 6.18).

This condition can be devastating, resulting in blindness and developmental delay.

Dandy–Walker complex

Cerebellar dysgenesis is fortunately rare, with an incidence of 1 in 30,000. It is responsible for between 4 and 12% of hydrocephalus.

Complete agenesis is far easier to diagnose since these cases are virtually always associated with a large cisterna magna and a clear communication with the fourth ventricle. Partial agenesis, often labeled as Dandy–Walker variant, is easy to "overcall" (with a tangential cut creating an illusion of a "nick"), especially prior to the twentieth week when the normal development of the inferior vermis is not yet complete. Beware of a defect having a "keyhole" configuration on coronal views. Recently, a compelling case has been made for demanding that the defect have a trapezoid-like shape to be labeled as a Dandy–Walker variant. Often a standard axial view will not tell the whole story and, if there is a suspicion of a vermal defect, a coronal slice will enable the examiner the opportunity to view both the superior and the inferior vermis (Figure 6.19).

The ideal way to nail down the diagnosis of partial vermal agenesis is to obtain a mid-sagittal view through the vermis, which is often best obtained with 3D. In this plane the vermis can be thoroughly scrutinized with regard to its size, configuration, and its position in the posterior fossa (Figure 6.20). In vermal abnormalities the vermis is elevated, which affects the angle of its long axis, and its bulk is often reduced by half. In complete agenesis there simply

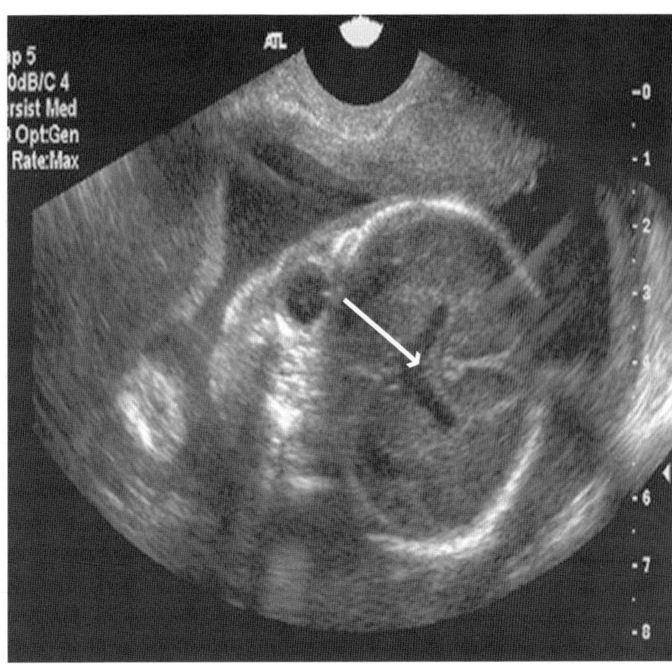

Fig 6.18 Septo-optic dysplasia. Note absent cavum, as marked by arrow.

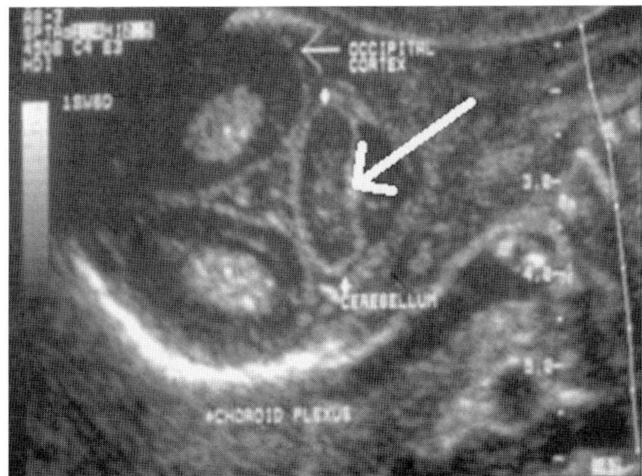

Fig 6.19 Normal posterior fossa coronal view. Arrow points to intact inferior cerebellar vermis.

will be a gap where the vermis is supposed to be and an obvious communication between the cisterna magna and the fourth ventricle (Figure 6.21).

Again, with Dandy–Walker variant a defect can be missed with an axial scan alone (Figures 6.22a and 6.22b).

If the vermal defect seems small, MRI can be used to confirm the diagnosis.

Mortality rates with Dandy–Walker syndrome can be as high as 24%, but often this is because of an elevated rate of associated extracranial anomalies (50–70%) such as polycystic kidneys, cardiac anomalies, and facial clefting. Subnormal intelligence has been noted in 40–70% of survivors.

Destructive intracranial abnormalities

Porencephaly simply refers to an area within the brain that is devoid of tissue. The term often is followed by the word "cyst," as in "porencephalic cyst." Actually, this absence of tissue can either be a primary developmental defect or can be acquired (pseudoporencephaly) secondary to a vascular accident, drug-induced effect (cocaine), or an infectious cause. The former tends to be bilateral and symmetrical, while the latter is unilateral or asymmetrical. An example of developmental porencephaly is schizencephaly in which clefts are seen connecting the lateral ventricles with the subarachnoid space through the area of the insula (Figure 6.23).

Hydranencephaly is the most severe variant of porencephaly. Here, little brain tissue is formed superior to the

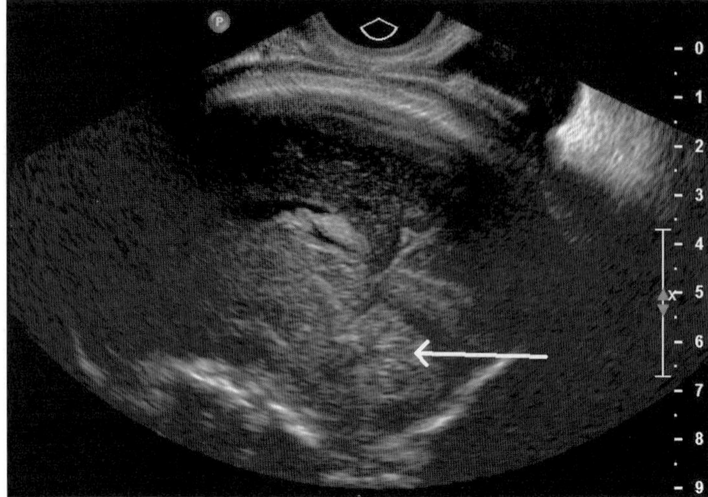

Fig 6.20 Normal alignment of posterior fossa on quasi-mid-sagittal view. Arrow points to cerebellar vermis.

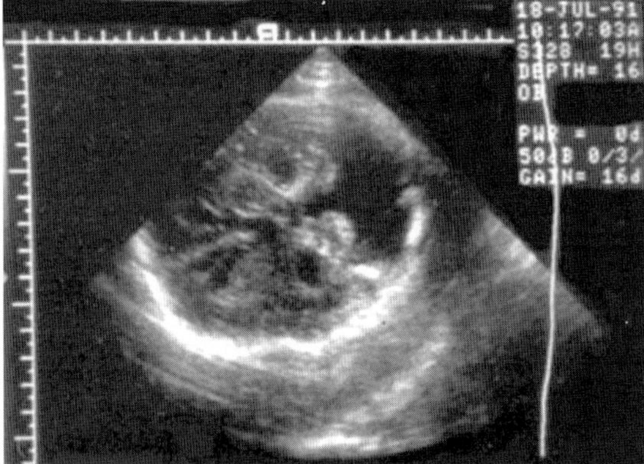

Fig 6.21 Complete agenesis of the vermis.

brainstem and the head seems almost completely filled with fluid in an otherwise normal appearing fetus.

It is unclear if this devastating condition is due to a massive vascular accident involving the internal carotids or to an infectious etiology.

Cerebral dysgenesis

This group of abnormalities involves inherent interference in neuronal migration and often evolves into a condition in which the fetus has a small head, a thin cortex, poorly developed sulci and gyri, and, ultimately, severe disability.

Microcephaly

Although simple biometry can alert the clinician to a possible problem, far more often than not, a small head circumference is a normal finding. In one study [5], if the head circumferences of infants were between 2 and 3 SDs below the mean, only 18% had mental retardation, but if the head circumference was more than 3 SDs below the mean, there was a 70% chance of retardation.

After a head circumference shows more than a 3-week discrepancy, a few simple steps will help to separate out the fetus with a problem. First, fetuses with pathologic microcephaly will have a sloping forehead secondary to a small frontal lobe, which can be indirectly assessed by a measurement made in the plane of the BPD from the back of the cavum to the inner table of the calvarium (Figure 6.24). This measurement is about 1–2 mm more than gestational age in weeks, up until 22 weeks. After this time the measurement is roughly the same as the TCD, the nomogram of which is in the Appendix. Also, a nomogram utilizing a measurement from the posterior margin of the thalamus to the calvarium (frontal thalamic diameter) is included in the Appendix as an alternative to assess the size of the frontal lobe. In pathologic microcephaly, these

(a)
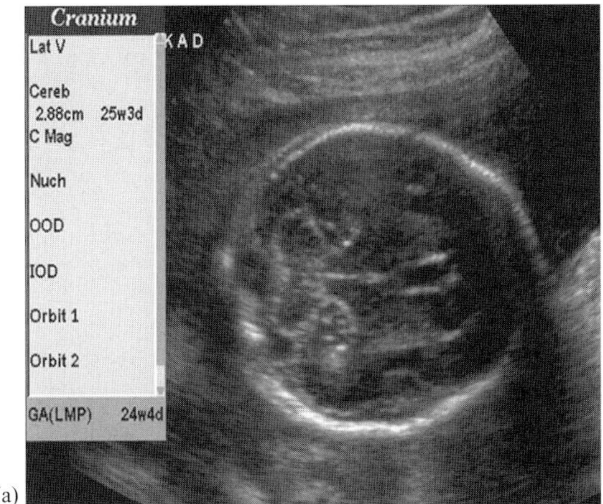

(b)
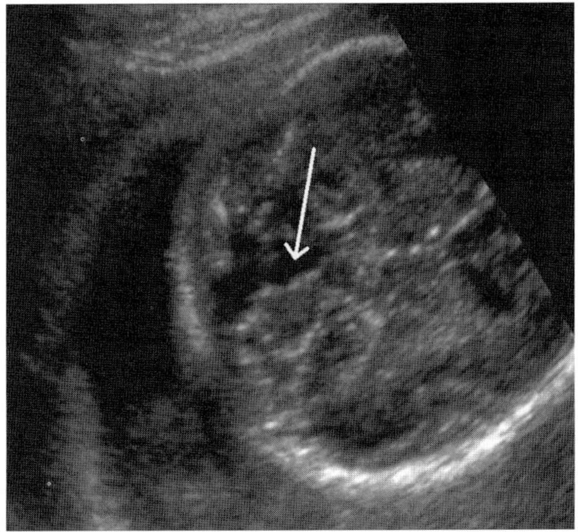

Fig 6.22 (a) Axial view showing seemingly a normal vermis. (b) In the same patient, a defect can be seen with a more coronal approach.

diameters are even smaller in weeks than indicated by the head circumference.

Second, the area in the mid-lateral portion, where the leptomeninges come together in the area of the insula, generally has a jagged box-like configuration (Figure 6.25). In cerebral dysgenesis, this outline is blunted, and in later pregnancy the gyri and sulci are less convoluted.

Infections

Ventriculomegaly is a very concerning sign in the patient with documented cytomegalovirus (CMV) infection. Unfortunately, the diagnosis is solidified when periventricular calcifications are noted (Figure 6.26). In reverse order, if one comes upon ventriculomegaly accompanied by periventricular calcifications, the very next step should be to explore an infectious etiology.

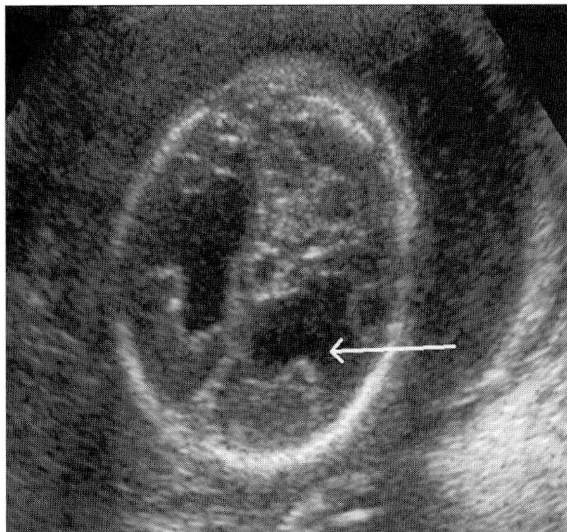

Fig 6.23 Schizencephaly. Typical cleft marked with arrow.

The advantage of 3D imaging

As indicated in the section on 3D, a search for the cause of every intracranial abnormality is enriched by 3D planar reconstruction. With all of the above conditions the greatest chance of clinching the diagnosis is through coronal and sagittal views, which can be obtained, using transvaginal sonography, through the anterior and posterior fontanelles of the fetus presenting as a vertex. Manipulation of 3D volumes, taken transabdominally or transvaginally, should further enhance the diagnostic investigation (Figure 6.27). Lastly, MRI can be extremely useful, especially in midline abnormalities and migrational disorders.

The fetal face

The new version of the AIUM/ACR guidelines for the standard ultrasound examination suggests that an attempt

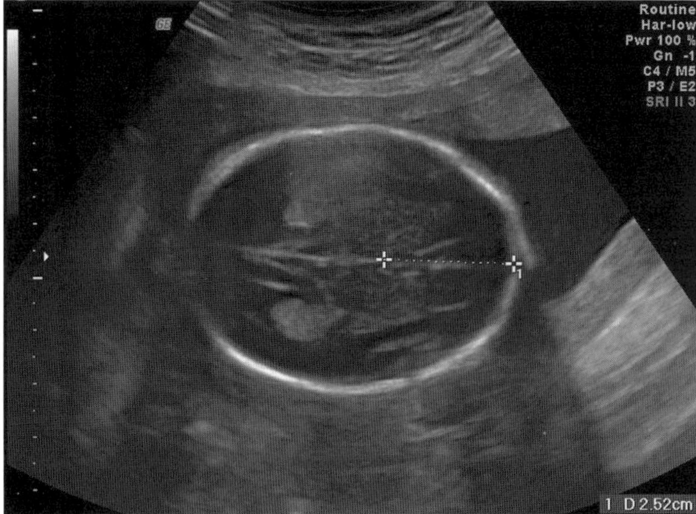

Fig 6.24 Frontal lobe.

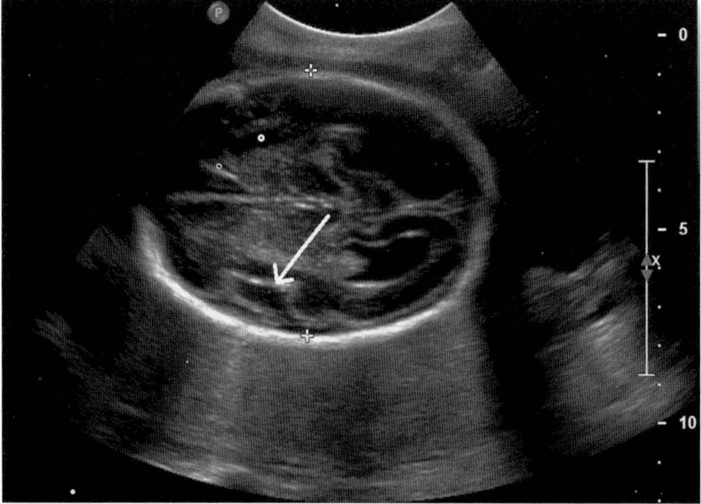

Fig 6.25 Box-like Sylvian fissure.

should be made to evaluate the fetal face. The most common method used today is designed simply to assess the integrity of the fetal lip by a coronal slice that isolates the nose, nostrils, philtrum, and mouth (Figure 6.28). If a cleft is suspected by noting an apparent communication between the nostril and the mouth (Figure 6.29) or by an inability to completely image the philtrum, it should trigger an in-depth evaluation of the fetal lip and palate.

The concept is to approach the nose, lip, alveolar ridge, and hard and soft palates from many angles with 2D and 3D methods. Cleft lip, cleft palate complex, in particular, lends itself perfectly to 3D investigation.

Our favorite method is to obtain a 3D volume with the fetus in a face up position so that the starting point for this sweep is a slightly angled mid-sagittal profile view (Figure 6.30). Once obtained, the volume information can be manipulated in a variety of ways. Initially, with planar reconstruction, one can come at the fetus with full frontal slices, moving through the upper lip, alveolar ridge, and then the hard palate. Stuart Campbell, one of the greatest contributors to the field of obstetrical sonography, reverses

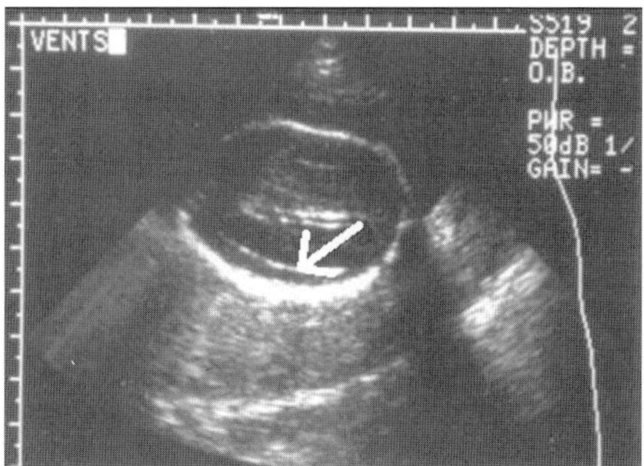

Fig 6.26 Intracranial calcifications.

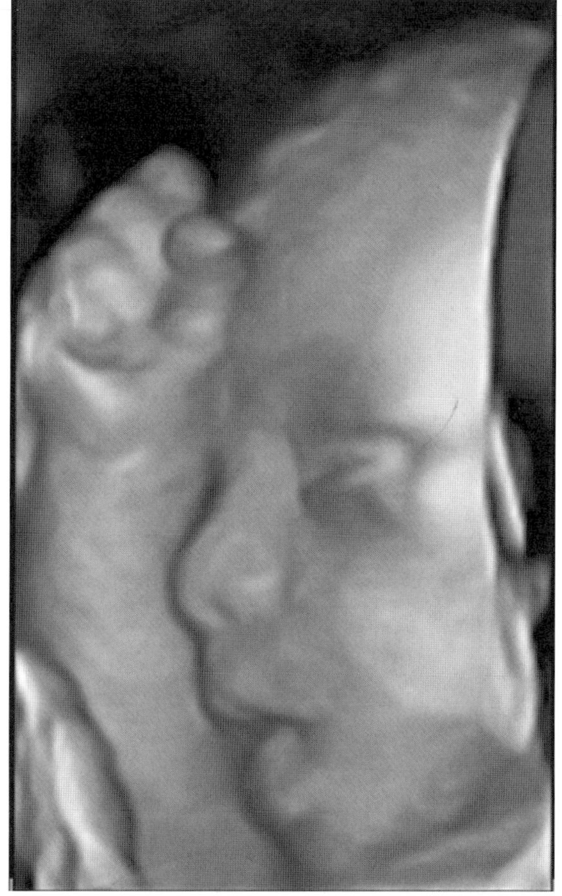

Fig 6.27 Rendered 3D image of fetal face.

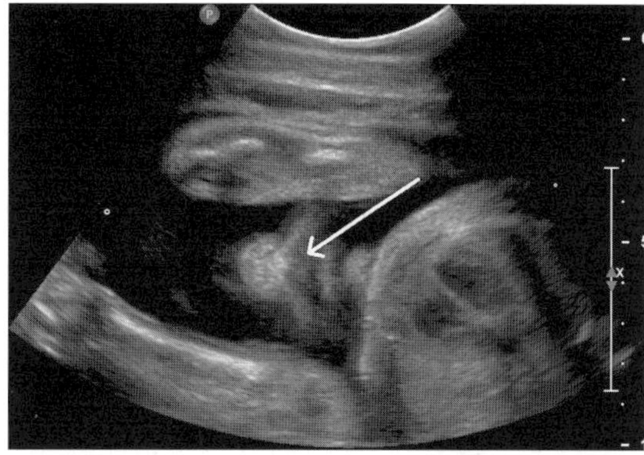

Fig 6.28 Upper lip.

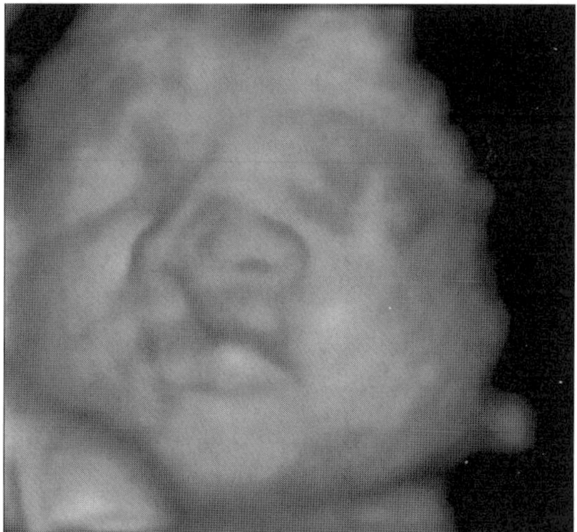

Fig 6.29 Cleft lip.

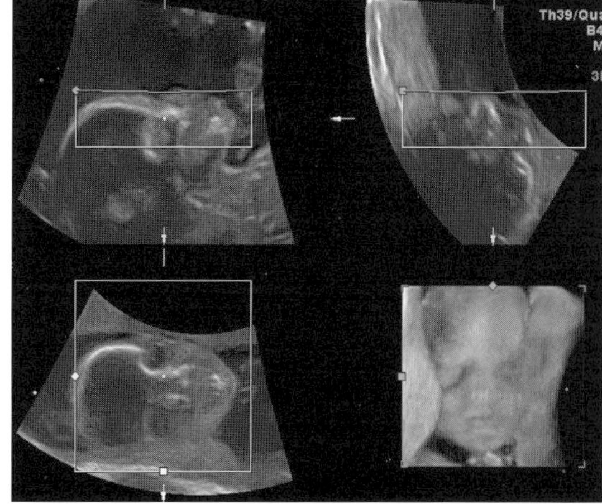

Fig 6.30 Standard 3D approach to lips and, further in, palate.

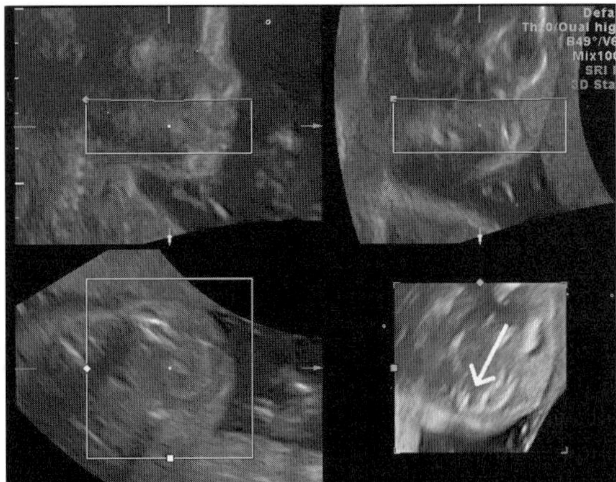

Fig 6.31 Approaching the palate from above with 3D. Arrow points to hard palate.

the format and comes at the fetus from back to front, soft palate first. Theoretically, based on the physics of ultrasound, it should make little difference in the image quality, but often it does seem to allow better visualization of the palate.

Another illuminating technique is to approach the target area with cross-sections from the nasal bridge down (Figure 6.31). This 3D "flipped" approach described by Platt, a prolific investigator who has done much to further the cause of ultrasound education, enables the investigator to make sure that the seemingly intact alveolar ridge is not actually the mandibular floor of the oral cavity. Manipulation in the rendering mode is very helpful in assessing gaps in bony versus soft tissue structures.

Cleft lip and palate complicates about 1 in 500 pregnancies. About 25% of the time it involves the lip alone, 50% of the time both lip and palate are involved, and in 25% of cases the palate is the only structure affected. This means that, since about 75–80% of fetuses with cleft lip will have an affected palate, one should thoroughly scrutinize this area before deciding the defect involves the lip alone, when the statistical deck is so loaded against it.

Clefts are most commonly isolated but can occasionally be associated with other anomalies and, if it is a midline defect, it is always accompanied by other anomalies or an abnormal karyotype.

If the cleft lip and palate are isolated, the prognosis for infants today is excellent; although, in general, the more tissue that is missing the more extensive will be the surgery and the longer is the recovery period. We have found the 3D surface rendered pictures to be very useful in preparing and counseling patients, and in communicating with our colleagues in pediatric surgery.

The fetal eyes

Rare conditions can affect the alignment and/or size of the fetal eyes. For example, in holoprosencephaly there is often hypotelorism, while in Apert syndrome and fetal alcohol syndrome there is hypertelorism. Although normative data for fetal eye size are available in the literature (see Appendix), a simple way to indirectly assess orbit size is to use the "one-third, one-third, one-third rule". In other words, each orbit is roughly of equal size and the distance between the two orbits is about the same size as either orbit (Figure 6.32).

These distances can be measured in the coronal plane (Figure 6.33) or in a cross-sectional slice at the level of the eyes, which includes the bridge of the nose (Figure 6.34). Again, use of the 3D rendering mode (thick slice—maximum transparency) will help the operator to distinguish calcified bony surfaces and to appreciate in the coronal plane the width of the metopic suture, which is often affected in syndromes affecting the eyes (Figure 6.35).

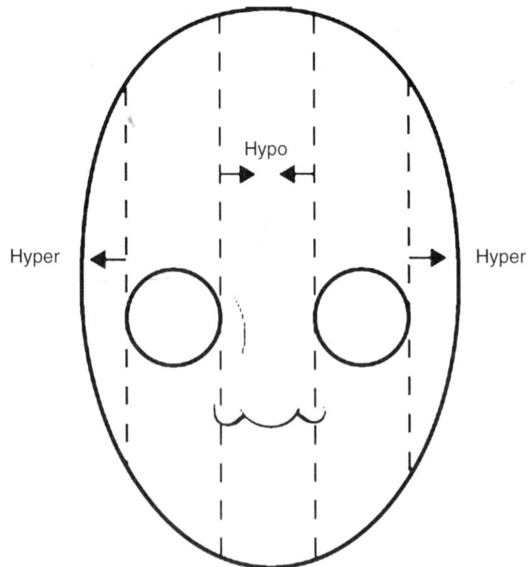

Fig 6.32 Way to assess orbital alignment.

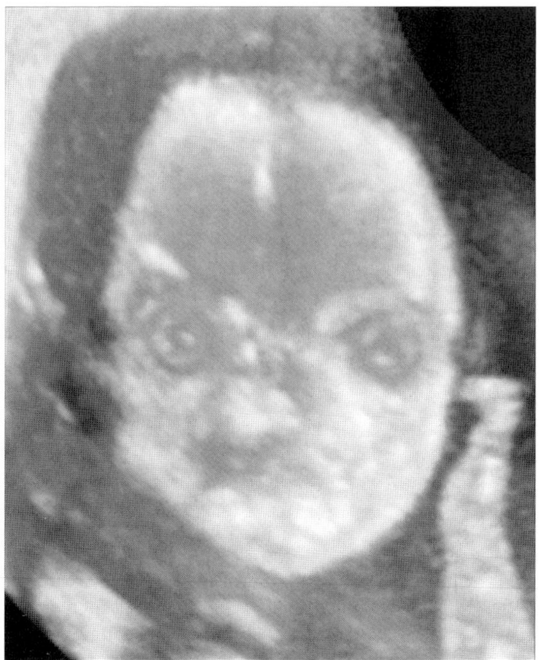

Fig 6.33 3D coronal view of the orbits for quantitative assessment.

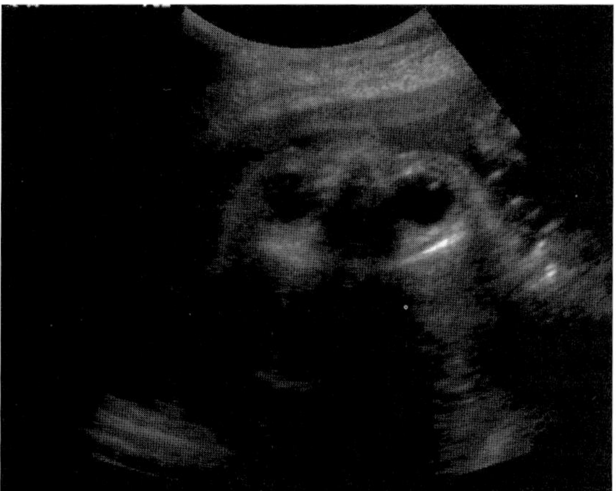

Fig 6.34 Cross-section through orbits.

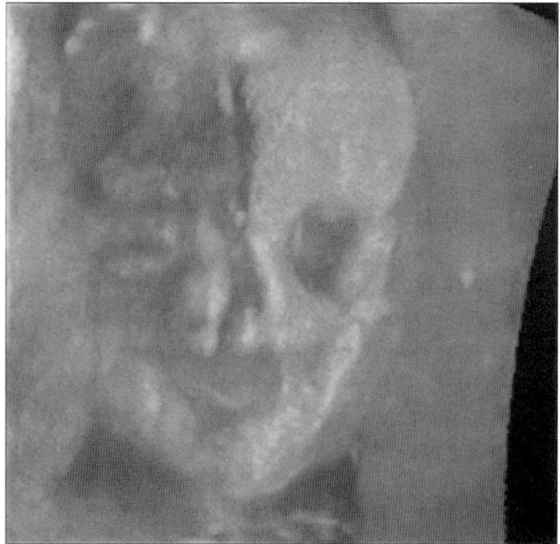

Fig 6.35 Metopic suture.

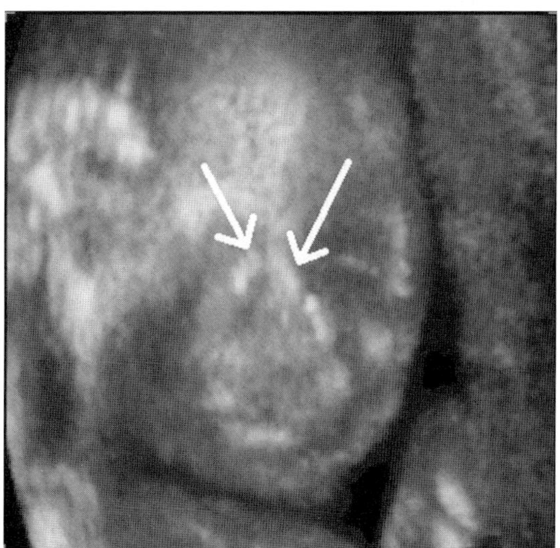

Fig 6.36 Arrows point to nasal bones.

The nose

As indicated later, the nasal bone is small or absent in some chromosomal abnormalities, such as trisomy 21 and trisomy 18, and in trisomy 13 it can be large and bulbous.

There are actually two nasal bones that come together in the midline, and this can be appreciated with 3D coronal views (Figure 6.36). However, the ideal way to evaluate the nose is to obtain a mid-sagittal profile, making sure that the beam approaches the nasal bone at 90° (Figure 6.37). In this way, one can also determine the presence of frontal bossing, seen in some conditions such as heterozygous achondroplasia.

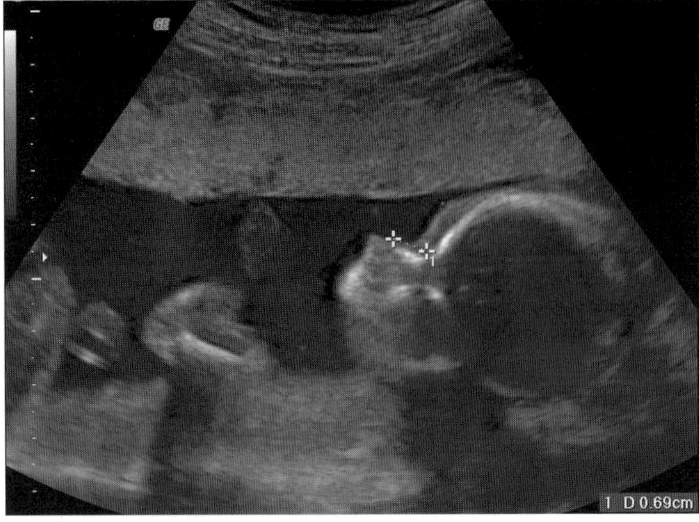

Fig 6.37 Nasal bone in second trimester.

The fetal chin

Micrognathia is a component of many anomaly syndromes, such as Apert syndrome, Pierre Robin sequence, Treacher Collins syndrome, and virtually always is a phenotypic feature of trisomy 18.

There are two excellent ways to appreciate chin size: to line up the profile in the mid-sagittal plane, where the bridge of the nose, the alveolar ridge, and the tip of the mandible are normally in a straight line (Figure 6.38). In micrognathia, the mandibular echo is not aligned and in most cases a simple visual assessment will suggest a depressed chin.

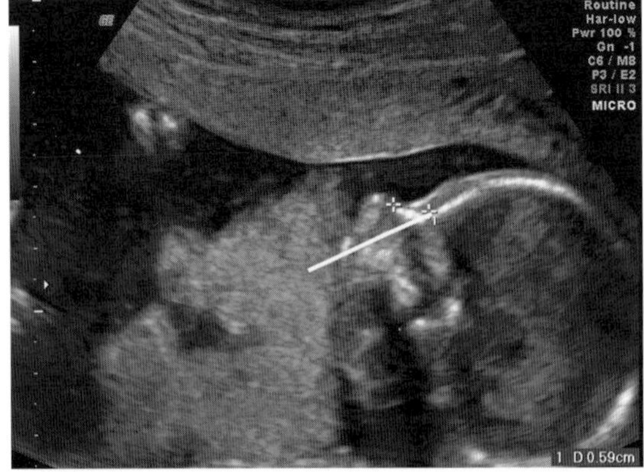

Fig 6.38 Normal chin alignment.

The most precise way to evaluate micrognathia is to measure the length of the mandible (Figure 6.39), as reported by Otto and Platt [6]. This is roughly the same size in millimeters as the transcerebellar diameter, or in the second trimester it is 1–2 mm larger than the menstrual age of the fetus in weeks (see Appendix). This also lends itself to 3D manipulation.

Case in point

Patient was referred at 20 weeks with a diagnosis of modest ventriculomegaly. The transvaginal examination of the intracranial anatomy revealed bilateral dangling choroid plexus, but the lateral ventricles did not exceed the cut (at 9 mm). The TCD was about 2 weeks behind dates, but the cisterna magna was not enlarged and the vermis was intact. The cavum appeared to be missing, seemingly leaving a communication between the frontal horns. Although it was not conclusive, a wisp of corpus callosum was fleetingly seen.

The MRI did not confirm the absence of the cavum but there was a suspicion of periventricular leukomalacia, which was not evident on ultrasound. Our differential diagnosis had included septal optic dysplasia, lobar holoprosencephaly, and partial agenesis of the corpus callosum with cerebral dysgenesis, and we predicted a very bleak outcome.

My observations involving the frontal portion of the brain led me in the wrong direction, even while the information was already at hand to make the right diagnosis. The infant was born with cerebellar hypoplasia and periventricular leukomalacia secondary to

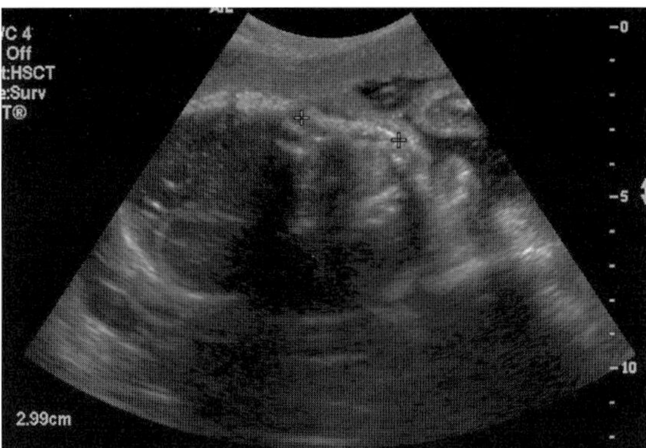

Fig 6.39 Mandible length.

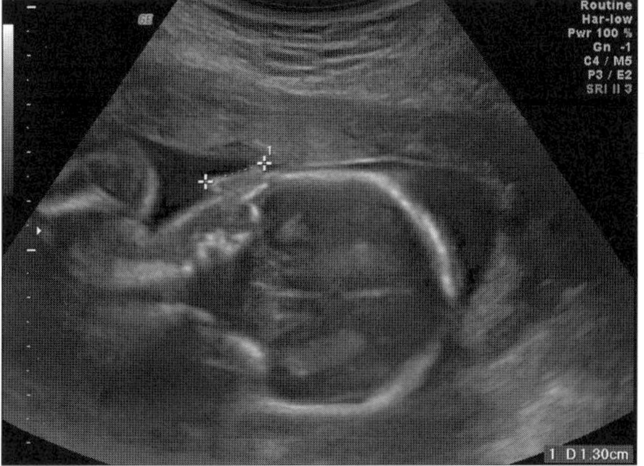

Fig 6.40 Coronal view of ear length.

CMV, which also had an effect on the frontal portion of the brain. The infant succumbed after a few days.

The fetal ear

Now the fetal ear can be fully examined with 3D surface rendering techniques. However, it is not part of the routine examination, and most investigators will only turn to the ear if they suspect a fetal syndrome in which the ear is a component. The fetal ear can be absent or extremely small, as in Treacher Collins syndrome, malformed, as in trisomy 18, simply small, as in Down syndrome, or low set, as in a variety of anomaly complexes.

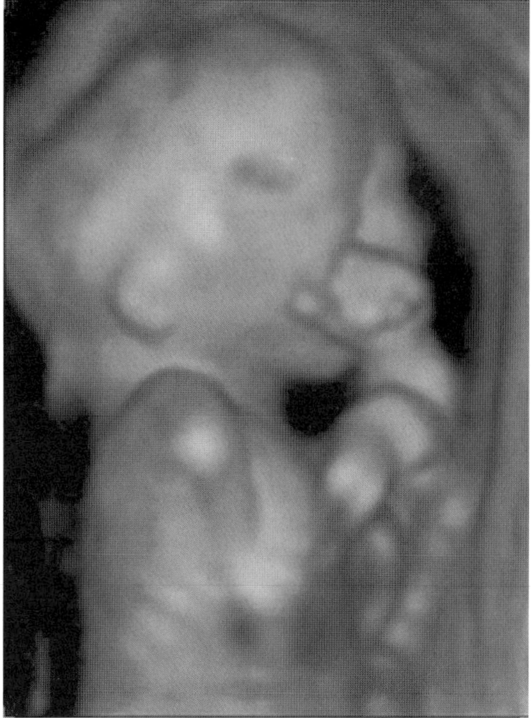

Fig 6.41 Fetal ear—surface rendered image.

The ear can be measured in the coronal plane with 2D (Figure 6.40) or straight on with 3D (Figure 6.41). Since one can never overestimate the diameter of the ear, it is important to obtain the largest measurement that can then be compared to normative data according to gestational age (see Appendix).

In AMA patients, we consider the ear to be a second-tier marker for Down syndrome, which we explore when we wish to make certain that another marker is truly isolated.

Another case in point

The patient was referred at 30 weeks with a diagnosis of fetal ventriculomegaly. This was her first pregnancy, which had been uneventful until the examination. Her scan showed dilated lateral ventricles, a dilated third ventricle, a normal appearing cortex, and what appeared to be a clot in one of the ventricles (Figure 6.42). It was clear from the patient's history that she was not a cocaine user, so we explored the next most common

(*Continued*)

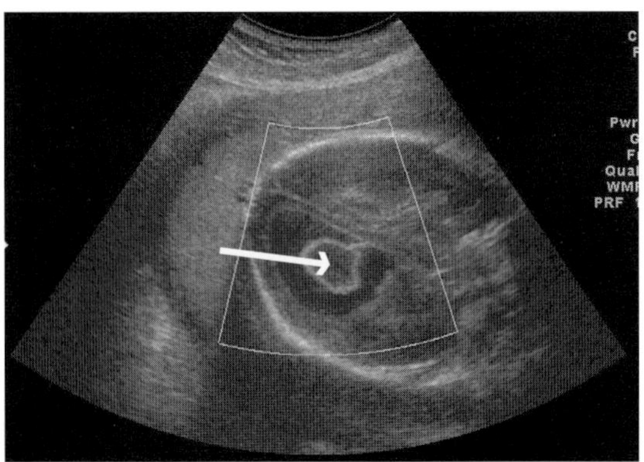

Fig 6.42 Dilated ventricle with intraventricular clot, marked by arrow.

reason for a fetal hemorrhage, alloimmune thrombocytopenia. She was positive for antiplatelet antibodies. We postulated that fragments from the clot in the lateral ventricle made their way downward to the aqueduct of Sylvius, which resulted in a secondary obstructive hydrocephaly.

She went into labor at 36 weeks of gestation and had a precipitous delivery of a normal size fetus that eventually died 3 days later. The fetal platelet count was 5000.

We counseled her that she had a 1 in 4 chance of this happening again, but, armed with the knowledge of this condition, and with proper early diagnosis and therapy, an affected fetus would have a reasonable chance of intact survival.

References

1 Goldstein I, Copel JA, Makhoul EI. Mild cerebral ventriculomegaly in fetuses: characteristics and outcome. Fetal Diagn Ther 2005; 20: 281–4.

2 Breeze AC, Dey PK, Lees CC, et al. Obstetric and neonatal outcomes in apparently isolated mild fetal ventriculomegaly. J Perinat Med 2005; 33: 236–40

3 Gaglioti P, Danelon D, Bontempo S, et al. Fetal cerebral ventriculomegaly: outcome in 176 cases. Ultrasound Obstet Gynecol 2005; 25: 372–7.

4 Pilu G, Hobbins JC. Sonography of fetal cerebrospinal anomalies. Prenat Diag 2002; 22: 321–30.

5 Martin HP. Microcephaly and mental retardation. Am J Dis Child 1970; 119: 128–31.

6 Otto C, Platt LD. The fetal mandible measurement: an objective determination of fetal jaw size. Ultrasound Obstet Gynecol 1991; 1: 395–400.

7 Examination of the fetal heart

Whole books have been devoted to the fetal heart and, because of the limitation of space and energy, I can devote to this topic this chapter, which will simply represent a pragmatic approach to screening for fetal cardiac abnormalities using the technology available today. Fetal echocardiography is a special skill unto itself, and once the practitioner decides that there is something amiss with the fetal heart, this should probably be best sorted out by those who do this for a living, and often will be responsible for the care of these fetuses after birth—pediatric cardiologists.

The original guidelines for a standard ultrasound examination suggested that a four-chamber view of the heart be obtained in every fetus. Later, there was a statement added to indicate that there should be an attempt made to evaluate both outflow tracts.

The four-chamber view

The outflows add icing on the cake, but the essential information comes from the four-chamber view. The standard approach is to use a cross-section of the chest above the diaphragm (Figure 7.1), although it can be done on occasion by an angled approach from under the diaphragm. I have found that the best way to find a starting point is to rotate the transducer in small increments until there is a full rib on each side of the heart within the image. In late pregnancy, when the ribs create a problem of acoustic shadowing, the transducer can be moved, without rotating, up or down a few millimeters to get through an intercostal space.

Once the best image is obtained, one quickly can run through the "four-chamber drill," which includes the following:

1 Check the cardiac orientation. The heart should occupy more of the left chest than the right, with the apex pointed toward the same side as the underlying stomach. Although a complete situs inversus may have little effect on some individuals, and, in fact, may be undiagnosed for years, some types of mixed situs can be associated with severe cardiac abnormalities, especially when accompanied by asplenia or polysplenia.

2 The angle of cardiac inclination is very important. Some abnormalities, such as transposition of the great vessels, sometimes escape diagnosis with a four-chamber view alone, but most of these will present with the heart rotated further to the left than usual. If one were to draw a line from the spine to an opposite point in the chest, and then draw another line along the long axis of the interventricular septum, the angle where the two lines meet should not exceed 60°, and never should exceed 90° (Figures 7.2 and 7.3).

3 A pericardial effusion (Figure 7.4) should alert the observer to the possibility of cardiac or extra cardiac abnormalities, such as fetal anemia or infection. One should be very careful not to mistake the hypoechogenic myocardium for an effusion. Also, there is always some fluid in the pericardial sac, and if one only sees the apparent effusion in the atrioventricular groove, this would not constitute a true pericardial effusion, which should extend down to the apex of the heart. By using M-mode, it is often possible to distinguish a pseudoeffusion from the real McCoy (Figure 7.5).

4 Inequity in chamber size should alert the practitioner either to a functional abnormality, such as in Down syndrome or an outflow obstruction (as in hypoplastic right or left heart syndrome) (Figure 7.6). The interatrial septum generally follows along the same axis as the interventricular septum, but it should be evaluated when blood is not flowing through the foramen ovale.

5 The interventricular septum should be unbroken throughout its length. There is some controversy as to the best way to investigate the integrity of the septum. In order to visualize its normal elongated triangular shape, one would utilize the axial resolution by cutting across the septum. This is particularly useful in diabetes

Obstetric Ultrasound: Artistry in Practice. John C. Hobbins. Published 2008 Blackwell Publishing. ISBN 978-1-4051-5815-2.

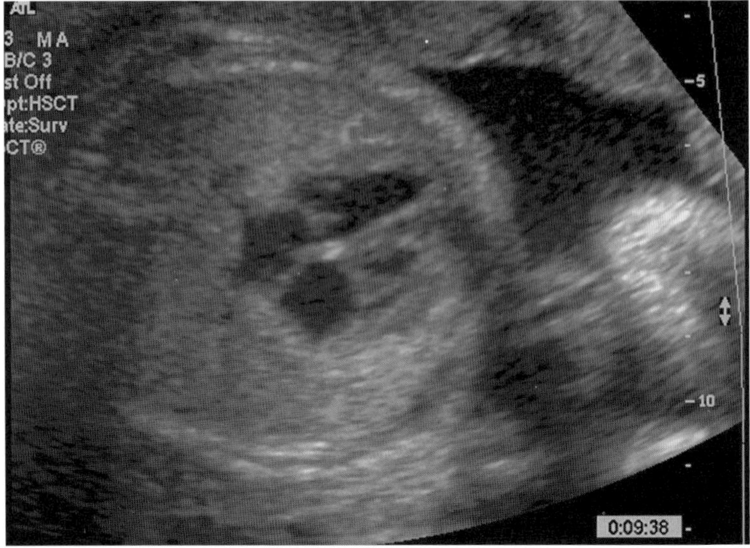

Fig 7.1 Subcostal four-chamber view.

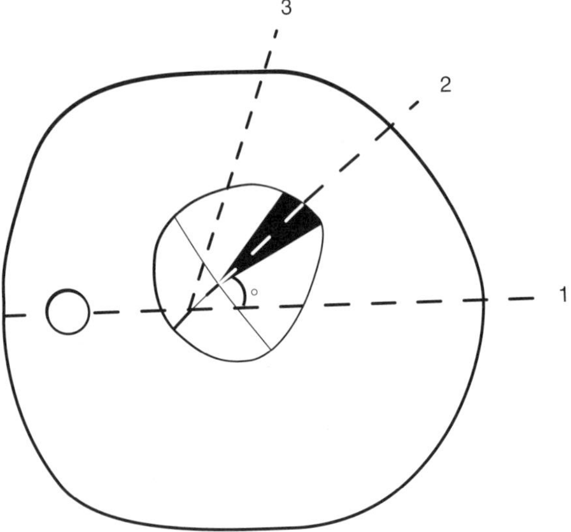

Fig 7.2 Way to quantify the degree of cardiac rotation. The angle between lines 1 and 2 should not exceed 60°. (1) Line drawn between spine (here at 3 o'clock) and a point on opposite wall of chest (here at 9 o'clock). (2) Line through interventricular septum. (3) Line showing where interventricular septum would be if there was levorotation.

since a clue to poor glucose control in the third trimester is an interventricular septum that is abnormally thick (Figure 7.7). For example, a cross-sectional diameter that exceeds 5 mm in the middle of the septum can represent a source of concern. Although some authors have advocated using an apical view to assess the interventricular septum, we feel that cutting across the septum has definite merit; especially when the defect is in the membranous portion of the septum. Also, there is an opportunity for creation of false positives when the ultrasound beam is running along the plane of the thin portion of the septum. It should be kept in mind that interventricular septal defects, especially if small, can be missed with 2D ultrasound alone. However, high defects in the membranous portion of the septum will often "light up" because of a bright, sometimes T-shaped condensation of echoes at the top of the septum (Figure 7.8). Generally, atrial septal defects are even harder to pick up unless accompanied by an interventricular septal defect, as seen, for example, in an atrioventricular (AV) canal defect (Figure 7.9).

A case in point

A 35-year-old patient was referred in at 18 weeks because of advanced maternal age. She had a reassuring quad screen with the risk of 1 in 1000 for Down syndrome. She was somewhat difficult to evaluate because of her obesity, but what caught our eye was a levorotation of the heart to about 80°. Interestingly, with transvaginal sonography we were able to perform the semblance of an echocardiogram, which showed a transposition of the great vessels. The point here is that in this patient in whom we could barely see the interventricular septum because of a 9-cm distance between

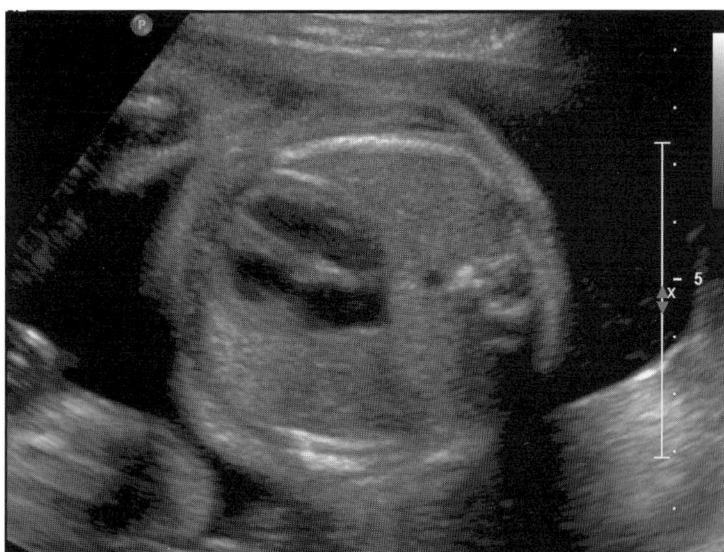

Fig 7.3 Four-chamber intercostal view with normal alignment of interventricular septum.

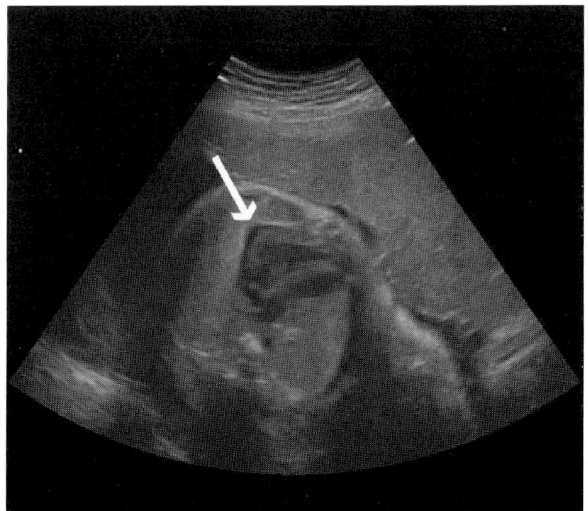

Fig 7.4 Pericardial effusion.

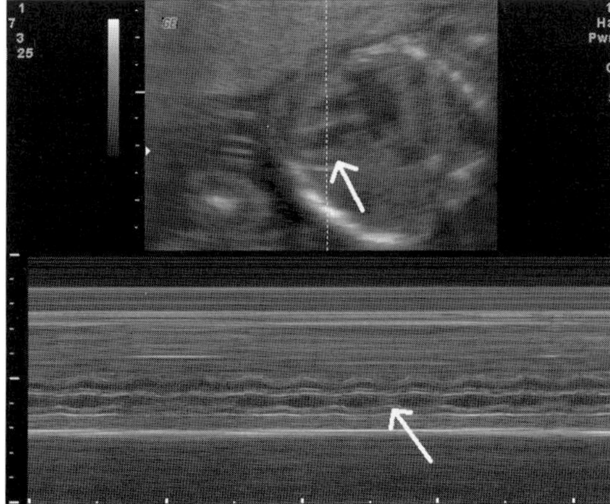

Fig 7.5 Pericardial M-mode of pericardial effusion. Arrow points to effusion.

the transducer and the fetal heart, the only clue to a possible problem was the angle of rotation. With some extra effort, this cardiac abnormality could eventually be diagnosed, though we might very easily have given up.

Outflow tracts

There are a number of ways to demonstrate the proper alignment of the outflow tracts. The most common method is to start with a four-chamber view and to rotate the transducer slowly in an arc that would eventually encompass a plane moving through a line drawn between the left hip and the right shoulder. So, for example, if the fetus is in a vertex presentation and on his/her left side, the rotation would be counterclockwise (Figures 7.10 and 7.11). The easiest way to get from here to the right outflow tract is to simply tilt the transducer toward the chin of the fetus (Figure 7.12).

Some studies have shown that, even with persistence, in about 10–20% of cases one still cannot get both outflow

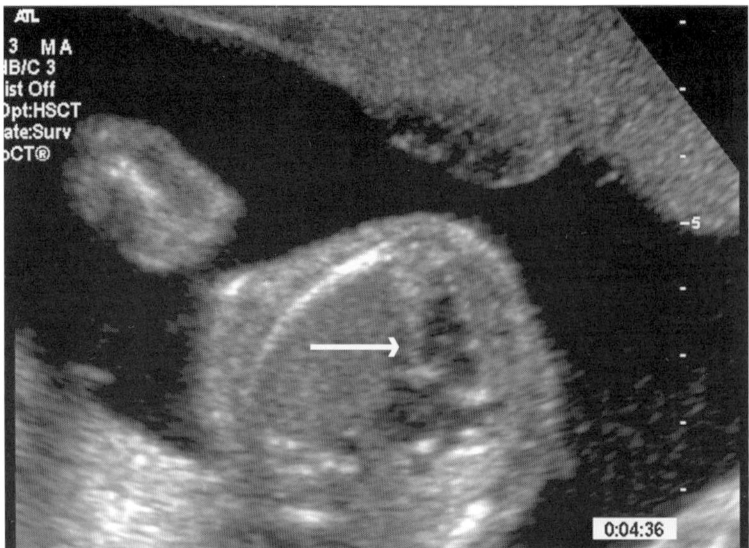

Fig 7.6 Unequal chamber size in hypoplastic left heart syndrome. Arrow marks small left ventricle.

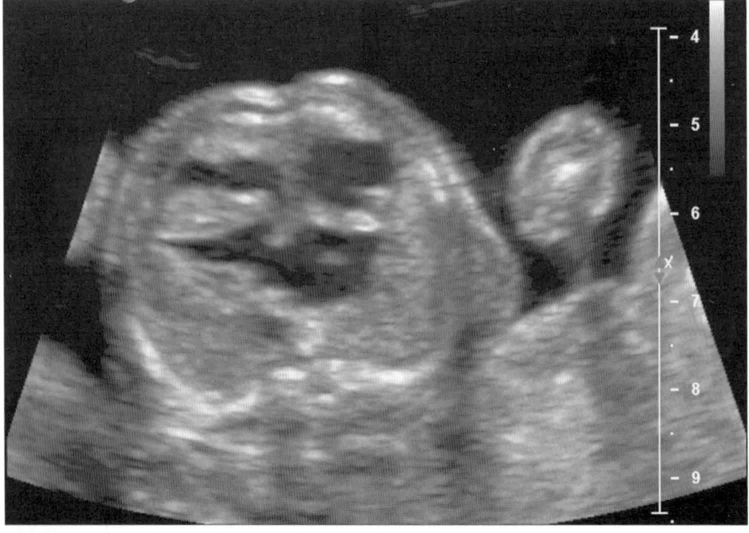

Fig 7.7 Thick septum with levocardia and levorotation.

tracts with this technique. If one is not doing a full fetal echocardiogram, the crossing of the great vessels can be appreciated by a short axis view obtained in such a way that the pulmonary artery is caught swinging around the aorta, often referred to as the "sausage and circle" view (Figure 7.13). A way to distinguish the right ventricle from the left involves the identification of the moderator band, seen only in the right ventricle. Also, one should easily separate out the pulmonary artery from the aorta by identifying the branching of the former vessel.

In addition to the four-chamber view, obtained at level 1 in Figure 7.14, other cross-sectional views, not specifically mentioned in the guidelines for performance of the standard ultrasound examination, are very useful in tracing out the cardiac anatomy. These are as follows: the five-chamber view, obtained on the cross-section about one "click" above the four-chamber view; the three-vessel view, obtained by moving the transducer transversely further cephalad; and a view just above this one, entitled the "tracheal view" [1,2].

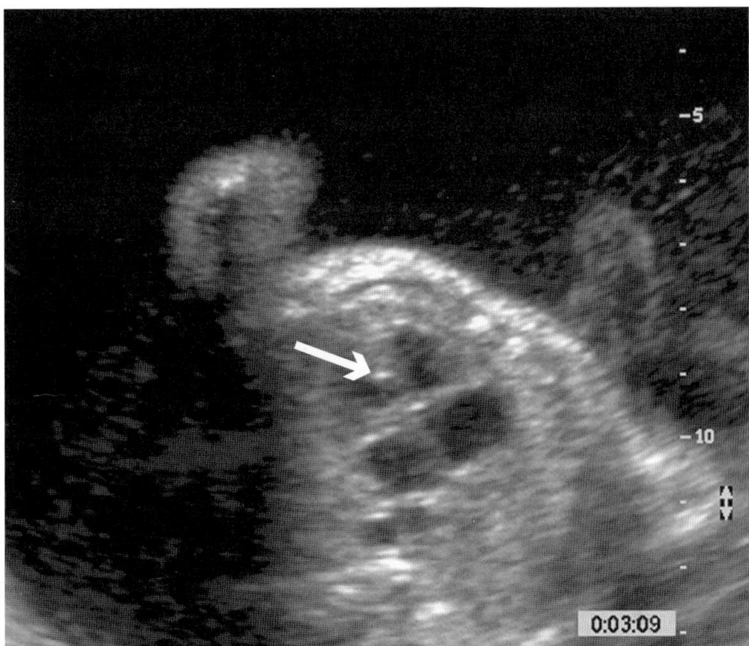

Fig 7.8 Arrow marks bright echoes from tip of defect in apical view of VSD.

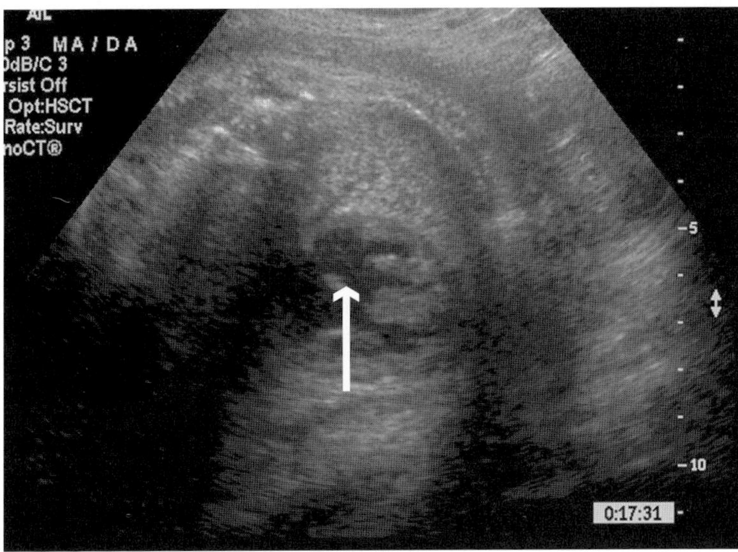

Fig 7.9 Arrow marks atrioventricular septal defect VSD.

Although capturing these views is currently not part of the standard fetal survey because it adds additional work to a sometimes time-consuming study, there are very exciting features of 3D and 4D ultrasound that make the evaluation of the heart less cumbersome, more accurate, and easier to teach. For example, a new multislice method can now enable the operator to create instantaneously displayed tomograms through the heart. This technique, entitled tomographic ultrasound imaging, "I" slicing, or simply, "multislicing" by different manufacturers, will allow each slice to be displayed on the screen, as designated by lines along the long axis target area (Figure 7.15). So with one

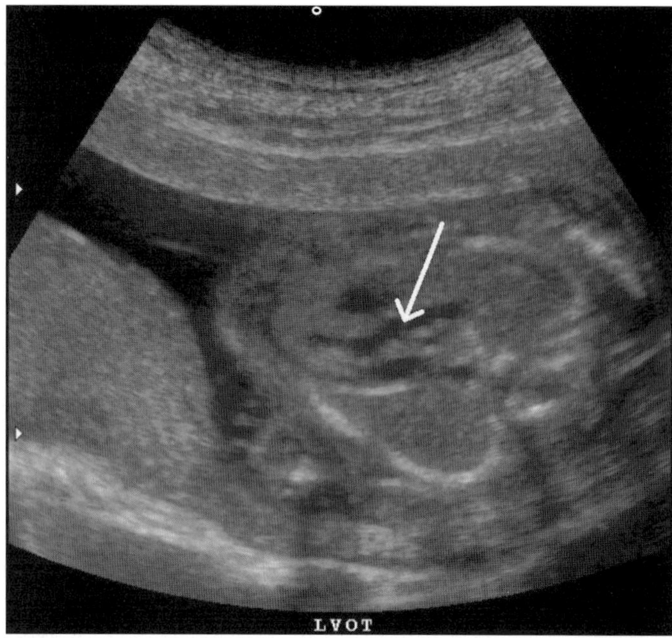

Fig 7.10 Left outflow tract.

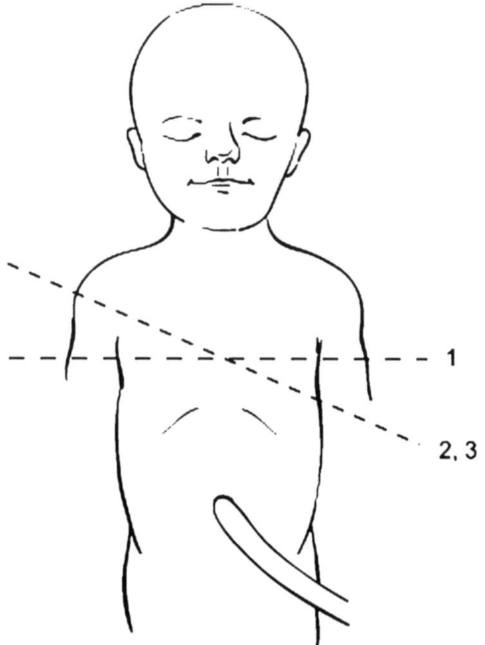

Fig 7.11 Method of obtaining views of the outflow tracts. (1) Plane of four-chamber view. (2) Plane to obtain left outflow (rotating transducer toward left hip and right shoulder). (3) Plane to obtain right outflow involves simply tilting transducer in plane toward fetal chin.

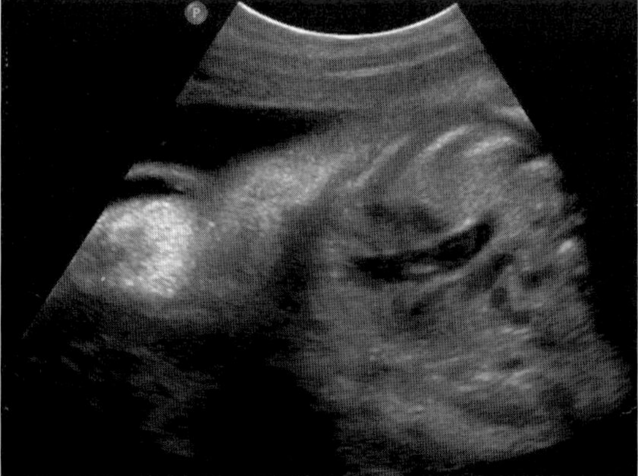

Fig 7.12 Right outflow tract.

cross-sectional sweep initiated in the plane of the four-chamber view, all four of the above-mentioned views in the sequence will be displayed simultaneously. This not only has "one-stop" diagnostic potential but also can have tremendous potential as a teaching tool.

Color Doppler

We always use color Doppler to rule out small interventricular septal defects. For years we used color Doppler

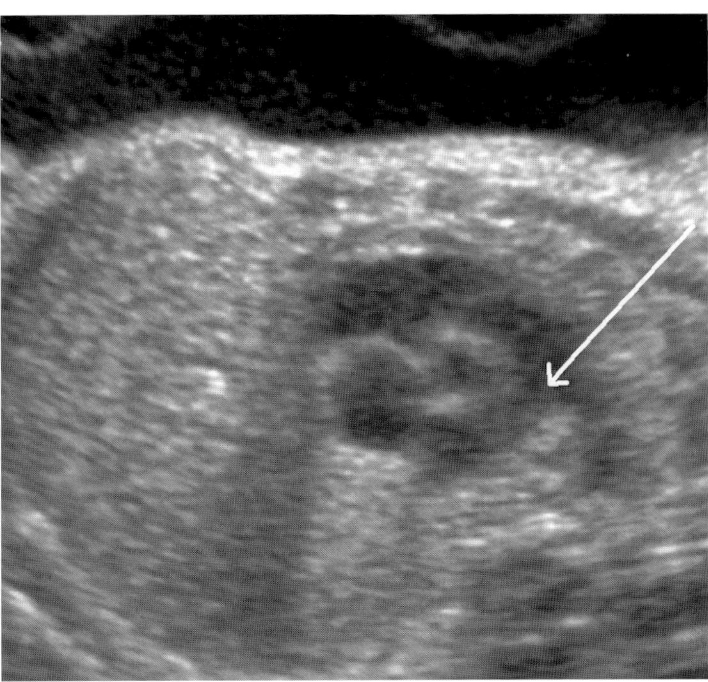

Fig 7.13 Short axis view. Arrow points to the splitting of the pulmonary artery.

only when we suspected a septal defect to be present, but now we are inclined to take the few extra seconds to do this in most patients. During diastole the ventricles fill equally (Plate 7.1). The AV valves close at the very end of diastole. If there is a septal defect, this is the perfect time for blood, with nowhere else to go, to move across an existing septal defect. Again, the cross-sectional intercostal view will allow the Doppler beam to be running along the pathway of the blood flowing through a potential septal defect. Since the pressures are nearly equal in the ventricles, blood can pass through a defect in both directions. During systole, one normally sees little color-related action in the right heart, other than blood crossing over it as it moves upward through the aorta from the left ventricle.

If all goes well during the evaluation of the four-chamber view, outflow tracts, and abbreviated color Doppler analysis of the ventricles, one can move on to other organ systems in patients in whom there is no suspicion, by history or initial findings, of a fetal cardiac problem.

The standard 2D examination has gotten bad press regarding its ability to identify cardiac anomalies. However, the addition of the outflow tracts to the standard cardiac evaluation will increase the pickup rate of cardiac anomalies. Also, the experience of the investigator has a major effect on the sensitivity of the examination [3]. DeVore, a true innovator in fetal echocardiography, has shown that the addition of color Doppler further enhances the yield, especially when screening for aneuploidy [4].

Newer techniques

Standard 3D and 4D methods

Of all the places for 3D technology, the fetal heart is the structure where it has most promise. However, seemingly with everything that is new and exciting, there are trade-offs. With static 3D ultrasound, the operator lines up an area of interest and initiates a 3D cross-sectional sweep through the four-chamber view of the heart. With modest manipulation, the standard display format will include the four-chamber view of the heart in the A (or x) plane, a cross-section perpendicular to, but running north to south to the above image in the B (y) plane, and an orthogonal section, again at right angles to the above plane, running east to west, in the C (z) plane (Figure 7.16). The A plane has the best resolution, similar to a standard 2D image, especially in the north–south axis, which represents the axial resolution. This is dependent almost completely upon the frequency of the transducer. The other two planes are dependent upon the lateral (east/west) resolution of the transducer, which is a function of how finely focused the beam is at the best focal distance. The C plane puts into play a third dimension (azimuthal) resolution of an ultrasound beam, the least reliable of the bunch—ergo, the fuzziest image. In 3D imagery, the lateral resolution is dependent upon the time required to make the sweep, which, in turn, is dependent upon the area covered while the machine is acquiring the volumes, often (today) at 6 per second.

Here is where there are more trade-offs. The more information you can cram into the volume, the better will be your lateral resolution. However, the longer the time taken during this sweep, the greater the chance of artifact created by contraction of the heart or by fetal movement during the prolonged acquisition time.

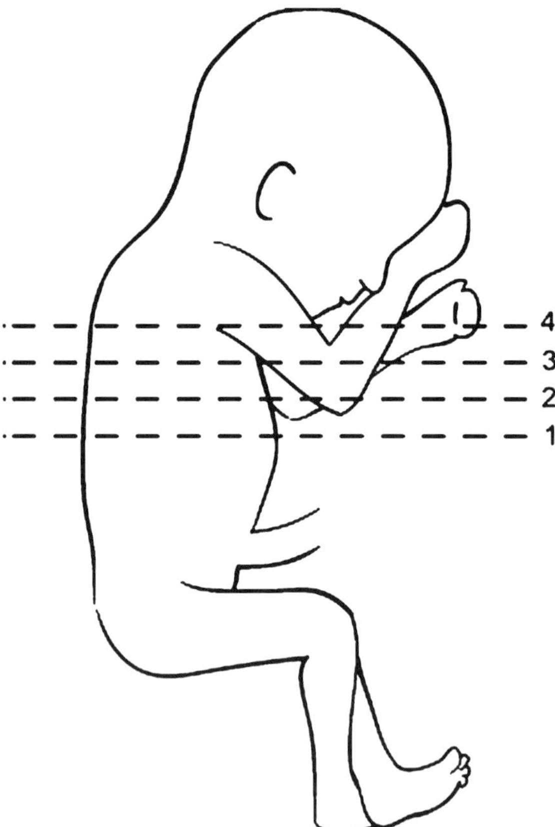

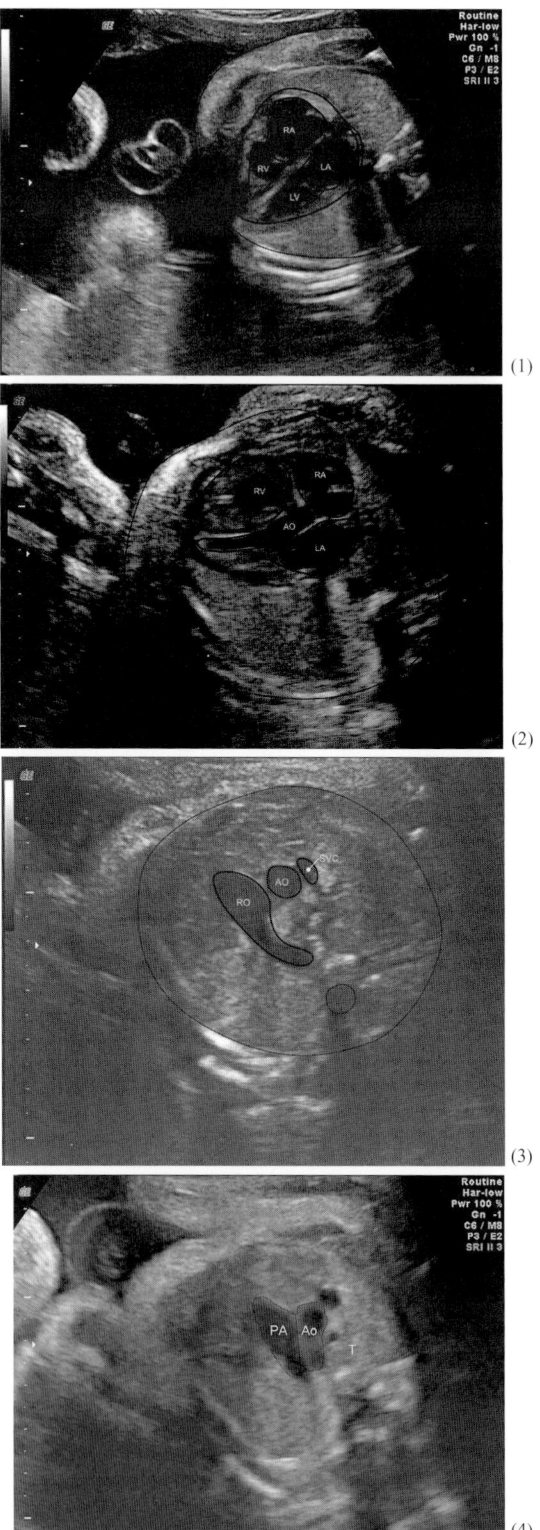

Fig 7.14 Method to obtain other useful views of the heart. (1) Four-chamber view at level 1. (2) Five-chamber view at level 2. (3) Three-vessel view at level 3. (4) Tracheal view at level 4.

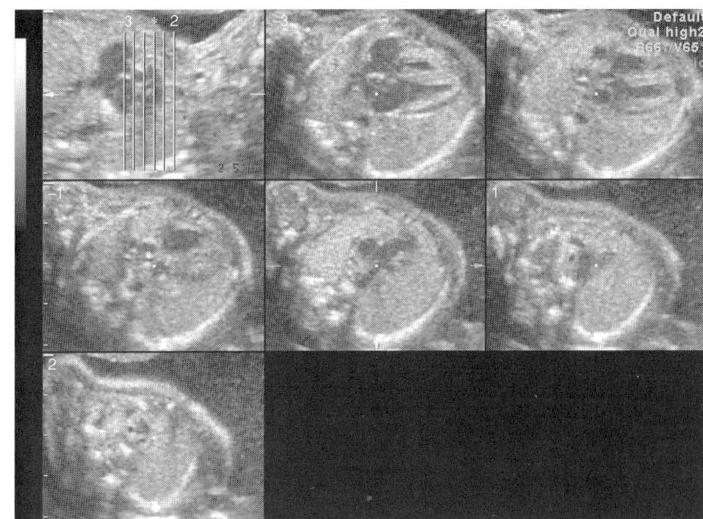

Fig 7.15 3D sweep using TUI with minus three representing four-chamber view.

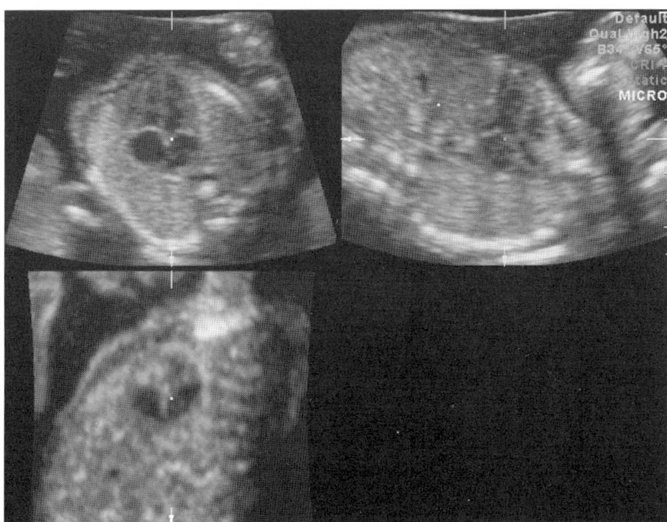

Fig 7.16 Standard 3D format for heart.

4D

Standard 4D technology has not been overly useful in imaging the fetal heart. Most mechanical array transducers will produce constantly refreshed images at a rate of about 6 volumes per second. Because the sweep speed has to be very fast, the resolution suffers when it is not. However, brand new matrix array technologies allow 4D volumes to be manipulated instantaneously, because they can generate very high repetition rates. The images generated from this methodology are remarkable.

Spatiotemporal image correlation

Here a single sweep through the heart lasting 7–15 seconds will produce a myriad of images that can be cobbled together to form a clip of an entire cardiac cycle. This allows the examiner to have information from the A, B, and C planes with very reasonable resolution in the normally inferior B and C planes. Also, with this technique color or power Doppler can be added to the images, greatly enhancing the ability to see small septal defects.

Last, as indicated above, matrix arrays have been recently developed that enable all of the many elements to

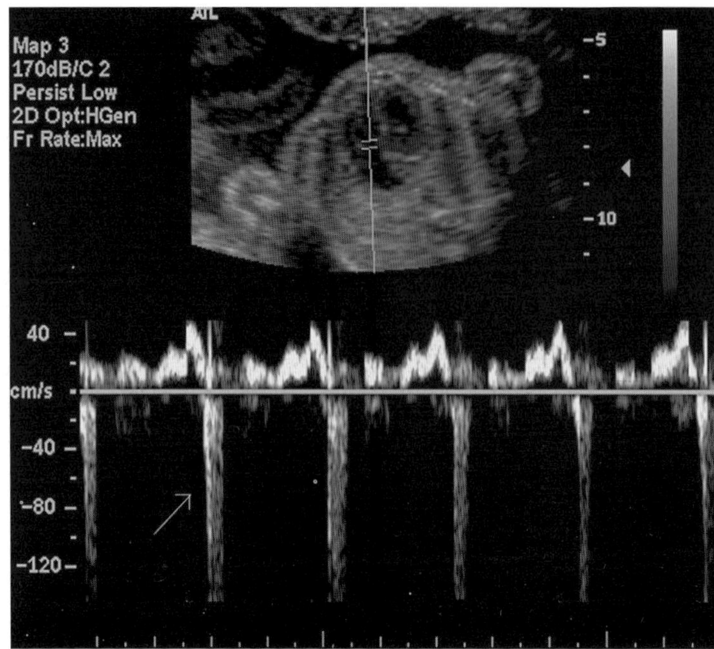

Fig 7.17 Tricuspid regurgitation of short duration.

fire simultaneously, creating a much higher volume rate (presently about 28 volumes per second). This should create the best of both worlds—excellent resolution with minimal artifact production.

Now, once these volumes are obtained, one can swing through any plane the operator desires using the x, y, and z rotation functions. DeVore describes a "spin" technique using the x and y functions to optimize the lateral resolution while tracing out, for example, the great vessels [5].

A transverse sweep from diaphragm to neck will allow the operator to select, through planar reconstruction, five cross-sectional planes that can be used as starting points for further rotational manipulation. By rotating mainly through the x and y axes, it is possible to track the pathways and length of the cardiac vessels while assessing their relationship to each other.

Pulse Doppler

With standard 2D guidance one can investigate with pulse wave Doppler any area within the heart—in essence, anything that moves within, going to, or leaving the heart. The areas we most often evaluate are the tricuspid valve (to look for tricuspid regurgitation—TR), the aorta (to search for increased peak velocities seen in coarctation), the mitral valve (to assess cardiac function by analysis of the waveform below it), and the pulmonary veins as they enter the left atrium (the identification of which effectively rules out anomalous pulmonary venous return).

In many structural abnormalities, often where the atrium is having trouble muscling blood through the tricuspid valve, the valve is not competent to keep blood from refluxing back into the right atrium during systole. This can be appreciated by color Doppler or by placing the pulsed Doppler cursor in the right atrium, just above the tricuspid valve. Regurgitation is noted with pulse Doppler as an upward deflection away from the ventricle during systole (Plate 7.2 and Figure 7.17).

The literature indicates that TR is rare in normal fetuses and some authors have suggested that when you do find it, it probably represents an atrial wall artifact. We have found that it is not unusual to have small amounts of TR in normal fetuses, and we are sure that it is not an artifact. However, it may not be appreciated with color Doppler, and, perhaps, it is only of clinical consequence when seen first with color Doppler.

Studies on abortuses with Down syndrome suggest an early, but probably temporary, aortic narrowing that could have a backward domino effect on flow through the tricuspid valve. As indicated later, the ductus venosus will

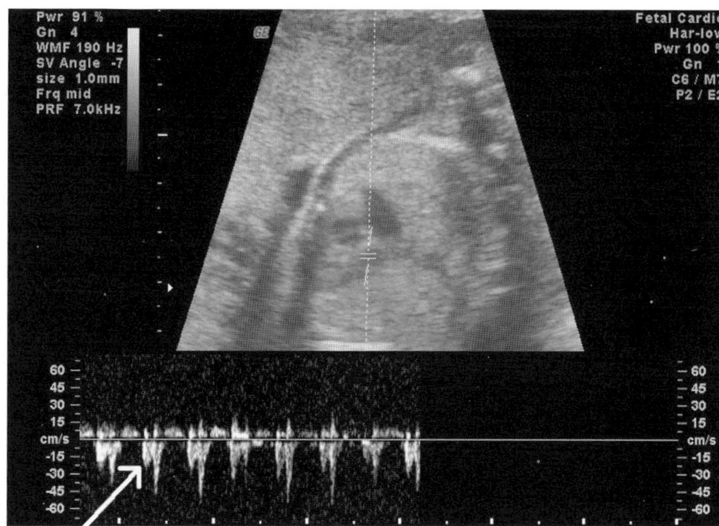

Fig 7.18 Points "E" and "A". The arrow is pointing to the "E" point and the larger defection is the "A" point.

often have low or reversed flow during atrial contraction in Down syndrome, especially in early pregnancy.

Coarctation of the aorta is a difficult condition to diagnose in utero because it probably represents a work in progress, and the area where the coarct occurs is difficult to pinpoint with ultrasound. We prefer to assess the waveform in the ascending aorta and arch with pulse Doppler. In normal circumstances, the peak velocity rarely exceeds 120 cm/s, but in coarcts, often it does.

The fetal heart is inherently "stiff," and a typically normal waveform obtained from a point just below the mitral valve will have a pattern that is dissimilar to that found in the adult; for example, the "E" point (representing early filling of the atrium) will be of lower amplitude than the "A" point (representing active contraction of the atrium) (Figures 7.18 and 7.19). As the fetal heart becomes compromised for whatever reason (infection or acidosis), the two points become equal in amplitude. Eventually, if the fetus gets into dire straits, the "E" point exceeds the "A" point in height.

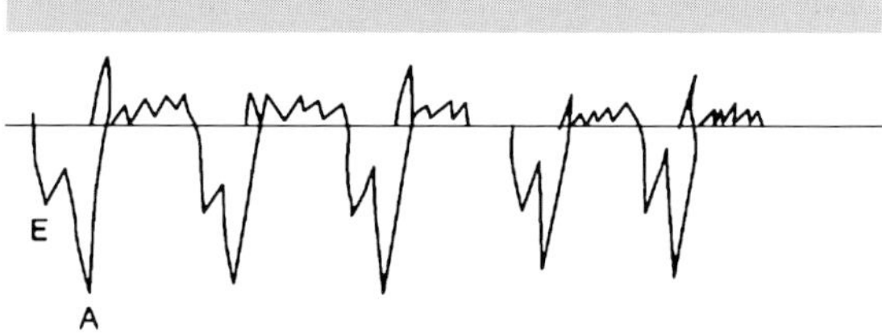

Fig 7.19 M-mode waveforms.

Abnormalities of cardiac rhythm

About once a week, we are referred a patient whose fetus has an irregular heartbeat as noted by a handheld Doppler device or during an ultrasound examination. The good news is that almost always it represents a fleeting finding, which is of little consequence. However, it is definitely worth exploring further, if only to reassure a patient who has been informed that her fetus has an "abnormal heartbeat."

Premature atrial contractions (PACs)

The most common irregularities that would fall under the category are PACs. Here the atria fire off early and some will be conducted through to the ventricle, causing it to contract prematurely. Alternatively, some may not be conducted or often there will be a combination of both phenomena. There is more than one way to sort out a seemingly confusing irregular rhythm. With M-mode the beam can be directed in such a way as to include the atrial wall, the interventricular septum, and the wall of the opposite side ventricle. With this view one can easily see when and how often the atrium and ventricle are contracting, and whether the latter is contracting in sync with the former (Figure 7.20).

Another method would be to focus on either the mitral or tricuspid valve with pulse Doppler. PACs would

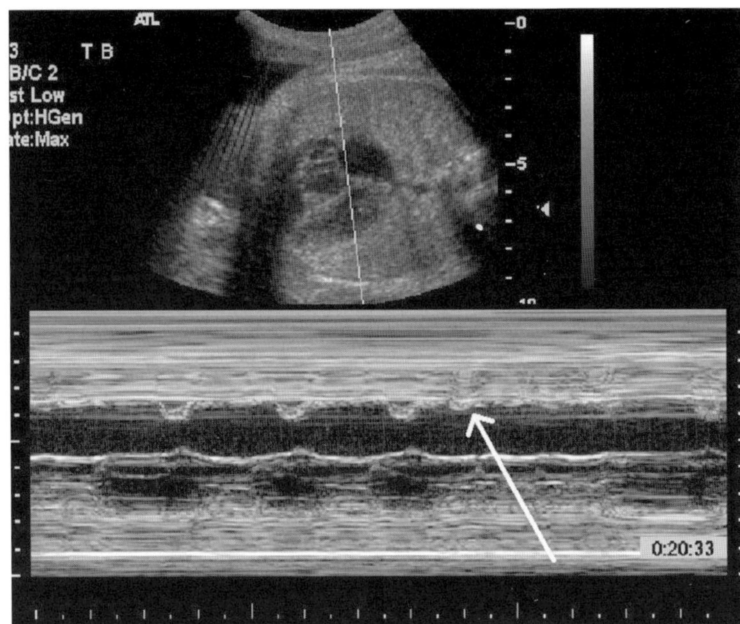

Fig 7.20 M-mode through right atrium and left ventricle. Arrow points to PAC.

result in a waveform that would show atrial contractions, designated by a point (as described earlier), followed by a spike-like deflection in the opposite direction, representing ventricular systole. PACs are virtually always innocuous findings and rarely develop into a serious arrhythmia. Only once have I seen a variation on this theme, bigeminy, segue into a supraventricular tachycardia (while I was watching).

PACs most often are triggered by caffeine. Many patients assume that caffeine only means coffee, but soft drinks and even chocolate can kick a susceptible fetal heart into PACs.

Supraventricular tachycardia (SVT)

This is fortunately a condition that is infrequently seen, but can represent a real problem for the fetus. A common theory to explain why this potentially serious situation, in which the fetal heart often beats at an ineffective rate of typically about 240, is that during the relaxation (repolarization) phase of the cardiac cycle an unexpected message from the atrium sets up a circular conduction "reentry" pathway that bypasses the AV node, giving the ventricle a life of its own. This results in a sustained tachycardia. Since the fetal heart cannot possibly fill and empty adequately at this speed, cardiac failure can result, along with hydrops, and, unfortunately, death if not corrected.

The diagnosis is made with M-mode and Doppler in the way described above, but in SVT, both atria and ventricles will be in sync, but contracting at the very high rate. These patients must be treated immediately because the lag time between initiation of SVT and hydrops can be only a few days.

The treatment in vogue for this condition is to start with the least noxious therapy—digoxin. By "digitalizing" the mother, AV conduction in the fetus will be slowed, hopefully breaking the cycle, in addition to allowing the heart to contract more efficiently. If this does not work, then bigger therapeutic guns will be necessary such as amiodarone, flecainide, and the latest favorite sotalol (a beta blocker). Obviously, hospitalization would be required because these may have undesirable maternal effects. Transmission of these drugs across the placenta, unfortunately, can be impaired in fetal hydrops. For this reason, we have attempted to inject digoxin and antiarrhythmics directly into the fetus on rare occasions.

Atrial flutter is a less common cause of tachycardia (making up 10–30% of them), but must be excluded, since the therapy differs. Of the two types of tachycardia, flutter is the most dangerous, because the atria beat at an extremely high rate (>350 beats/min), resulting in a very unpredictable and inefficient ventricular rate, and there is a suggestion that it is more resistant to therapy.

In an effort to cut down on confusing "noise," some older fetal heart rate monitors may not pick up either tachycardia because they have a built-in "blanking period," cued immediately after systole, during which time the machine will not print out input from the transducer. Therefore, with a tachycardia of 240, for example, every other beat will be missed, causing the machine to halve the heart rate to an unexciting 120. However, this can be averted by leaving the auditory function of the machine on, which will allow the operator to listen to the true fetal heart rate.

Another case in point

The 35-year-old patient was sent in from the mountains for a fetal evaluation because on the Doppler check the fetal heart was irregular. This was her second pregnancy and her previous obstetrical history was unexciting. She denied intake of any caffeine-containing items (with the exception of about twice a week ingestion of chocolate candy bars).

Her fetus's cardiac examination was confusing. No structural abnormalities were noted, but the fetus flipped from one rhythm to another. About half the time the fetus was in normal sinus rhythm and the remaining time the fetus spent having PACs, some of which were conducted and some of which were not. One M-mode vignette had a short episode of what seemed like a 2-to-1 heart block. The latter finding stimulated us to look for specifically responsible antibodies in the mother, which were negative.

Her care was transferred to the university because of the difficulty in monitoring the fetus during labor in the face of this irregular rhythm. Frankly, since we did not have an operational oxygen saturation monitor, we had no creative ideas regarding management of her labor. Fortunately, at term, her fetus spontaneously converted to a normal sinus rhythm and she delivered without event.

Bradycardia

Intermittent bradycardia in the second trimester will happen many times in the life of every fetus and it occasionally occurs when someone is listening. It is predominantly a second trimester phenomenon and, although the fetal parasympathetic system is immature at this point, the sudden irregular drop in heart rate has every earmark of being mediated through the vagus. It may respond to patient positioning, and rarely lasts more than 30–45 seconds, which seems like an eternity while one is watching. Early in my career I saw this for the first time after I had just done an amniocentesis, and I was sure I had caused it (it is one of the few instances when an obstetrician, and not the fetus, may pass meconium). Again, this is generally a normal finding.

Heart block is not an innocuous finding. In this rare condition, the messages traverse sluggishly from the atria to the ventricle, as in first- and second-degree heart block, or do not get through at all, as in complete heart block, resulting in the ventricle beating at its own rate of 40–60 per minute. Although the contractility of the ventricle is not directly affected, occasionally the heart does not contract frequently enough to perfuse the fetus, and the cardiac output, which not only is a function of the stroke volume but also the heart rate, suffers. Therefore, this can be a lethal abnormality.

Complete heart block is seen in patients with lupus-like antibodies, particularly anti-Ro and La (SSA or SSB), which slow conduction through the AV node. Other causes would be an anomaly that would interfere with the conduction pathway, such as large septal defects or marked dilation of the atrium, as in the type of disruption occurring in tricuspid atresia.

In utero treatment has been met with inconsistent success. Attempts to raise the fetal heart rate with betamimetics, such as terbutaline, have been discouraging, although treatment with corticosteroids has seemed to work in some fetuses where the above antibodies may have been responsible for the slowed conduction.

Early delivery often is the only answer in fetuses not tolerating their intrauterine environment, but infants with this condition will still represent major therapeutic challenges to the pediatric cardiologist after birth. Unlike the tachycardias, where our brethren cardiologists would prefer that we solve the problem in utero (if possible), little can be done other than to tread water until the fetus is old enough to have any chance of surviving.

Congenital abnormalities of the heart

About 8 per 1000 fetuses will have a structural cardiac abnormality, and in many cases a prenatal diagnosis of a cardiac defect will impact positively on the outcome for these fetuses, mostly by forewarning the providers involved in the immediate care of the neonate.

The two major categories representing a "loaded deck" for cardiac anomalies are a family history of cardiac abnormalities and patients with diabetes. In general, the recurrence rate for most cardiac anomalies is about 3–4% if the parent or sibling has one. However, there are some anomalies involving the left side of the heart, especially the aorta, which have recurrence rates of up to 15%. With the exception of the left heart abnormalities, when a defect does recur it may not surface as the same anomaly. The good news is that generally there is more than a 95% chance that the fetus of a parent or sibling with congenital heart disease will not have a defect.

Diabetes is a condition that predisposes the fetus to cardiac abnormalities, but this is wholly dependent upon the glucose control of the patient during cardiogenesis. For example, true gestational diabetics do not have an increased rate of cardiac anomalies, and those known diabetics going into pregnancy with fasting glucoses that are normal have a low rate of cardiac anomalies. Also, using glycosylated hemoglobin (HbA1C) as an indicator of long-term glucose control, those patients with values below 6 mg% have the same risk of a fetal cardiac abnormality as the overall population. On the other hand, those with levels above 12 mg% have a 25% chance of fetal cardiac abnormalities.

Among other possible predisposing factors to fetal cardiac anomalies would be exposure to medications known to be teratogenic to the heart. Lithium is notorious as a possible cause for Epstein's anomaly (tricuspid atresia). However, in our experience the relationship has been overplayed. Awhile back at Yale, Kleiman and Copel, a formidable diagnostic team, created a half-day clinic during which fetal echocardiograms were performed on seemingly hundreds of patients who were on this antidepressant medication. When we did not find any affected fetuses, we moved on to a more productive use of our time. Despite this experience, one cannot completely dismiss an association between lithium and tricuspid atresia, and these patients should have a fetal echocardiogram at about 18–22 weeks of gestation.

Another patient often benefiting from a comprehensive cardiac evaluation is the pregnant mother with a Down syndrome fetus. These fetuses have a 30% chance of having a major cardiac anomaly. Since the presence of a cardiac anomaly may impact on the quality of life of a fetus, already affected by the trisomy itself, many parents wish to have this information while weighing their options. Also, in continuing pregnancies, these fetuses will need special neonatal attention.

As indicated in the section on AMA, any patient whose fetus is at risk for cardiac anomaly would benefit from a nuchal translucency (NT) evaluation between 11 weeks and 13 weeks 6 days. The current thinking is that up to 50% of those fetuses with a cardiac abnormality will have an increased NT (above 2.5 mm). Conversely, a normal NT can help to reassure the "wired" patient in any of the above categories until a full fetal echocardiogram can be undertaken later in pregnancy.

Again, since it would take many pages to deal with every structural cardiac anomaly that a fetus could have, and most of these abnormalities would not be encountered by a sonographer or sonologist in a lifetime, I have chosen to concentrate on the more common problems affecting this organ. For more, I will refer the reader to textbooks that concentrate on the fetal heart.

Again it is strongly recommended that a pediatric cardiologist be brought in as early as a possible fetal cardiac abnormality (involving structure or rhythm) is suspected.

Yet another case in point—this time involving fetal chest

Patient was referred from a city in southern Colorado when an ultrasound scan showed a uniformly bright mass in the fetal left chest, deviating the heart to the right. Although the cardiac dextro rotation initially got our attention, a full fetal echocardiogram showed no obvious structural abnormalities. The right lung was compressed somewhat by the malaligned heart. Interestingly, in the apex of the left chest a triangle of nonbright tissue was seen and, with 3D planar reconstruction and VOCAL (virtual organ computerized aided analysis) manipulation (see the chapter on 3D), it was possible to quantify the volume of the lung mass as well as that of the opposite lung.

Initially, we thought the mass was a classic microcystic CAM, but when we identified what seemed like a feeder vessel emanating from the aorta, we strongly suspected this to be an extra lobar sequestration.

The volume of the mass increased slowly over the next month, but there was no evidence of hydrops or cardiac compromise. The opposite lung diminished in size over a 3-week period, but then the mass size plateaued and the opposite lung increased in volume. At 36 weeks, the patient was induced and the infant had no respiratory difficulty in the nursery. A diagnosis of CAM was made and at the time of surgical removal it was clear that the lesion had regressed in size.

In our review of the literature, we were surprised to find some reported cases of bona fide CAM that had feeder vessels from the aorta, which we thought was the hallmark of the extra lobar sequestration. Although in utero surgical intervention was contemplated early on, the mass became less aggressive and a plan of careful observation was adopted instead when there was no evidence of hydrops. We found the ability to do volume measurements through 3D techniques to be invaluable in tracking not only the mass but the size of the contralateral lung.

References

1 Yagal S, Arbel R, Anteby EY, et al. The three vessels and trachea view (3VT) in fetal cardiac scanning. Ultrasound Obstet Gynecol 2002; 20: 340–5.

2 Ryu JM, Kim MY, Choi HK, et al. Three-vessel view of the fetal upper mediastinum: an easy means of detecting abnormalities of the ventricular outflow tracts and great arteries during obstetric scanning. Ultrasound Obstet Gynecol 1997; 9: 173–82.

3 Tegnander E, Eik-Nes SH. The examiner's ultrasound experience has a significant impact on the detection rate of congenital heart defects at the second-trimester fetal examination. Ultrasound Obstet Gynecol 2006; 28: 8–14.

4 DeVore GR. Trisomy 21: 91% detection rate using second-trimester ultrasound markers. Ultrasound Obstet Gynecol 2000; 16: 133–41.

5 DeVore GR, Polanco B, Sklansky MS, Platt LD. The 'spin' technique: a new method for examination of the fetal outflow tracts using three-dimensional ultrasound. Ultrasound Obstet Gynecol 2004; 24: 72–82.

8 Fetal spine

Open spina bifida

The prevalence of this condition has decreased somewhat from 10 years ago, when it was found in about 1 in 1000 births. One reason for this downward trend is the liberal use today of folic acid, which will prevent some fetuses from developing neural tube defects. For example, the recurrence rate of neural tube defects is about 4%, but if the patient is on folic acid from the beginning of pregnancy until 28 days postconception, when the neural tube is closed, the recurrence rate is only 1.5%. Another reason that the incidence of this condition at birth has dropped is that screening with maternal serum alpha-fetoprotein (MSAFP) and improved ultrasound diagnosis of spina bifida have been effective in identifying most fetuses with this condition in the second trimester.

As indicated above, the neural tube closes between 20 and 28 days postconception, and the level of the defect varies according to when, during this window, the process is arrested. Spina bifida occulta is not uncommon and may go unnoticed because the full thickness of skin over the bony defect prevents the complications seen in this condition.

Open spina bifida comes in two forms: a meningocele, in which a sac devoid of neural tissue has herniated through the open defect, or a myelomeningocele, which contains tissue. In general, the level of the defect predicts the consequences after birth for the infant, which would include at least bowel and bladder dysfunction with lower defects and difficulties in ambulation and paralysis with larger higher defects.

Because of the effect in the posterior fossa, most often hydrocephaly is an accompaniment to this condition—requiring ventriculo-peritoneal shunting at some time after birth. The supra tentorial effect of spina bifida, until recently, has been blamed on a secondary effect from the mid-brain herniation, but now there is a suspicion, by the occasional presence of heterotopia, of a parallel effect on this area, rather than one that occurs "in series."

The reason that the diagnosis of open spina bifida can be clinched in a high percentage of those in whom the condition is suspected is that virtually every fetus with it will have disruption of the posterior fossa. There are two theories as to why this occurs. First, tethering of the spinal cord occurs at the level of the defect, where the cord becomes stuck to a placode, disallowing the cord to move freely upward through the spinal canal as the fetus lengthens out over time. When this upward movement cannot occur, something has to give, and the cerebellar vermis gets pulled downward into the foramen magnum (Arnold–Chiari 2 malformation). The alternative theory, the one used by the fetal therapists to justify attempts at in utero repair of this condition, is that large amounts of spinal fluid are lost through the defect, thereby sucking the structures in the posterior fossa down into the foramen magnum.

Whatever the reason, the important message is that in seemingly every case of open spina bifida, even in the low sacral defects, the posterior fossa is affected—thereby creating a diagnostic starting point for the investigation of any fetus suspected of having an open spina bifida. The findings include the following: (1) a "banana sign" in which the deviation downward of the vermis gives a banana-like shape to the cerebellar hemispheres (or, more precisely, a plantain-like configuration) (Figure 8.1); (2) complete obliteration of the cisterna magna in essentially every instance; or (3) a lemon-shaped calvarium in which there are temporal indentations of the fetal skull (Figure 8.2). This occurs in approximately 75% of cases in the second trimester, but not in the third trimester.

In this condition, the spinal findings are more subtle than the cranial findings and an unsuspecting observer can easily miss the defect with a standard examination. The common practice today is to obtain a longitudinal

Obstetric Ultrasound: Artistry in Practice. John C. Hobbins. Published 2008 Blackwell Publishing. ISBN 978-1-4051-5815-2.

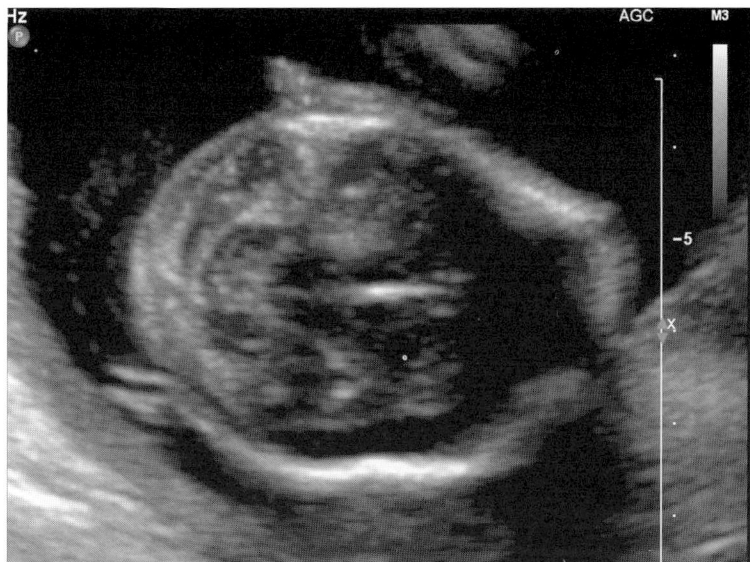

Fig 8.1 Banana sign of cerebellum with obliteration of the cisterna magna.

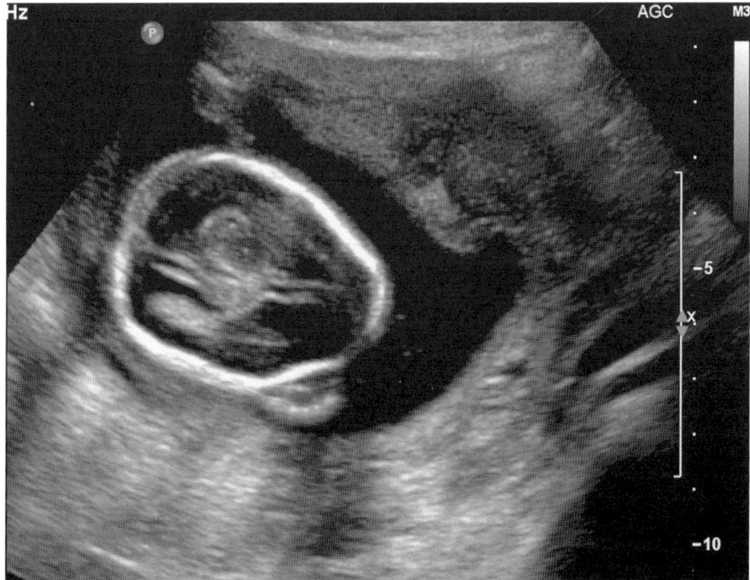

Fig 8.2 Lemon-shaped head.

image of the spine to demonstrate normal coronal alignment of the two lamina (Figure 8.3), or to assess a normal relationship between each spinal body and its companion lateral element in mid-sagittal view. The usual ritual continues with one-shot cross-sections of the spine at the thoracic, lumbar, and sacral levels, which are scrupulously documented (Figure 8.4)

There are three ossification centers in the fetal spine—the spinal body and the two lateral elements (pedicles or lamina) (Figure 8.5). In spina bifida the spinal process, which is not ossified, is missing, as well as the skin. Also, the two lamina diverge, and with today's equipment the often thin walled sac can be seen herniating through the defect on cross-sections or sagittal views (Figure 8.6).

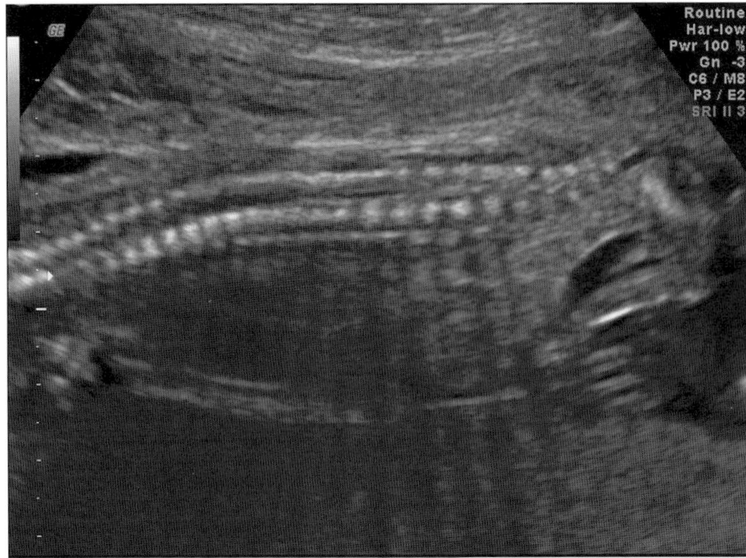

Fig 8.3 Sagittal view of the spine.

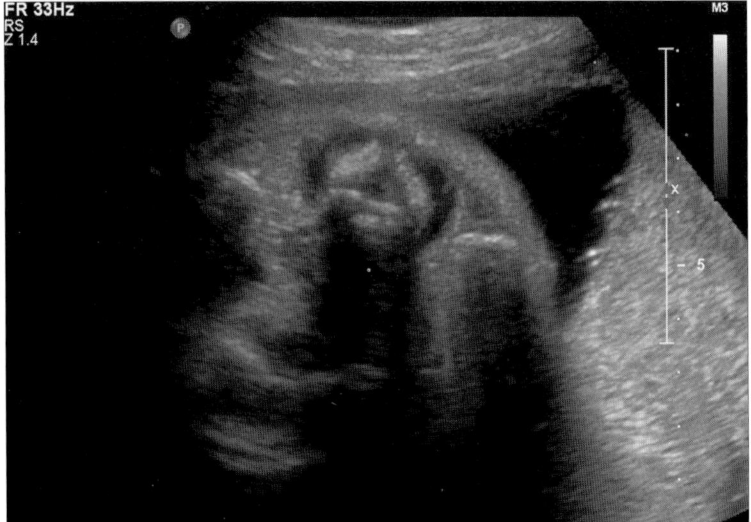

Fig 8.4 Spine cross-section: two lamina and spinal body.

Today, it is the task of the sonographer/sonologist to identify the exact level of the defect, since this is extremely important information to pass on to patients in early pregnancy who are wrestling with their options. We have found the transvaginal route to be extremely useful in breech fetuses and we will also always use 3D ultrasound to pinpoint the level and extent of the lesion with planar manipulation and rendering. This can be done first by obtaining a coronal view in which the L1 spinal body can be labeled by its position immediately adjacent to the twelfth rib (Figure 8.7, lower left image). Then, with rotation through the Z plane, one can identify the defect and count the number of spinal bodies between the superior margin of the defect and the labeled spinal body (Figure 8.7, upper left and upper right images). Surface rendering does not add much to the ability to pinpoint the

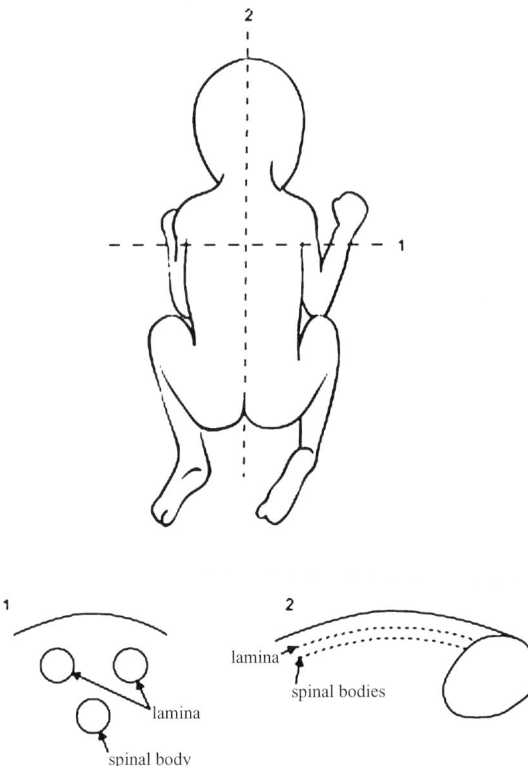

Fig 8.5 Schematic of longitudinal and cross-section through spine.

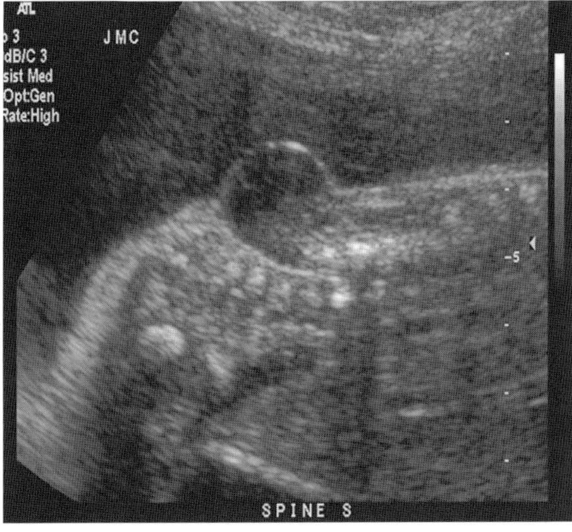

Fig 8.6 Low spinal defect.

location of the defect, but can characterize the appearance of the defect (Figures 8.8a and 8.8b). The multislice technique (Figure 8.9) brings into play in one fell swoop all of the imaging facets noted above.

Today most patients in North America are screened for neural tube defects with MSAFP. In fact, in California a law exists that every pregnant patient should be offered this type of testing. Alpha-fetoprotein is a fetal product that gets into the amniotic fluid in high concentrations through the meninges, which in spina bifida are uncontained by a full thickness of skin. For some reason, high concentrations of amniotic fluid AFP result in higher levels of maternal serum AFP, and about 85% of fetuses with open defects will be screened in with elevations above 2.5 MoM (multiples of the median).

The court of last resort, however, is the detailed ultrasound examination as described above, and the recent diagnostic track record from centers of experience is impressive. For example, in one center 2257 high-risk patients were evaluated with a detailed ultrasound examination [1]. One thousand seven hundred fifty-seven patients were referred because of an elevation in MSAFP and the remaining patients were referred because of a family history. Two hundred four had amniocenteses, but these were predominantly because of advanced maternal age. Sixty-eight fetuses in the study had neural tube defects and 66 of these were diagnosed with ultrasound alone (97%). In two cases, the ultrasound was suspicious but the investigators decided to do an amniocentesis for further confirmation. Parenthetically, in this sampling there were 17 cases of ventral wall defects, all diagnosed with ultrasound. The sensitivities for both neural tube defects and ventral wall defects was 100%.

The main reason that we still concentrate on longitudinal views of the spine is to screen for segmental spinal abnormalities producing scoliosis, a diagnosis that can be suspected by an angulation of the fetal spine. This type of abnormality is one of few where I feel that 3D plays an essential role in the ultimate diagnosis. The method involves manipulation of a 3D volume, preferably initiated in the mid-sagittal view, into a coronal image in which the lateral elements are lined up with the spinal bodies. When hemivertebrae are the cause of the malalignment, the missing lateral element can be identified by a 2-for-1 appearance across the level of the spinal body (Figures 8.10a and 8.10b). Also, in this plane the angle of the spine can be quantified. If more than one segment is involved, or if the spine takes the jog of greater than 30°, the chances of a major life-altering effect are, unfortunately, far greater.

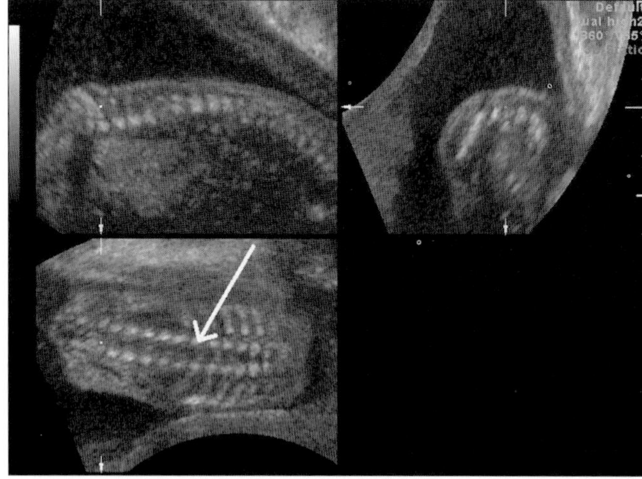

Fig 8.7 3D ultrasound. Arrow marks twelfth rib. Spot is on S1 segment.

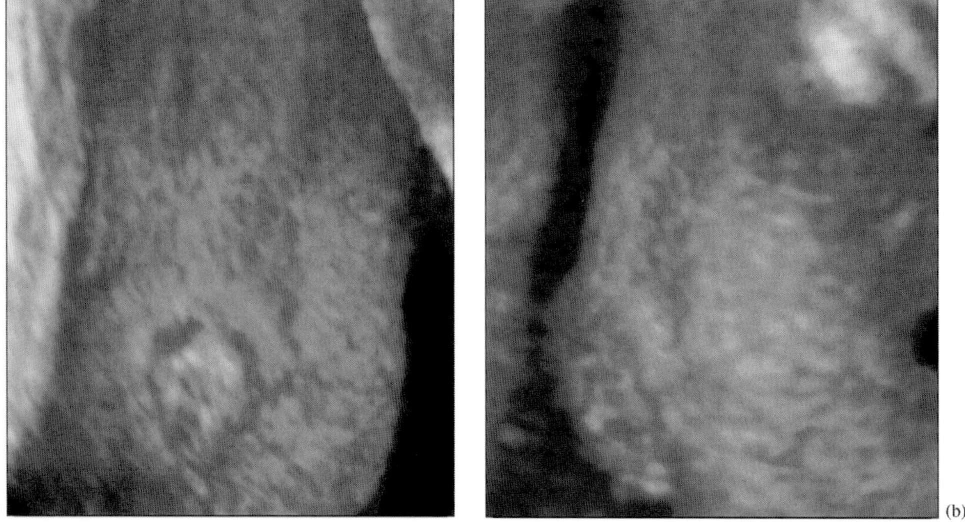

Fig 8.8 (a) A straight-on view of the defect with neural tissue involved. (b) Lateral surface rendered view shows the shallowness of the defect.

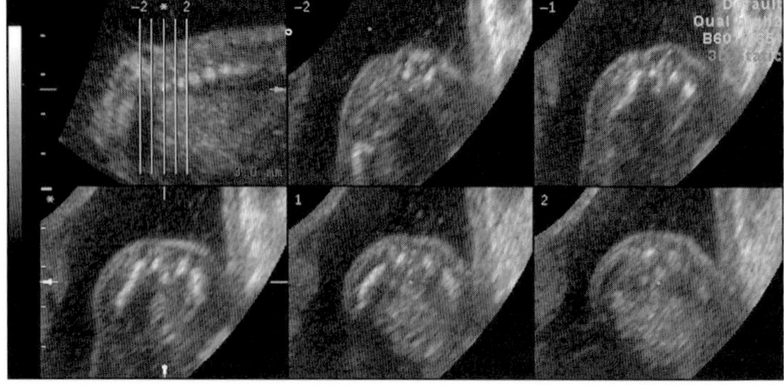

Fig 8.9 Multislice image of defect. Upper level of defect corresponds with minus 1.

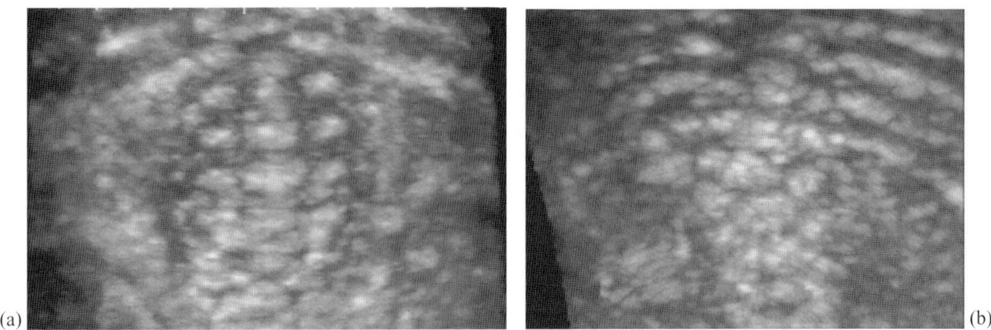

(a) (b)

Fig 8.10 (a) Spine: normal alignment at 34 weeks. (b) Fetal spine hemivertebra causing abnormal alignment.

Refrence

1 Lennon CA, Gray Dl. Sensitivity and specificity of ultrasound for the detection of neural tube and ventral wall defects in a high-risk population. Obstet Gynecol 1999; 94: 562–6.

9 Fetal abdomen

The existing guidelines indicate that the stomach, bladder, and kidneys need to be evaluated, as well as the ventral wall of the fetus.

First, there are normative data in the literature regarding stomach size at different times in gestation. However, any attempt at quantification represents consumption of time that has little clinical payoff. In most circumstances, there should be enough fluid in the stomach to enable its visualization after about 14 weeks. If the stomach is not seen, or is very small, then either a bolus of fluid was recently dumped into the intestines, the fetus regurgitated some fluid back into the amniotic cavity, or there is a fetal problem, which, fortunately, is the least likely possibility.

Tracheal esophageal fistulas (TE fistulas) come in two varieties: a blind ending of the esophagus (Figure 9.1a) or a high communication between the esophagus and the trachea, accompanied by a lower interconnecting channel back to the esophagus (Figure 9.1b). In the former condition the stomach will always seem empty, while in the latter, the stomach will simply be very small. After 16 weeks both are always associated with polyhydramnios. The only other possibility is that the fetus has a condition that interferes with swallowing such as a neuromuscular disorder, which is a very rare occurrence and also associated with polyhydramnios.

In essence, since polyhydramnios is the factor that separates abnormal from normal, a small or absent stomach is a finding that could cause little concern, if unaccompanied by a generous amniotic fluid volume. Nevertheless, a follow-up should be scheduled for a month in case the small stomach represents a heralding sign of trouble to come.

In most cases a TE fistula is a diagnosis made by exclusion, but one investigator with remarkable patience has documented on real time the reverse flow in the esophagus during swallowing. It should be emphasized that the predelivery diagnosis of TE fistula can avert the severe complications stemming from aspiration when the condition is unrecognized at birth.

GI obstruction

Dilated bowel loops should alert the clinician to the possibility of an intestinal obstruction anywhere along the GI tract. Upper GI obstructions are almost always associated with polyhydramnios, while obstructions involving the colon are not. Duodenal atresia is associated with Down syndrome in about 20% of cases, and when a typical "double bubble" is noted (although usually not until the second trimester), a fetal karyotype should be high on the diagnostic "to do" list (Figure 9.2).

Lower obstructions include volvulus, intussusception, and meconium ileus, often secondary to cystic fibrosis. 3D planar reconstruction and MRI can help to pinpoint the location of the obstruction, but even if the diagnosis is refined, the management of all these intestinal obstructions is to await delivery, after selecting the delivery site based on the capabilities of the center and the comfort level of the pediatricians.

If meconium ileus is suspected, cystic fibrosis testing of the mother can be useful in excluding this diagnosis. Also, the finding of an intact gallbladder (Figure 9.3) lessens the possibility of cystic fibrosis since in cystic fibrosis inspissated material will prevent the gallbladder from filling in about 75% of cases.

Echogenic bowel (EB)

Like other markers for aneuploidy, this finding, in isolation, is an enigma. However, the difference between EB and, for example, echogenic intra cardiac focus (EIF) is

Obstetric Ultrasound: Artistry in Practice. John C. Hobbins. Published 2008 Blackwell Publishing. ISBN 978-1-4051-5815-2.

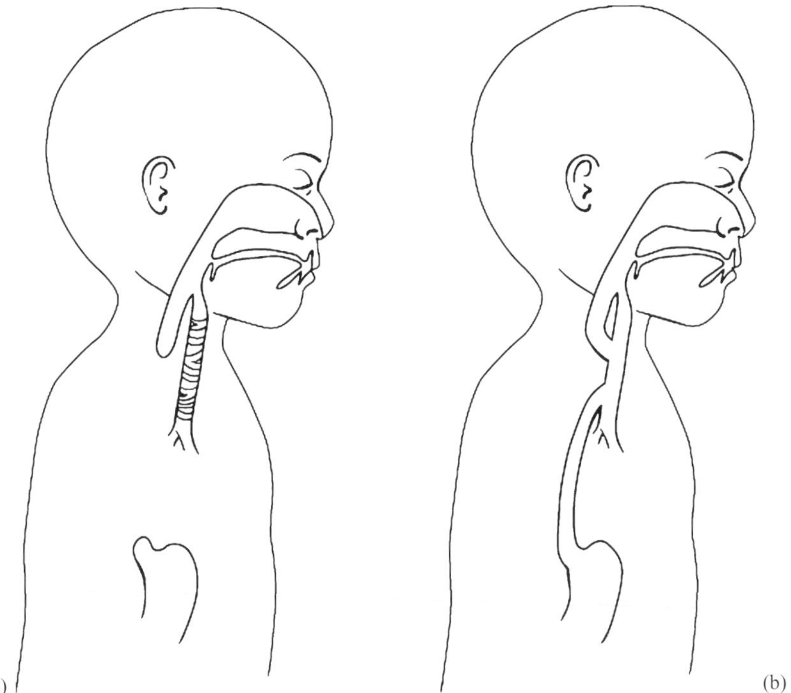

Fig 9.1 TE fistulas. (a) Blind pouch. (b) Communicating fistula by way of trachea.

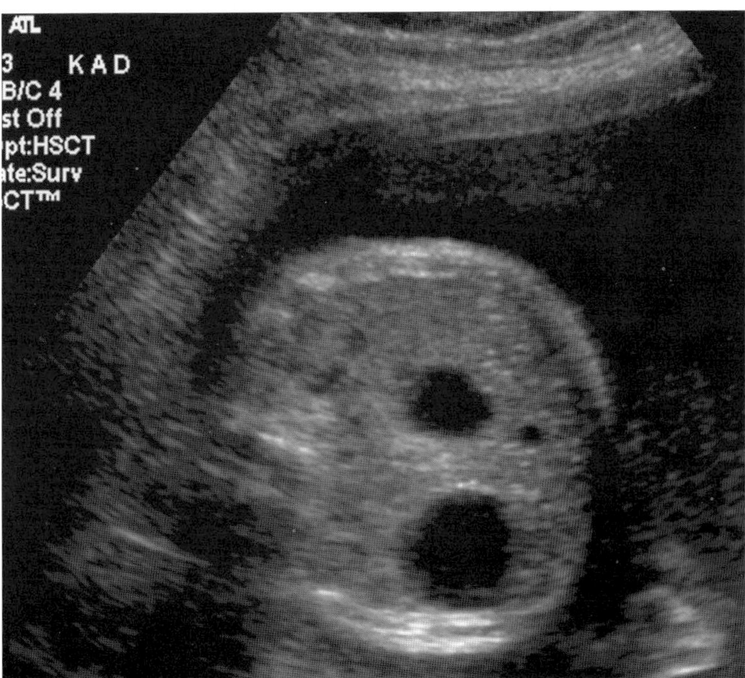

Fig 9.2 Double bubble in duodenal atresia.

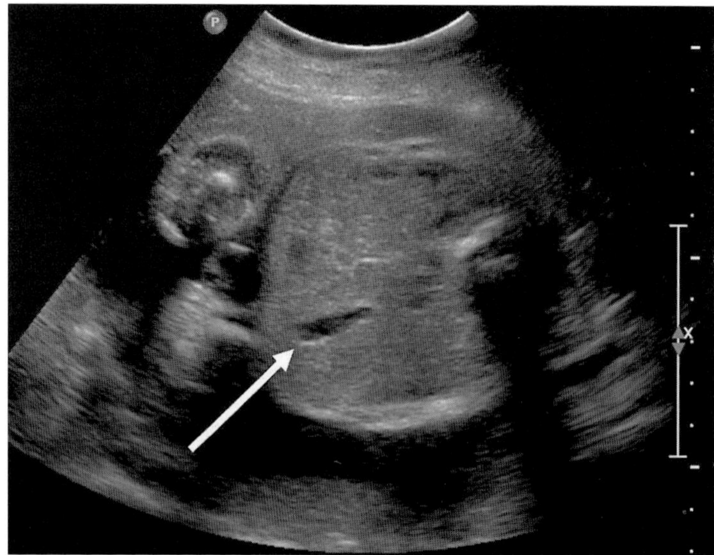

Fig 9.3 Fetal gallbladder.

that the former finding is much more frequently a sign of fetal abnormality. As with EIF, the diagnosis should depend upon the brightness of the bowel being at least as intense as adjacent bone (Figure 9.4). Some have advocated grading the echogenicity according to brightness, but I feel this adds little clinically to the "all or none" approach. Also, like EIF, it is dependent upon the frequency of the transducer and postprocessing.

EB occurs in between 0.2 and 1.4% of pregnancies, and, in addition to being a normal variant it represents a "mixed bag" of possible etiologies. Fetal bowel lights up for a variety of reasons. For example, if there is an overabundance of peritoneal fluid (pre-ascites), there is an acoustic mismatch between the bowel wall and the adjacent fluid (as in Down syndrome), or if there is bowel wall edema (as in infection or some types of obstruction or IUGR), the bowel will appear hyperechogenic. Last, if the lumen contains echogenic material, such as swallowed blood, the bowel can appear to be quite bright.

Let's explore the possible etiologies for EB. It is one of the better markers for Down syndrome. In one series [1], involving 680 cases of EB, 4.3% had aneuploidy and 2.5% were associated with Down syndrome. If the finding was isolated there was a 1.6% chance of Down syndrome. Since the likelihood of this condition increases fivefold in the face of this finding, many have advocated amniocentesis, even when the finding is isolated.

Another possible avenue to explore is cystic fibrosis. The carrier rate in Caucasians is about 1 in 25, representing a risk for cystic fibrosis of 1 in 2500 in the overall population (since there is a 25% chance of a fetus having cystic fibrosis if both parents, with previously unknown carrier status, are carriers). That risk rises appreciably when fetal EB is noted. The study above, with rather large numbers, indicated that 3.1% of fetuses with EB in parents of unknown carrier status will have cystic fibrosis. Certainly, based on these figures, one should discuss carrier testing in the mother as a first diagnostic step.

Intrauterine infections can be a cause of EB, making up about 3% of fetuses presenting with this finding. EB is also seen in between 4 and 18% [2] of IUGR, and often precedes the realization that the fetus is growth restricted. The addition of elevated MSAFP to IUGR and EB represents a dangerous diagnostic trifecta, being associated with a very high rate of stillbirth and neonatal death [3].

Last, EB is seen in at least 1 in 5 patients who have blood products in the amniotic fluid. Since the prognosis for these fetuses, who simply swallowed the hemepigments is excellent, one almost hopes that this is the cause of the finding.

If none of the above conditions is present in the fetus or excluded in the infant, one study shows no long-term effects in children who had isolated echogenic bowel in utero [4].

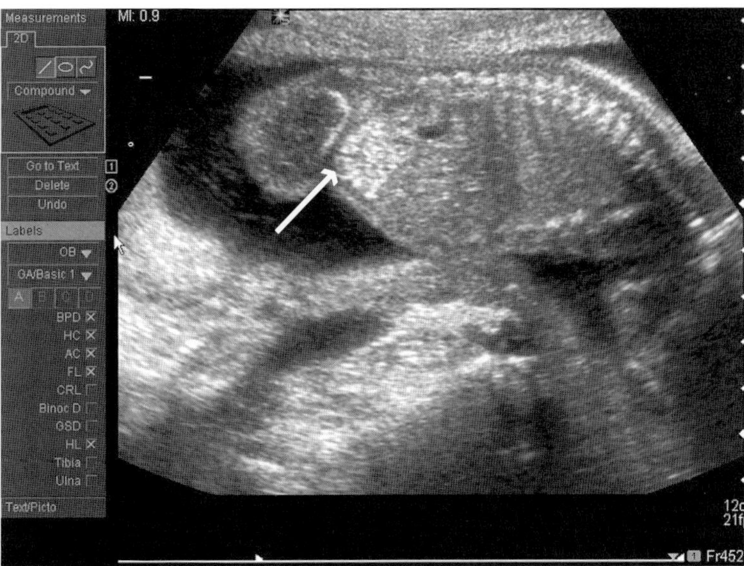

Fig 9.4 Echogenic bowel marked by arrow.

Ventral wall defects

As indicated earlier, prior to the twelfth week of gestation bowel normally herniates into the umbilical cord, but by the beginning of the second trimester, this channel will have closed over in all cases.

This section will deal with two types of herniations that can occur, omphalocele and gastroschisis, both of which can be diagnosed early in pregnancy.

Omphalocele

In this condition, which complicates 1 in 2500 pregnancies, varying components of the abdominal cavity herniate through the umbilicus into the umbilical cord. In smaller omphaloceles, modest amounts of bowel are contained within an intact sac into which the umbilical cord inserts. Larger defects will include liver and bowel (Figure 9.5). This condition can be isolated and of modest size with little long-term impact, or it can be part of an anomaly complex such as Meckel–Gruber syndrome or Pentalogy of Cantrell (in which cardiac anomalies, diaphragmatic hernia, and thoracic defects accompany the ventral wall defect). Frequently, omphaloceles may be associated with chromosome abnormalities such as trisomy 13, and generally these represent the more modest herniations. For this reason, we recommend offering amniocentesis to patients whose fetuses have this condition.

The prognosis depends upon whether the defect is an isolated finding, the extent of the defect, or whether bowel is obstructed secondary to kinking.

Unless the fetus has a "giant" omphalocele, the surgical treatment after birth is straightforward and, in many cases, the outcome is more dependent upon the immediate neonatal care than the operation itself. This represents another example of how the prenatal diagnosis of a fetal condition can affect outcome.

We follow these patients every 4–6 weeks with ultrasound, but I am not sure that our reasoning for this is valid, since, even if there is evidence of intestinal kinking, our colleagues in pediatric surgery indicate that they would rather deal with a large pulmonically mature neonate with the bowel obstruction than a preterm baby with any type of problem. Also, as opposed to gastroschisis, kinking seems to be less of a problem when the sac is intact.

Gastroschisis

This ventral wall defect is generally located below and to the right of the umbilicus, allowing small bowel to protrude through and into the amniotic cavity, where the loops are uncontained by a membrane. This defect

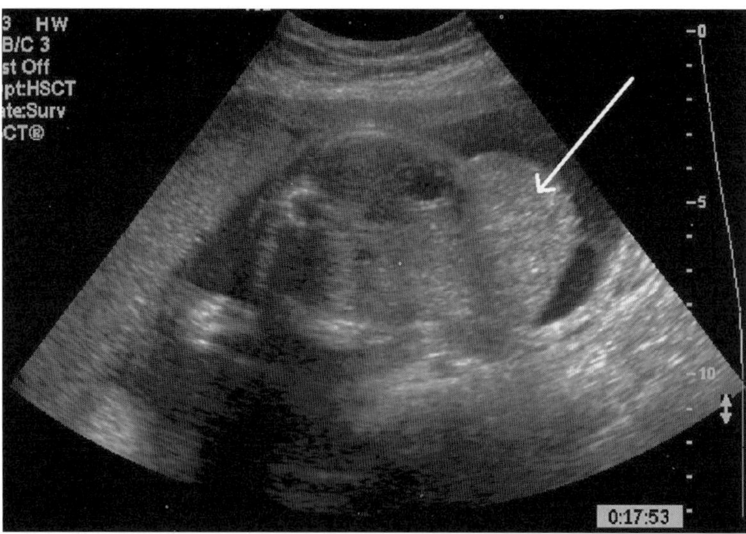

Fig 9.5 Large omphalocele. Arrow points to liver jutting into amniotic cavity.

in the abdominal wall may be due to an early localized interruption of the blood supply to the affected area. It is our impression that the quoted prevalence of 1 in 1000 represents a gross underestimation of the problem, which, in our experience occurs half the time in fetuses of teenagers.

The diagnosis is made by finding free-floating loops of bowel adjacent to the umbilical cord insertion. The bowel can twist, resulting in dilated loops (Figure 9.6). The fetal abdominal circumference almost always is small, causing the estimated fetal weight to be below the 10th percentile in over 50% of cases. Also, oligohydramnios is common in this condition (for reasons other than brain sparing).

Although infants respond beautifully to surgery with only rare complications, the greatest threat to fetuses with this condition is the surprising increase in intrauterine demise, which, in most cases, is unexplained.

Both ventral wall defects should be identified with a basic fetal survey, but often the scan is preceded by a quad screen productive of a high MSAFP. The mechanism for the elevation is similar to that in neural tube defects in that the AFP crosses readily from the extruded bowel mesentery into the amniotic fluid, raising the level of AFP in the maternal blood.

As with omphalocele, the prenatal diagnosis allows the provider to make delivery plans to optimize outcome. I feel that if gastroschisis is clearly isolated, karyotyping is not necessary (as it is with omphalocele). However, these fetuses should be followed with serial ultrasounds to monitor the status of the fetal bowel and amniotic fluid. We have found that, by using umbilical artery Dopplers and daily fetal movement counts, fetal well-being can be monitored adequately. As to the route of delivery for these patients, common sense would suggest that it is not a good idea to drag the delicate exposed bowel through an unsterile birth canal. However, no nonrandomized studies have shown a better outcome if these fetuses are delivered by cesarean section, and randomized trials have been impossible to get off the ground because of difficulty in recruitment.

Two other types of ventral wall defects are worth mentioning. A body stalk anomaly (limb body wall complex) is a lethal anomaly involving a large ventral wall defect, limb reduction abnormalities, an extremely short umbilical cord, and, often, a hockey stick shaped angulation to the spine. Occasionally, this is mistaken for another anomaly complex, amniotic band syndrome, which can be associated with clubbing, amputations, encephaloceles, and large ventral wall defects.

The mechanisms are different, but the diagnosis of amniotic band syndrome can be made by noting a normal umbilical cord length, adequate amniotic fluid, and, although not always, the demonstration of band-like structures in the uterine cavity, sometimes entangling the fetus.

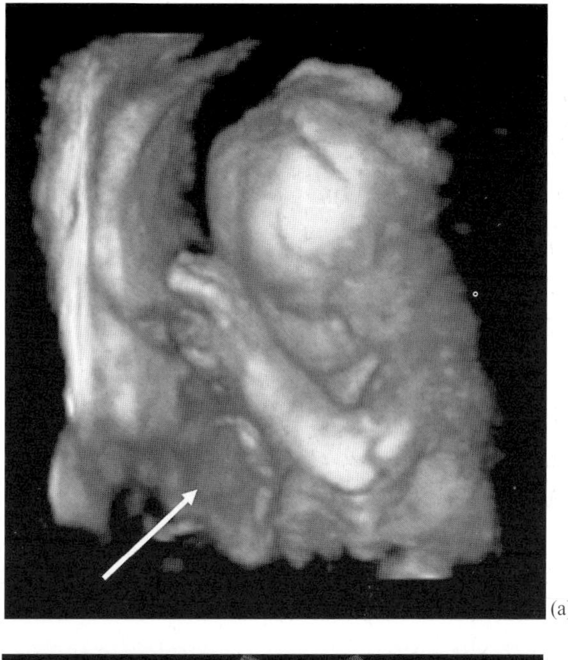

(a)

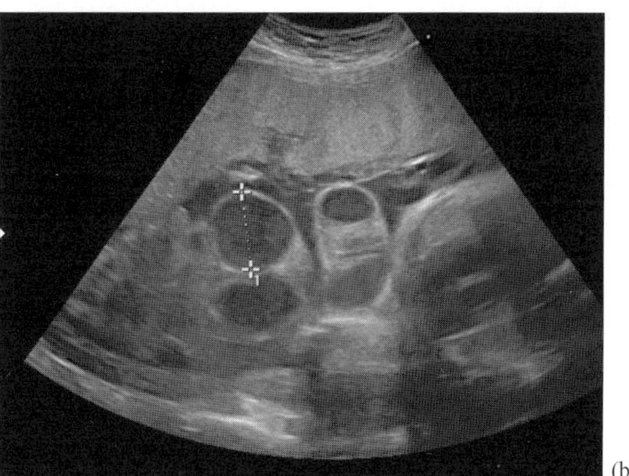

(b)

Fig 9.6 (a) 3D image of fetus at 24 weeks with gastroschisis. Arrow points to extruded bowel. (b) Same fetus at 34 weeks with dilated bowel in amniotic cavity.

References

1 Simon-Bouy B, Mueller F. French Collaborative Group. Hyperechogenic fetal bowel and down syndrome: results of a French collaborative study based on 680 prospective cases. Prenat Diagn 2002; 22: 189–92.

2 Rochon M, Eddleman K. Controversial ultrasound findings. Obstet Gynecol Clin North Am 2004; 31: 61–99.

3 Achiron R, Seidman DA, Horowitz A, et al. Hyperechogenic fetal bowel and elevated serum alpha-fetoprotein: a poor fetal prognosis. Obstet Gynecol 1996; 88: 368–71.

4 Patel Y, Boyd PA, Chamberlain P, et al. Follow-up of children with isolated fetal echogenic bowel with particular reference to bowel-related symptoms. Prenat Diagn 2004; 24: 35–7.

10 Fetal kidneys

Obstructive and dysplastic renal abnormalities have been covered elsewhere, so this small chapter will deal only with the most common, and, unfortunately, vexing renal finding—pyelectasis.

Pyelectasis

Pyelectasis occurs in between 0.3 and 4.5% of pregnancies, and the diagnosis depends upon the cut-off used to define the condition. Most investigators will use an anterior/posterior diameter of the renal pelvis of equal to or greater than 4 mm through the second trimester, but others will up the ante to 5 mm (Figure 10.1). Between 20 weeks and term the definitions vary even more. We simply use a threshold of 7 mm after 28 weeks of gestation. All investigators agree that the measurement should be made with the calipers placed on both inner margins.

First, let's discuss the problems associated with making the diagnosis of mild pyelectasis. Six years ago we enticed 20 patients with fetal pyelectasis and 3 patients whose fetuses were without pyelectasis to have measurements of the renal pelvis made every 15 minutes for 2 hours [1]. Seventy percent had at least one measurement during this time that was in the normal range (less than 4 mm). Three patients with fetuses with initially normal renal pelves had one measurement during the 2-hour period that exceeded 4 mm. The point here is that pyelectasis can wax and wane to a point where accuracy becomes almost laughable if the diagnosis is of the "mild" variety.

When the renal pelves are generous in size, then the next step should be to approach both kidneys longitudinally, looking for evidence of lengthening of the renal pelvis (about 1.5 cm), and most importantly for evidence of calicectasis (Figure 10.2). If this is found, there is a greater chance that the sometimes-fleeting finding of pyelectasis has greater meaning. However, calicectasis is more suggestive of obstruction downstream than aneuploidy.

Bilateral pyelectasis is two times more common in males. The usual course of pyelectasis is that it either regresses or stays the same (70% of the time), or gets worse (in 30% of cases). If pyelectasis persists into the third trimester, there is a 40% chance of nephropathy in the infant. If the pyelectasis is only seen in the second trimester, 12% will have significant nephropathy after birth. In a long-term follow-up study [2] 75 children were followed over a 4-year period after the in utero ultrasound showed pyelectasis. In the 42 with mild pyelectasis (AP of less than 10 mm) only 5% required surgery and there were no neonatal deaths or chronic renal failure. Unfortunately, in the 30 children in the moderate group (10–20 mm after 30 weeks), 37% required surgery and 13 had a neonatal death. If severe (greater than 20 mm after 30 weeks), 33% required surgery and 33% died. A very recent study showed simply that a 15-mm threshold after 30 weeks was the best prognostic cut-off regarding the need for surgery.

Now, to concentrate on intrarenal problems initially surfacing as pyelectasis, the presence or absence of a dilated ureter(s), bladder, or urethra will help to pinpoint the site of an obstruction. As indicated in another section, the diagnosis of ureteropelvic junction obstruction is hard to miss in the fetus with unilateral hydronephrosis, a normal-sized bladder, and a ureter that is not dilated. If the bladder is of normal size and ureter is dilated, then the obstruction is likely to be at the site of the ureterovesico junction. However, if both renal pelves are modestly dilated, with everything else in the system being unremarkable, the most likely diagnosis, other than this being a normal variant, is ureto-vesical reflux, a condition that is more common in males.

Unfortunately, mild pyelectasis represents yet another finding that raises the possibility of Down syndrome. As indicated in another section, yes, it can be a marker

Obstetric Ultrasound: Artistry in Practice. John C. Hobbins. Published 2008 Blackwell Publishing. ISBN 978-1-4051-5815-2.

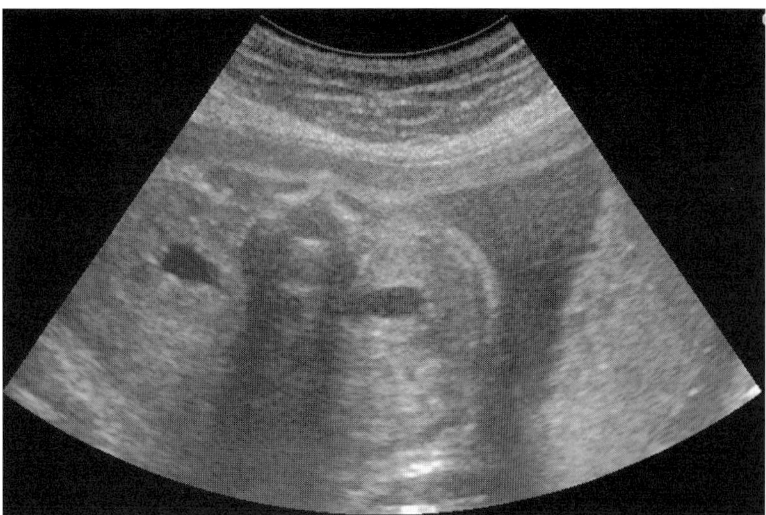

Fig 10.1 Modest bilateral pyelectasis.

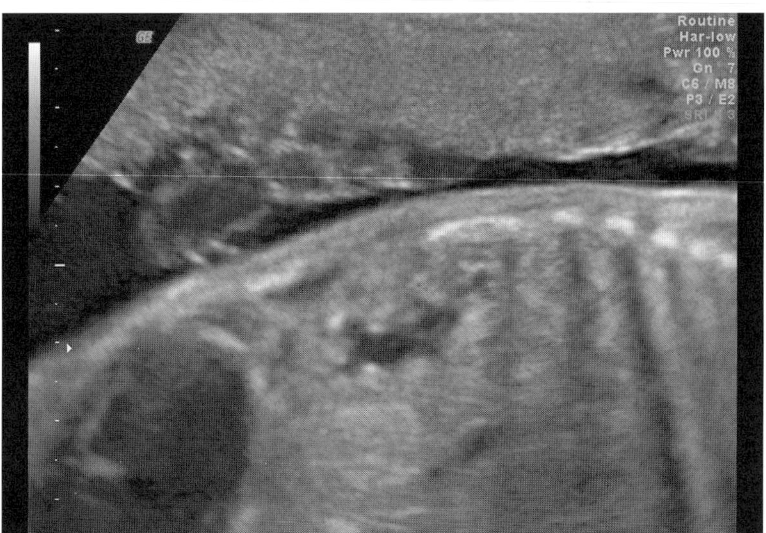

Fig 10.2 Mild calicectasis.

for Down syndrome, but it is a weak one. The finding should cue the clinician to do a thorough screen for ultrasound markers for Down syndrome. However, if isolated, my take on the literature is that even meta-analysis data, suggesting increased likelihood ratios for this finding, do not have the statistical power to adjust a patient's risk upward; especially if she is at low risk for fetal Down syndrome by age and/or quad screen.

A case in point

This case represents a very typical progression of mild pyelectasis. The patient was referred at 19 weeks of gestation because during a standard ultrasound examination the fetal renal pelves were noted to be bilaterally dilated (5.5 and 5.8 mm). Five weeks later we obtained

(*Continued*)

measurements of 5.5 and 6.0 mm. The kidneys were not enlarged, there was no evidence of caliectasis, and the amount of amniotic fluid was normal. In addition, the ureters and bladder were not enlarged. The patient was 28 years old and her quad screen gave her a risk of Down syndrome of 1 in 2000.

She was counseled that this could be a normal variant, or early signs of reflux. She was asked to return at 28 weeks.

At that time the renal pelves measured 5.0 and 5.5 mm and there were no other remarkable findings. Since this now represented a normal examination, it was indicated to the patient that reflux was less likely. As a precautionary measure she was booked for another examination at 36 weeks (to determine if neonatal assessment was worth pursuing), and this time the renal pelves both measured 4 mm. It could well be that the last ultrasound was unnecessary, but there was no doubt that if the trend in this patient had worsened, this infant would have needed further study, most likely invasive, in the neonatal period. Although the measurements between 19 and 28 weeks were essentially the same, they did not increase in parallel with overall growth of the fetus (which was great news).

References

1 Persutte WH, Hussey M, Chyu J, et al. Striking findings concerning the variability in the measurement of the fetal renal collecting system. Ultrasound Obstet Gynecol 2000; 15: 186–90.

2 Broadley T, McCugo J, Morgan I, et al. The 4 year outcome following the demonstration of bilateral renal pelvic dilatation on prenatal renal ultrasound. Br J Radiol 1999; 72: 265–70.

11 Fetal limbs

Many syndromes involve the fetal long bones, hands, and feet, and it seems that half of our patients want to know "does the baby have all its fingers and toes," which is apparently more important than the heart or the head. In any case, they are not, and only recently has there been a push at least to demonstrate the presence of four limbs as part of the standard ultrasound examination. The exclusion was not an oversight, and probably represented a way to protect the sonographer/sonologist from being sued. However, based on the idea that more lawsuits would be averted if one looks for a severe limb abnormality than are caused by an inability to recognize one, this brief task has now been incorporated into the guidelines for the standard ultrasound examination.

Examination of the fetal limbs

Measuring the fetal femur length has always been a part of the standard biometric examination, and many centers have added the humerus to their biometry. However, the distal bones are often ignored. My suggestion is that an attempt be made to image both tibia and fibula in the same plane, cutting across the lower leg in such a way that the image should not normally include a substantial portion of the foot, but rather only the ankle (Figure 11.1). This simple task will assure the observer that both bones are present and that a clubfoot is not.

Although we had not made a special effort to image the downside femur (the one not measured), we do now after having missed a unilateral femoral aplasia on an early ultrasound examination.

Visualizing the distal arm bones adds extra time to the examination, especially if one were to include the hands in the task, but anyone either having missed a radial aplasia or who has picked up a lobster claw deformity is now likely to be in the "I do it" category. Certainly, the hands should be one of the first areas to scrutinize when any type of fetal abnormality is found since they are involved in so many syndromes and aneuploidies (Figure 11.2).

Clubfoot (talipes equinovarus)

This is the most common abnormality to affect the limbs (Figure 11.3). From newborn statistics one would estimate it to complicate about 1 per 1000 births, but the in utero studies cite a prevalence of clubfoot is about 1 in every 250 pregnancies. Fifty percent of these abnormalities are bilateral and are associated with other anomalies much of the time.

Clubfoot can be part of an aneuploidy complex (most commonly trisomy 18) or can result from fetal crowding, for example, secondary to oligohydramnios. The condition can result from lack of fetal movement (as in neuromuscular disorders or neural tube defects), or can be secondary to amniotic bands. Last, it can result from a connective tissue disorder (such as arthrogryposis).

In isolated form, the genetics of this condition are very interesting, but puzzling. For example, the recurrence rate is 2% if an affected sibling is a male and 5% if the affected sibling is a female. If two family members have it, the recurrence rate is as high as 20%. What is particularly fascinating is that identical twins will share clubfoot far more often than fraternal twins. It is also clear that fetal crowding, even for a short time, can cause the abnormality. At least three studies have shown that early amniocentesis is associated with at least a 10-fold risk of clubfoot, and if temporary vaginal leakage of fluid occurred after the procedure, the risk was about 15%.

There is little in the literature regarding the identification of clubfoot in low-risk patients but it is clear that there is less than a stellar identification rate for this condition in this setting, and the false positive rate exceeds 10%, mostly because normal limbs can briefly

Obstetric Ultrasound: Artistry in Practice. John C. Hobbins. Published 2008 Blackwell Publishing. ISBN 978-1-4051-5815-2.

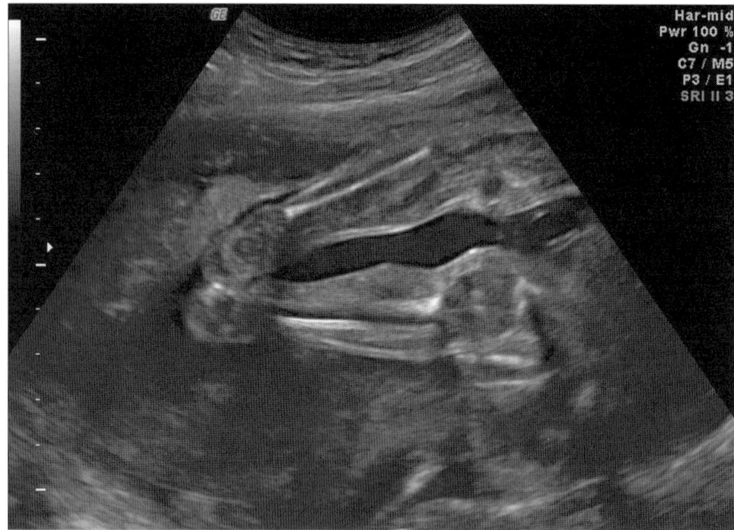

Fig 11.1 Normal alignment of both lower legs.

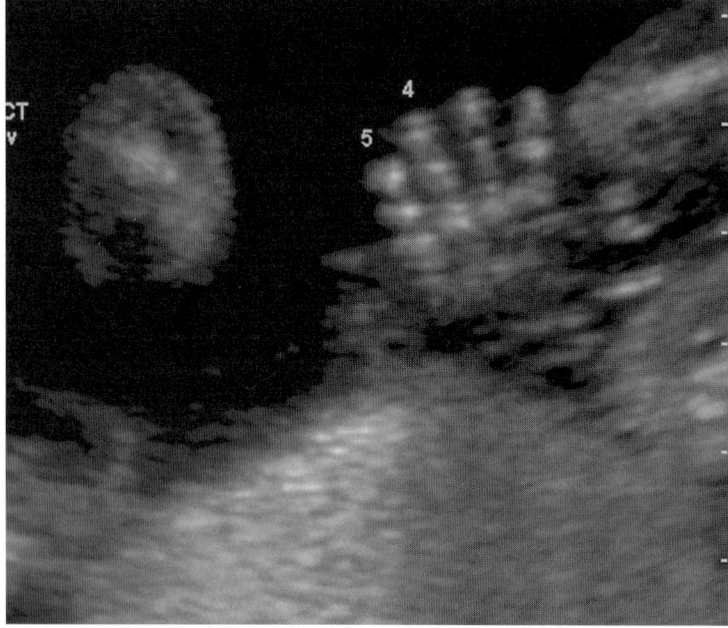

Fig 11.2 Normal hand.

stray into a cramped area at the same time someone is doing an ultrasound examination.

When one finds a clubfoot, a thorough anatomy survey should be undertaken to rule out associated anomalies. Also, with gentle manipulation of the fetus it should be easy to write off the initial finding as simply a positional event.

As to karyotyping, the overwhelming majority of aneuploidy cases found to be associated with clubbing have been in trisomy 18, a condition that should

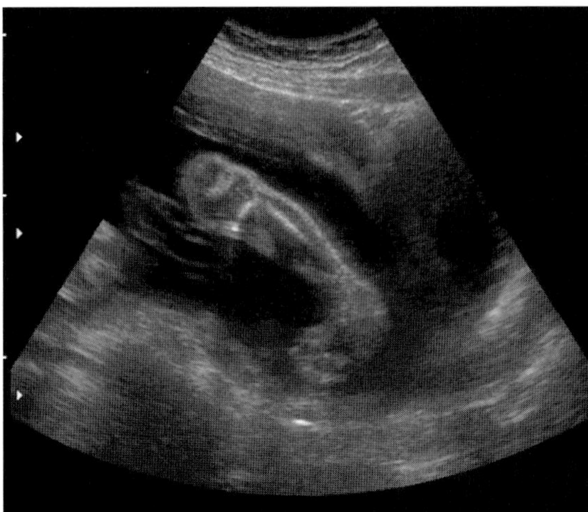

Fig 11.3 Clubfoot.

beexcluded with ultrasound alone. Obviously, if clubbing is clustered with other fetal anomalies, karyotyping should be strongly considered.

The good news here is that isolated clubbing generally can be remedied in infancy with little long-term impact on the affected individual. The majority of infants with clubfoot can be treated conservatively with casting and splinting, and those requiring surgery are the ones in whom the foot is markedly angulated inward and upward, something that can be appreciated before birth with ultrasound.

Short-limb dysplasias

Here is a situation where a rare finding, short limbs, can be a component of more than 175 extremely rare conditions, making the task of narrowing down the diagnosis particularly daunting. Lumped together, the incidence is 2.3–7.6 per 10,000, and about one-third of these are lethal. Since whole textbooks have been devoted to these types of problems, I will deal only with the most common of these, but first a few words on some essential elements of the workup.

The tip-off to a possible problem comes when, during a standard ultrasound examination, a femur is found to be more than 2 standard deviations below the mean for gestation. This usually translates into at least a 2.5- to 3-week discrepancy (with dates) in the second trimester, and more than a month's discordance in the third trimester. Even though this difference possibly could represent a normal variant, it should trigger the sonographer/sonologist to measure all other long bones. If shortening occurs only in the proximal bones (femur or humerus), this would represent rhizomelic shortening. If the effect is mainly on the distal bones (tibia, fibula, radius, ulna), then this would indicate the shortening to be mesomelic. If all of the bones are affected, this would fall under the category of micromelia.

While addressing these bones, it is important to evaluate their configuration, looking for bowing or evidence of fractures. Also the degree of relative mineralization can be appreciated by the ability of the bone to cast an acoustic shadow. In addition, the hands and feet should be carefully evaluated for unusual alignment and number of the digits. The foot length itself is useful as a reference, as it should be about the same size as the femur.

Once the limbs are thoroughly scrutinized, the next step can be the chest. Some of the lethal abnormalities are associated with a very small fetal chest. An abdominal circumference to thoracic circumference ratio can be useful, as well as a longitudinal scan, simply looking for a bell-shaped chest.

While in the neighborhood, it is important to assess the length of the ribs, which are quite short in some skeletal dysplasias, most of which are lethal. This can be done in a rather simple way. The ribs encircle about 66% of the chest parameter [1] (Figures 11.4 and 11.5). In short rib dysplasias the ribs are often extremely short, occupying less than 40% of the circumference of the chest at the level of the four-chamber view of the heart.

An important portion of the fetal anatomy on which to focus in short-limb dysplasia is the fetal face. With 2D and 3D ultrasound one can appreciate clefts or frontal bossing, seen to a certain extent in all fetuses with achondroplasia.

Other areas of the fetal anatomy survey that deserve special attention are the fetal heart, affected in many of the most serious dysplasias, and the fetal kidneys, which are abnormal in a few.

A three-tiered approach is often required. Tier 1 involves the finding of short limbs. Tier 2 represents a fact-finding search of the entire fetus. Once the fetus has been comprehensively surveyed, this would be the time to take stock of what has turned up during the tier 2 investigation. This is where the Internet or textbooks on skeletal dysplasias can be helpful if the diagnosis does not

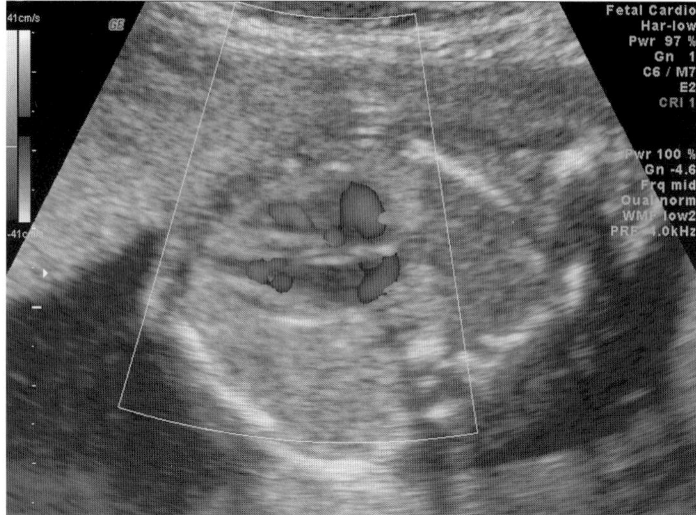

Fig 11.4 Ribs. Note in this echocardiogram that the ribs enclose about 60% of the chest perimeter.

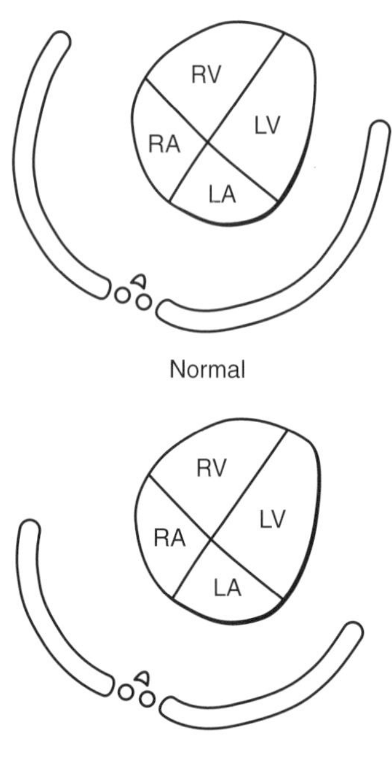

Fig 11.5 Short rib dysplasias.

immediately pop out from the information at hand. This research and, sometimes, consultation with a pediatric dysmorphologist, will tailor the direction of the last bit of fine-tuning required to make the diagnosis, representing tier 3. This might involve further 3D views of the fetus, an MRI, or an amniocentesis to look for various growth factors that have been noted in some diagnosable dysplasias.

Again, for the sake of brevity, I will only deal with the few individual skeletal dysplasias that most frequently confront the clinician. Many of these have subtypes to which someone has attached a surname (immortalizing these individuals through a form of academic cloning).

Heterozygous achondroplasia

This condition occurs in 1 in 15,000 pregnancies, and, although its pattern of inheritance is by the autosomal dominant route, it most always (80%) emerges as a spontaneous mutation in unaffected parents. It is the most common nonlethal short-limb dysplasia. Interestingly, the rhizomelic shortening of the limbs is not significant enough to raise concern until the end of the second trimester. The major diagnostic features are short bowed femurs, a large head, frontal bossing, hypoplasia of the mid-face, and trident hands (Figure 11.6).

These individuals generally have normal intelligence, and are at risk of upper airway obstruction and spinal cord compression in the first year of life. Virtually always cases spring from two mutations in the *FGFR-3* gene, and can be identified through amniocentesis. Most of the time, however, the diagnosis can be made through the pattern of ultrasound findings alone.

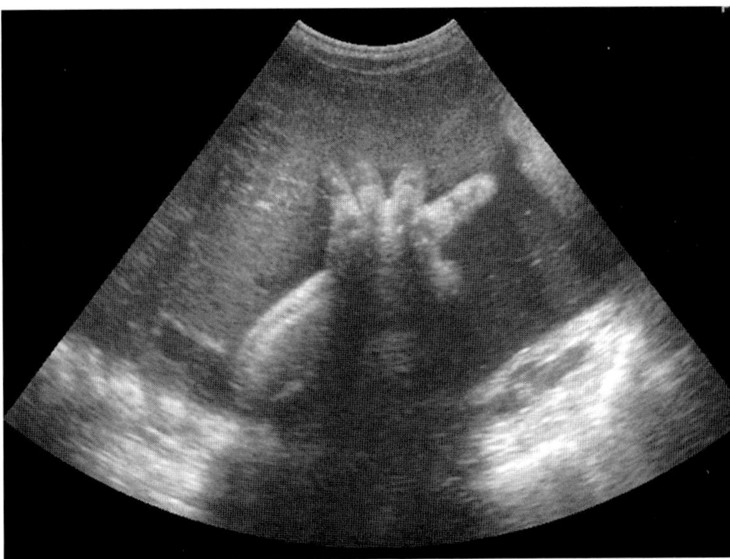

Fig 11.6 Trident hand from fetology.

Thanatophoric dysplasia

This is a uniformly lethal disorder and has the most striking features on ultrasound. The limbs are micromelic and the fetal cranium is often large. The chest is narrow and the ribs are short (Figure 11.7). There is a long trunk, and polyhydramnios is always noted.

There are two types of this dysplasia. Type 1 is characterized by flat vertebral bodies and the generally well-known "telephone receiver" shaped femurs (for those left to remember what a telephone receiver looks like). Type 2 variety has straighter femurs and a normal spine, but the classic feature is a cloverleaf skull (craniosynostosis).

Like achondroplasia, this can be diagnosed with fetal growth factor analysis, but the combination of a very small chest, very small limbs, and polyhydramnios should make this the easiest of the short-limb dysplasias to diagnose.

Achondrogenesis

This is a severe type of short-limb dysplasia that is manifested by a severe micromelia, distended abdomen (often because of ascites), hydrops, and, depending upon the subtype, absent or markedly decreased vertebral ossification. Type 1A (Houston–Harris) achondrogenesis is inherited through an autosomal recessive pathway. Affected fetuses have severe micromelia, flipper-like limbs, poorly ossified calvaria, and rib fractures.

Type 1 B (Fracarro) is a condition in which the ribs and head are normally ossified, but the long bones are triangular in shape and the spine is demineralized. This is caused by a mutation in the sulfate transporter gene.

Type 2 (Langer–Saldino). This could be labeled as a type of hypoachondrogenesis and the manifestations are less severe and therefore the diagnosis can be elusive. However, the diagnosis can be made through DNA studies.

Hypophosphatasia

All the above achondrogenesis syndromes can be mistaken for hypophosphatasia in which demineralization is a feature. This lethal abnormality stems from decreased activity of the alkaline phosphatase isoenzyme and can be diagnosed through amniocentesis. Affected fetuses will have hypoplastic, fragile bones, and the defining diagnostic finding—a very thin malleable cranium that is indentable and does not cause an acoustic shadow. However, in general, in hypophosphatasia the spine is not as poorly mineralized as seen in the achondrogenesis.

Osteogenesis imperfecta (OI)

There are four types of OI, each with its own features and impact on the life of the affected individual. Type 2 is lethal, while type 1 is the mildest variant.

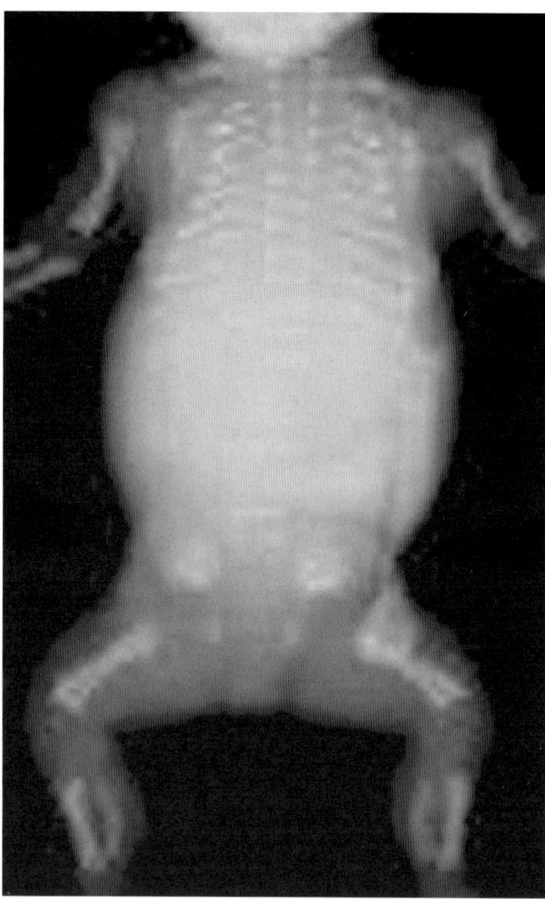

Fig 11.7 Abortus with thanatophoric dysplasia.

Here is a condensation of the characteristics of each subtype.

Type 1
Autosomal dominant
Normal stature
Blue sclera
Hearing loss in 50% of cases

Type 2
Autosomal dominant and autosomal recessive
Short long bones
Multiple fractures
Beaded ribs
Indentable cranium
Blue sclera

Type 3
Autosomal dominant or recessive
Short stature and variable deformities
Dental problems
Hearing loss possible
Scleras are not consistent

Type 4
Autosomal dominant
Normal sclera
Short or normal stature
Mild to moderate bone deformities
Dental problems

Progressing from worst to best prognosis, the progression is 2, 3, 4, 1.

Type 2 is the most common type of OI. The areas on which to concentrate are the fetal cranium, which will create no or minimal acoustic shadowing, creating a unique ability to see the near contents of the fetal cranium (Figure 11.8). The skull usually is indentable with the weight of the transducer alone. Multiple fractures of the long bones, especially the femur (Figure 11.9) are noted, and the beaded ribs are apparent on ultrasound or MRI.

Miscellaneous dysplasias

Diastrophic dysplasia is associated with the short tubular long bones, early calcification of the intercostal cartilage, micrognathia, and the classic tip-off, hitchhiker thumbs.

Chondroectodermal dysplasia (Ellis-van Creveld syndrome) is a short-limb dysplasia that has been seen more commonly in the Amish population in the USA. Cardiac anomalies frequently accompany the condition and polydactyly is the feature that helps sort out a confusing clinical picture.

Camptomelic dysplasia is a rare but, ultimately, lethal condition that affects many organ systems, as well as the fetal limbs. Almost two-thirds of fetuses will have a cleft lip and or palate. One-quarter will have a cardiac anomaly and one-third will have hydronephrosis. The diagnosis can be strongly suspected when tibial bowing is noted and the diagnosis can be made by amniocentesis.

Other long bone anomalies

Some skeletal anomalies involving the long bones are not associated with shortening. These can affect the fetal limbs

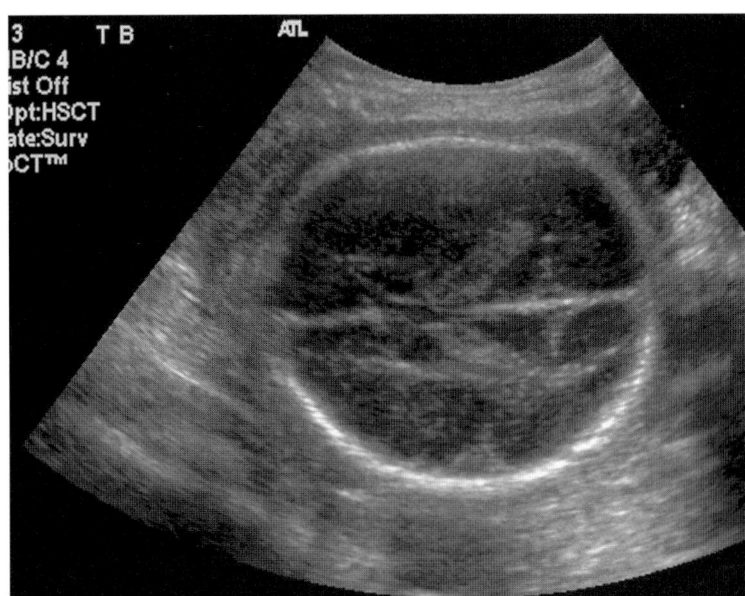

Fig 11.8 Osteogenesis imperfecta: head flattened by transducer pressure.

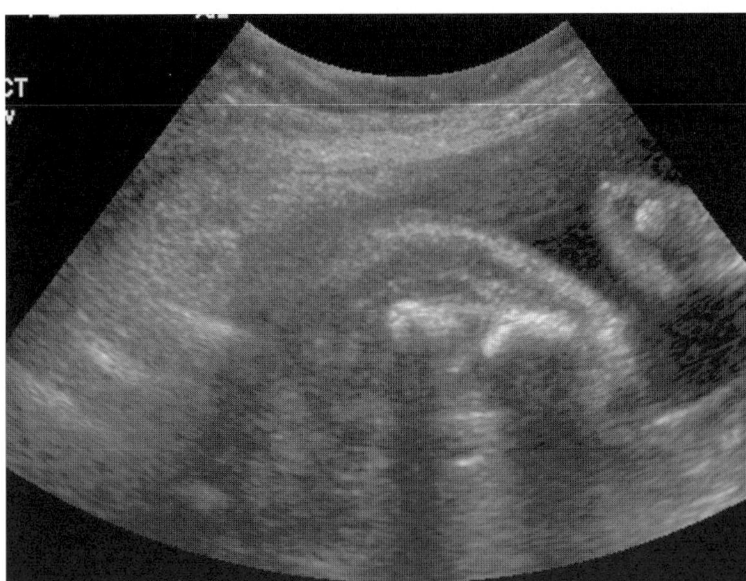

Fig 11.9 Osteogenesis imperfecta fracture of the left femur.

in a variety of ways. For example, amputation can occur in amniotic band syndrome, or an isolated transverse limb defect can emerge (with an incidence of 6 per 10,000). Various bones can be missing, such as femoral (Figure 11.10), tibial, or radial aplasia. The latter is seen occasionally in association with a syndrome, thrombocytopenia absent radius syndrome. Last, limbs can be deformed in a variety of arthrogrypotic syndromes due to contractures or lack of fetal movement. Conditions falling into this category would be arthrogryposis multiplex congenita, multiple pterygium syndrome (Figure 11.11), or severe prolonged oligohydramnios.

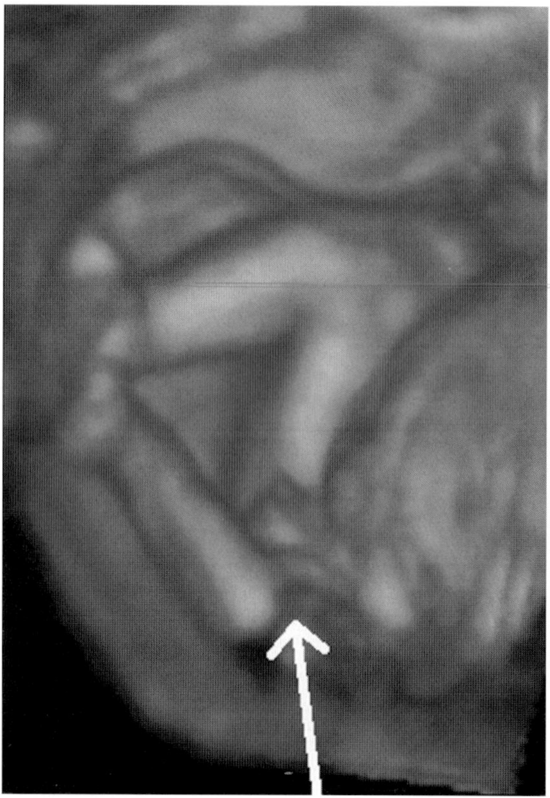

Fig 11.10 Missing femur.

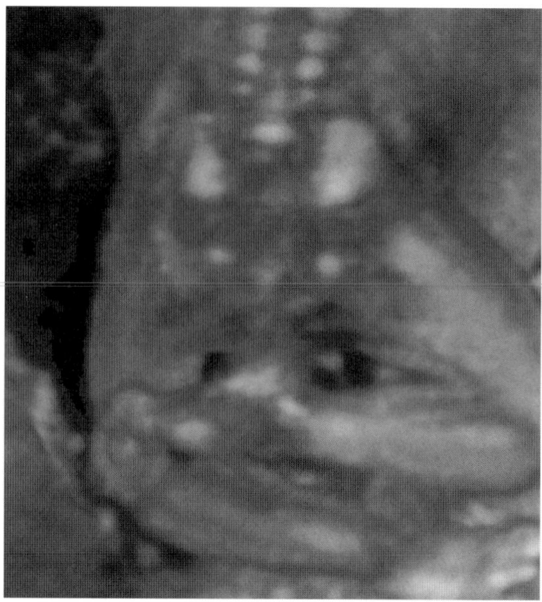

Fig 11.11 Arthrogryposis. Note that lower limbs are frozen in "lotus position."

Again, the differential diagnosis list is sometimes extensive for these types of skeletal dysplasias, and the ultimate diagnosis may evolve from many revisits to the ultrasound laboratory, and often will require a collaborative effort with more than one specialist. Sometimes the true diagnosis will only become clear long after birth. However, the diagnostic process can only be started by the alert sonographer/sonologist, realizing that something is not quite right with the limbs.

A case in point

An 18-year-old primigravida was referred in because during an ultrasound evaluation in her doctor's office there was a suspicion that her fetus had a clubfoot. The fetus was in the breech presentation, making it somewhat difficult to evaluate the lower extremities transabdominally, but it opened up an opportunity for a transvaginal approach. The latter examination showed both feet to be seemingly frozen in a lotus position. On a later 3D transabdominal ultrasound examination, the lower extremities were mapped out, and on 4D little movement was noted in the knee joints and ankles (Figure 11.11).

A diagnosis of arthrogryposis was made and various possible causes were explored. The fetus appeared to be swallowing, and there was no evidence of polyhydramnios. The upper extremities (the least, the hands, and wrists) actively moved.

We narrowed the diagnosis down to arthrogryposis congenita multiplex (a wastebasket category) or multiple pterygium syndrome, both of which are devastating. The fetus was born with a latter condition and, unfortunately, died soon after birth.

Reference

1 Dugoff L, Thieme G, Hobbins JC. Skeletal anomalies. Clin Perinatol 2000; 27: 979–1005.

12 Multiple gestations

Over the last 15 years, the incidence of twins has doubled from 1 in 80 to 1 in 40 pregnancies and the rate of higher order multiples has increased by 400%. While comprising 21% of low birth weight babies and being responsible for 13% of infant mortality, twins generally make up 25% of most newborn special care units' census. This concerning increase in multiple gestation can be chalked up exclusively to assisted reproductive technology (ART). Twins, in general, have higher perinatal mortality and morbidity rates than singletons, but those twins from ART have even greater elevations of preterm birth (PTB) and cerebral palsy than twins from spontaneous conceptions.

If that is not enough to get our attention, the cost of twins should. Contemporary figures show that perinatal expenditures for a set of twins are 6 times those of a singleton. About 1 in 10 identical twins and 1 in 20 fraternal twins will be delivered at 32 weeks or less. The average hospital expenditure for twins delivered at 30–31 weeks is \$170,000, and if delivered at 28 weeks or less, the figure is \$500,000. At the rate at which health-care costs are escalating twins could suck up an impressive portion of our obstetrical health-care budget.

Although peer pressure does not seem to be even weakly effective in keeping six fertilized eggs from being implanted in some desperate women, we can do our part in utilizing ultrasound to diminish morbidity and to consolidate costs.

Zygosity

Before tackling the major problems confronting twins it is important to discuss the importance of determining zygosity, since the incidence of the above problems is substantially higher in identical twins (Table 12.1).

About one-third of spontaneously conceived twins are from a single egg; the remaining stem from two fertilized eggs. The overwhelming majority of twins conceived through ART (ovulation induction or in vitro fertilization, IVF) are of double egg variety for obvious reasons, but one does encounter occasionally a monozygotic placentation in these patients.

One indirectly determines the zygosity (which is a diagnosis made after the fact by examination of the placental membranes or through human leukocyte antigen (HLA) typing of the infants), by the number of chorions present in the separating membranes. That said, it has been occasionally stated that about 20–30% of monozygotic twins will separate early enough to result in a single placenta, dichorionic/diamniotic (di/di) type of picture. Nevertheless, whether or not this is fact or fiction (and would have to be proven by today's sophisticated HLA-type testing) it is likely that these types of identical twins behave the same as fraternal twins with regard to a diminished risk of adverse pregnancy outcome, when compared with mono/di identical twins.

The earlier in pregnancy one assesses zygosity, the more accurate is the answer. For example, at 6–7 weeks' gestation dichorionic twin sacs are clearly separated by a substantial band of tissue (Figure 12.1) compared with monozygotic twins that appear early as a single cavity with a thin membrane separating the two twin units (Figure 12.2).

In both monochorionic/diamnionic (mono/di) and di/di twins there are virtually always two yolk sacs, although a recent article suggests that in very rare circumstances only one yolk sac has been seen in a mono/di situation. However, the justifiably concerning monoamnionic twins are always associated with only one yolk sac and, therefore, the early investigation of yolk sacs is warranted in all early twin pregnancies.

Often two separate placentas can be outlined, which will tip off the observer to a di/di pregnancy in the second trimester and zygosity should be obvious. As D'Alton has pointed out, the ultrasound clues include (1) assessment of the thickness of the separating membranes, (2) counting the number of these membranes, and (3) the presence or

Obstetric Ultrasound: Artistry in Practice. John C. Hobbins. Published 2008 Blackwell Publishing. ISBN 978-1-4051-5815-2.

Table 12.1 Outcomes of twin pregnancies undergoing ultrasound screening for nuchal translucency at 10–14 weeks (likelihood ratios). (From Sebire NJ et al. [1], with permission from Blackwell Publishing).

	Monochorionic	Dichorionic	*P* value
Number pregnancies	102	365	
Fetal loss prior to 24 weeks (%)	12.2	1.8	<0.05
Perinatal mortality (%)	2.8	1.6	<0.05
Preterm delivery prior to 32 weeks (%)	9.2	5.5	<0.05
Birthweight below 5th percentile (both twins%)	7.5	1.7	<0.05
Birthweight discordancy below 25% (%)	11.3	12.1	NS

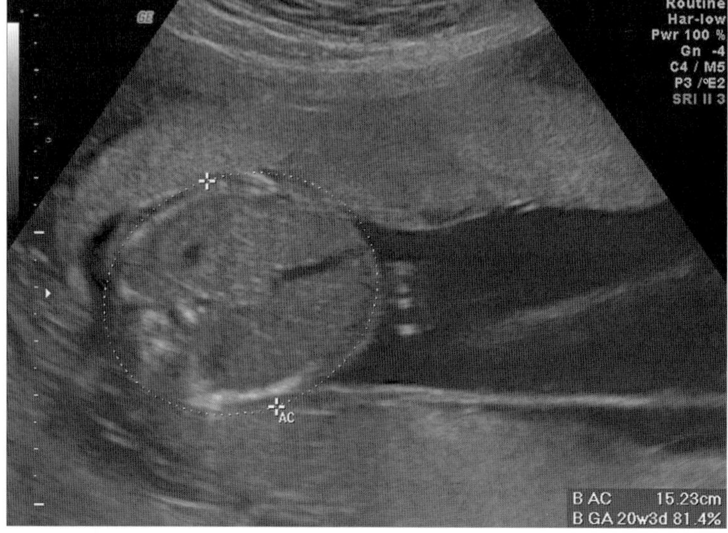

Fig 12.1 Thick separating membrane.

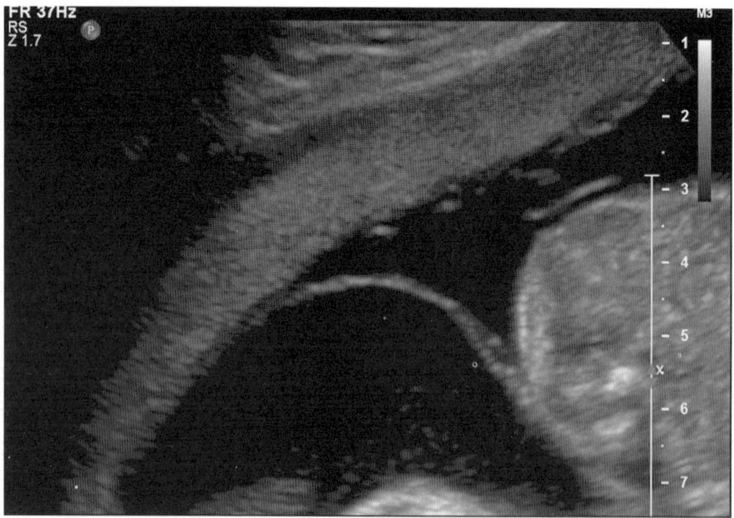

Fig 12.2 Thin separating membranes with, seemingly, only two layers.

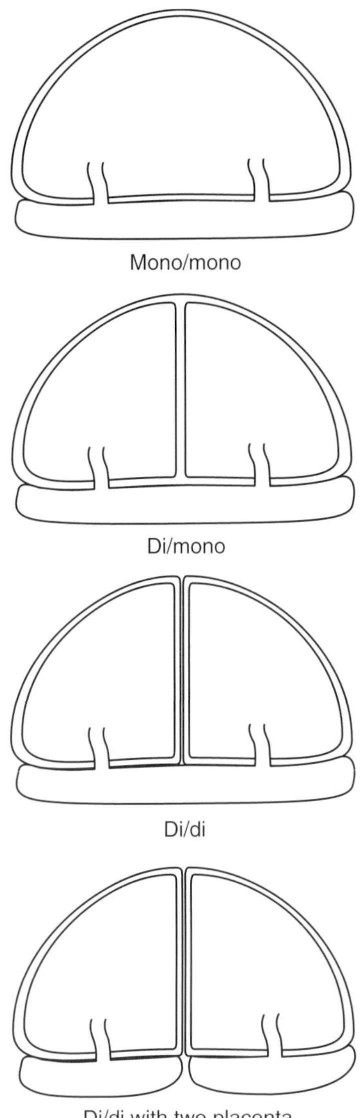

Fig 12.3 Twins: different types of placentation.

absence of a "twin peak." Obviously, gender determination will also be of help.

When concentrating on the separating membranes, one keeps in mind that di/di twin sacs are separated by four membranes (Figure 12.3); a fact that has stimulated many sonologists to count the layers in the separating membranes. Also, since four membranes are thicker than two, if the diameter of the separating membranes exceeds 2 mm, this is synonymous with a di/di setup. It is important to note that if using this approach one should employ the superior axial resolution of the transducer by having the angle of insonation with the membranes as close to 90° as possible. Also, the depth and zoom feature should be utilized to magnify the area of interest (Figure 12.4).

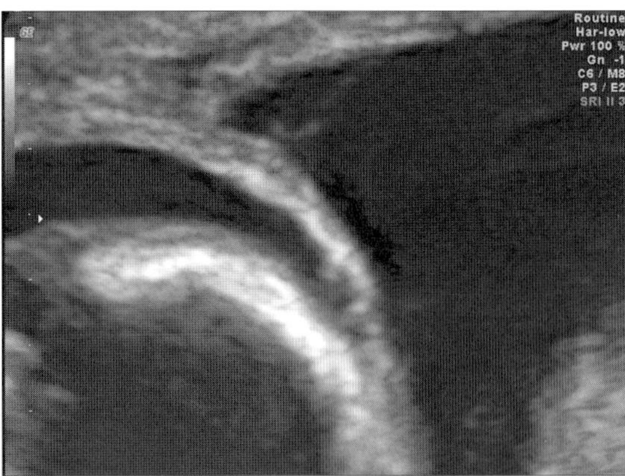

Fig 12.4 Magnified view of separating membranes in twins.

In dizygotic twins, the membranes come together at their junction with the middle of the placenta or at the placental edge in such a way as to form a "lambda" sign. This has been labeled a "twin peak" (Figure 12.5), and can be clearly distinguished from the T-shaped configuration seen in mono/di twins (Figure 12.2).

In the third trimester, the ability to use the membrane feature in a same-sex single placenta backdrop diminishes in accuracy because the membranes are stretched thin and even the twin peak is somewhat attenuated. In these cases we will apply the "boing" test. After approaching a magnified free portion of the membranes

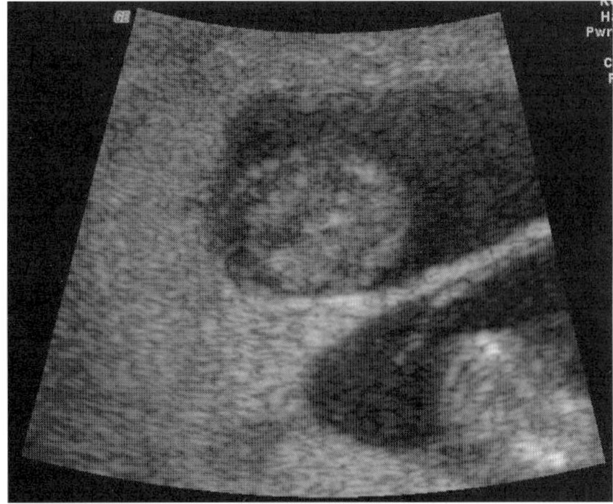

Fig 12.5 Twin peak.

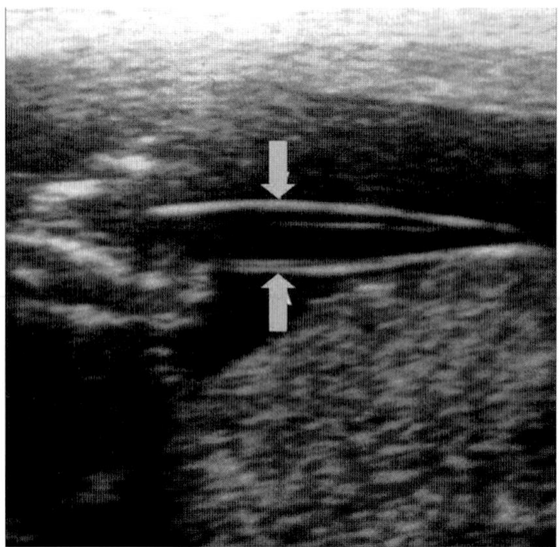

Fig 12.6 Fetal membranes can be counted during "boing" test.

the transducer is quickly but gently pushed toward the membranes, creating a fluid wave that causes the membranes to separate, thus making them accessible to counting. This is done by freezing the image immediately after "bopping", and bringing the stored images back one by one (Figure 12.6). Any count exceeding 2 indicates di/di twins.

As indicated above, twins are more susceptible to complications than singletons, but the "big three" are:

1 Anomalies
2 PTB
3 Twin discordance (IUGR—intrauterine growth restriction).

Twin anomalies and aneuploidy

Approximately 2.8% of singleton fetuses will have a major congenital anomaly, but in twins the anomaly rate is over 6%. One reason for the higher rate of anomalies and aneuploidy in twins is simply because one is drawing two tickets in the lottery instead of one. However, there is more to the story, especially since identical twins have a higher rate than fraternal twins. Some of these abnormal fetal conditions are specific to multiple gestation such as, obviously, conjoined twins, twin reversed-arterial perfusion (TRAP) sequence, and twin-to-twin transfusion syndrome (TTTS). However, others are shared by singletons, but at a higher prevalence in twins. These include cardiac anomalies, neural tube defects (NTDs), facial clefting, clubfoot, intestinal atresia, and cystic hygromas.

One reason the risk of twin aneuploidy is far higher than in singletons is because another predisposing factor is added to the mix—advanced maternal age (AMA). Half of the patients with twins have them because of ART, and a substantial percentage of those are AMA, creating a loaded deck for age-related aneuploidy, such as trisomy 21 and 18. Table 12.2 breaks down the risk of Down syndrome (DS) according to maternal age. Some AMA patients are pregnant with donor eggs from younger women, and the donor's age should, obviously, be used to calculate the risk for aneuploidy for each twin.

Plan for identification of anomalies (aneuploidy) in twins

Those patients pregnant from ART are a captive audience and their pregnancies are available for evaluation early on, while spontaneously occurring pregnancies most often show up for care late in the first trimester or sometimes well into the second trimester.

An ideal approach would be to examine the fetuses transvaginally as early as possible in the first trimester to assess the zygosity, crown–rump discordance, and twin viability. Then the best time to screen for aneuploidy with nuchal translucency (NT) is between 11 and 13 6/7 weeks, at which time crown–rump length (CRL) can be evaluated to further nail down gestational age. NT is also useful at this time to screen for cardiac anomalies and in monozygotic twins, to pick up early signs of TTTS.

The addition of first trimester biochemistry (PAPP-A and beta hCG), which is now commonly offered (and covered by most insurance) in those of AMA, would be helpful in all twins. If the NT is below 2 mm in women below age 30 and/or below 1.5 MoM (based on age and CRL), and the biochemistry is reassuring, then her risk should drop appreciably for aneuploidy.

Although NT screening usually is done transabdominally, a transvaginal examination in twins is especially useful during this 11 to 13/6 week window, because many anomalies can at least be suspected through the superior views afforded by this method. These would include NTDs, ventral wall defects, limb abnormalities, and, after 13 weeks, some renal abnormalities (renal agenesis and lower urinary tract obstructions). At least 50% of the time, four-chamber views and outflow tracts can be imaged (at

Table 12.2 Risk of Down syndrome of at least one affected twin.

Maternal Age	Singleton	Dizygotic (2× age risk)	Monozygotic* (same as age risk)
30	641	320	641
31	610	305	610
32	481	240	481
33	384	192	384
34	303	151	303
35	237	118	237
40	69	34	69

*This is the same for one or both fetuses being affected.

least in the presenting twin), and discrepancies in amniotic fluid volume can be appreciated. If all of these areas check out as normal, the next ultrasound stop for these fetuses will be in the second trimester.

Second trimester of anomaly screen

As indicated in detail later, a genetic sonogram consists of a standard sonogram and a search for markers for aneuploidy. If this is reassuring, then the risk of aneuploidy drops by at least half (or by a likelihood ratio based in a center's sensitivity for DS), and the chances of a major abnormality diminishes by at least 80% in experienced hands. Particular attention should be paid to the anomalies most prevalent in twins.

Although Timor-Tritsch, one of the foremost sonologists over the last three decades, has made a compelling case for an early (14–16 week) transvaginal scan in all pregnant patients, most others would push for this anomaly search to be after about 17 weeks by a transabdominal approach, when the larger fetal organs, such as the heart (which then is about the size of a quarter, instead of a dime at 14 weeks), lend themselves to better visualization. Of course, combining the two approaches would be ideal.

Biochemical testing through the commonly used quad screen is very useful, although currently some labs will not quantify the specific risk of aneuploidy (or NTD) because of the theoretical effect of masking that a normal twin will have on the results when the other twin is affected with aneuploidy. Perhaps a more valid reason for this reluctance is that most labs rarely have enough data on twins to generate a valid algorithm.

Preterm birth

On average, twins are delivered at 37 weeks. About 5% of dizygotic twins deliver prior to 32 weeks, while about 10% of identical twins deliver before this time—when neonatal morbidity, together with the extra attention prematurity requires, escalates. There is recent evidence to strongly suggest that a nonreassuring cervical length at 20–24 weeks will identify at least half of those twin pregnancies delivered at ≤32 weeks. Better yet, the technique has been shown to be an excellent excluder of preterm delivery, allowing providers to use cervical length for twin surveillance into the third trimester.

Here is the story. Souka et al. [2] have shown that, when compared with singletons from the same population [3], the average of cervical length between singletons and twins at 20–24 weeks is about the same (38 mm), but in those programmed to deliver at ≤32 weeks, the average cervical length in twins is 2.5 cm versus 1.5 cm in singletons (Table 12.3). However, if the cervical length in twins exceeds 2.5 cm, the likelihood of *not* having a very early delivery at less than 28 weeks is 98.6%, and at less than 32 weeks is 95.3%. Although the general feeling has always been that heightened perinatal care, in general, enhances perinatal outcome in twins, unfortunately nothing specific such as bed rest, prophylactic tocolytics, or cerclage have been shown to be of benefit. In fact, one meta-analysis [4] of the effect of bed rest in twins (irrespective of cervical length) shows a higher rate of PTB and neonatal morbidity. The tendency today is to overtest and to overrestrict high-risk patients, especially those with multiple gestations. The finding of an adequate cervical length should allow the clinician to pursue a more mellow approach to the management of twins, which would include abandoning

Table 12.3 Cervical length in predicting spontaneous preterm delivery: singleton versus twin gestations.

	Singletons [3]	Twins [2]
Spontaneous preterm delivery at ≤ 32 weeks	1.6%	8%
Median cervical length	38 mm	38 mm
5th percentile	23 mm	19 mm
1st percentile	11 mm	7 mm
Best cervical length cut-off	15 mm	25 mm
Sensitivity at ≤ 32 weeks	58%	47%
Risk spontaneous preterm delivery	4%	33%
Spontaneous preterm delivery with cervical length below cut-off	Exponential	Linear

commonly used, yet less informative, serial digital examinations.

So unless the patient has a history that would suggest incompetent cervix, a single CL, measured between 20 and 24 weeks, should be invaluable in laying out a plan of management for every set of twins. If the CL is greater than 2.5 mm, then the patient's chance of delivering at 32 weeks or more is about 96% [5] and these patients can be left alone to enjoy, at that point, a singleton-like pregnancy (unless other mitigating circumstances emerge later). Unfortunately, it is unclear what specifically to do for those with short cervices, other than to step up surveillance.

A few years ago, based on little data, some authors were advocating empirically performing cerclage procedures in twin patients with short cervices. The group who initially suggested this later backed off after showing no benefit to this practice. Today, a randomized trial in twins with enough numbers to attain adequate statistical power to answer that question seems impossible to accomplish, so as of this writing, there appears to be little evidence available to indicate that doing a cerclage in a multiple gestation patient with a short cervix has appreciable benefit.

Twin-to-twin discordance (TTD)

Most textbooks indicate that a twin weight discordance of greater than 20% is associated with adverse outcome. However, rather than assume the sky is falling when the estimated fetal weights (EFWs) are discordant, let's take a more selective, pragmatic, approach.

In fraternal twins, it is common to have more than 20% discordance in twin weight and it can only be due to genetic predisposition, inequity in the supply lines, or a combination of both.

After reviewing our data (unpublished), we found that the only real trouble stemming from discordancy happens when at least one twin has an EFW that is below the 10th percentile. This resulted in an average time of delivery of 33 1/2 weeks and days spent in the newborn special care unit, on average, of 24 days, compared with discordant, but AGA, twins who, on average, were delivered at 35.7 weeks and spent, on average, 6 days in the nursery. Interestingly, if the twins were SGA but concordant, their outcomes were no different than concordant AGA twins.

Further analysis of our data also showed that discordant twins, in whom the disparity in twin weights occurred prior to 30 weeks, fared more poorly than those whose discordance occurred after 30 weeks, the latter group having neonatal courses that were similar to those of concordant AGA twins.

The combination of observations suggests that occasionally in fraternal twins one placental unit gets shortchanged during the second (branching angiogenesis) and/or third stage (nonbranching angiogenesis) of placental development, and the smaller twin becomes growth restricted. These twins simply act like singleton IUGR fetuses, and should be monitored in the same way with ultrasound.

Most importantly, if one were to combine simple biometry at 20–24 weeks with cervical length measurements by TVS, one has the ability to earmark twins with the early discordance for further monitoring, and to lighten up on those in whom there is no discordance at this time, perhaps revisiting the biometry at 30 weeks.

Interestingly, we have observed an early difference in waveforms from the umbilical arteries of soon to be growth-restricted twins, suggesting (by the increased impedance) a deficiency in the villus circulation of some portion of the small fetus's placenta. Also, we have

Table 12.4 Sonographic staging classification of TTTS. (From Quintero RA et al. [6], with permission from Elsevier.)

Stage I	The bladder of the donor twin is still visible; Doppler studies are still normal
Stage II	The bladder of the donor twin is not visible (during the length of the examination ~1 hour); Doppler studies are not critically abnormal
Stage III	Doppler studies are critically abnormal in either twin, characterized as absent or reverse end diastolic velocity in the umbilical artery, reverse flow in the ductus venosus, or pulsatile umbilical venous flow
Stage IV	Ascites, pericardial or pleural effusion, scalp edema, or overt hydrops present
Stage V	Demise of one or both fetuses

observed that umbilical vein volume flow in the smaller twin is less than expected even before the small twin is labeled as SGA.

All of these observations point toward a one-sided supply line problem for the discordance, and its clinical aftermath, that renders management problematic, because there is often an innocent AGA bystander, who can suffer from an early delivery carried out because of his/her sibling's deteriorating condition.

Obviously, if the twins are truly dizygotic, then TTTS can be ruled out as a cause of TTD.

Monozygotic twin discordance

Twin discordance in identical twins immediately catalyzes thoughts of the dreaded TTTS. However, this potentially devastating setup occurs in only 10% of monozygotic situations, and often it is mild or treatable. Since identical twins comprise only 1 in 240 pregnancies and 10% of these are complicated by TTTS, only 1:2400 pregnancies would fall into this category. Yet, this condition has gotten great attention in the literature. Still, by far the most common reason for twin discordance in identical twins is inequity in the placental delivery system.

Here are ways to sort out the cause of discordant monozygotic twins. In TTTS,

1 early polyhydramnios is virtually always present in the recipient's compartment;

2 eventually the degree of oligohydramnios in the donor twin's sac is far greater than in garden-variety IUGR, and the fetal bladder is much smaller;

3 first trimester NT is generally increased in the recipient twin, while this is not a feature of placentally mediated discordance.

In TTTS, the communication across the placenta through small artery/artery, venous/venous, or the more common artery/cotyledon/vein anastomoses results in one twin sending a small amount of blood across to the sibling with each beat of his/her heart. The donor twin becomes growth restricted and often anemic, while the recipient is polycythemic and macrosomic. The smaller twin, having a depleted blood volume, produces less urine, and oligohydramnios ultimately develops. The recipient produces large amounts of urine, and, when cardiac function falters secondary to an overloaded circulatory system, polyhydramnios is the rule.

Quintero has created a staging system to quantify the severity of TTTS (Table 12.4), which is based on the amount of fluid in each sac, the presence or absence of a bladder, Doppler waveform analysis, and hydrops.

Various treatment modalities have been described in the literature. However, the two methods that are most commonly used are laser ablation of the communicating vessels and therapeutic amnio reduction. Over the last 7 years the competition for the best technique has been played out in the literature. As of now, the laser ablation method seems to have better outcome with regard to intact perinatal salvage by the end of pregnancy. However, the procedure is associated with its own immediate problems of premature rupture of the membranes and preterm labor. Interestingly, some cases of TTTS respond to only one amnio reduction procedure and other cases will remain stable without any intervention.

For the above reasons, it is most important to make sure that the etiology of twin discordance in mono/di twins is TTTS by documenting the essential diagnostic features of this syndrome before attempting intervention. Again, at the time of this writing, laser ablation seems to be the better method in the long run for some carefully selected patients with TTTS.

Conclusion

The tendency today is to overtest and to intrude too much into the lives of most patients with twins. Unfortunately, triplets or more need almost constant attention, and are excluded from the algorithm below. However, in most sets of twins by using some simple ultrasound steps, a cost-effective and minimally intrusive plan can be drafted for patients with twins that make sense without compromising safety.

Schedule for twins

First trimester

A. Very early scan (6–10 weeks)
   - Viability
   - Determine zygosity
     - Membranes
     - Yolk sacs
   - CRL

B. Early screen (10–13 6/7 weeks)
   - CRL
   - NT
   - Nasal bones
   - Obvious anomalies
   - The zygosity—if first scan

C. Second trimester (16–18 weeks)
   - Biometry to look for early discordance
   - Major anomalies
   - Markers for aneuploidy (in any at-risk patient)
   - Add quad screen

D. Late second trimester (20–24 weeks); preferably 1 month after previous scan
   - Biometry
   - Anomaly survey—concentrate on fetal heart
   - Amniotic fluid amount in each sac
   - Cervical length
   - *Then*
     - If no discordance in biometry
     - If cervical length >2.5 cm
     - If no anomalies
   - Repeat basic ultrasound every 6 weeks until delivery unless EFW of one twin plateaus

The case in point

The 22-year-old patient in her first pregnancy was referred when her ultrasound examination at 12 weeks revealed twins. These were conceived spontaneously. Since the bulk of our twin referrals seemed to be in women of advanced maternal age undergoing infertility treatment, this was somewhat refreshing. The first scan showed concordant twins of appropriate size and the CRLs were within one day of each other. A single anterior placenta was noted, and there was a clear twin peak leading into thick separating membranes.

The twins grew in parallel until the twenty-second week when twin A's estimated fetal weight was in the 50th percentile, and twin B's estimated fetal weight was in the 20th percentile. By 30 weeks, twin B's weight was at the 10th percentile and twin A was in the 50th percentile.

We began Doppler investigations and at 33 weeks the umbilical artery in twin B had very low end diastolic flow (S/D ratio of 8) and there was brain sparing with an MCA S/D ratio of 3. Oligohydramnios was present in twin B. Dopplers and fluid in twin A were always normal.

At 34 weeks the umbilical artery of twin B had absent end diastolic flow, and there was a progressive worsening trend in the ductus venosus waveform during atrial contraction.

We bailed! Since twin A was in a breech presentation, she was delivered by cesarean section. Twin A weighed 2200 g and twin B weighed 1600 g. Although twin B spent 2 weeks in the nursery to beef up, both babies flourished eventually and now have met their developmental milestones.

This is a case of discordance in di/ di twins, one of whom had classic placentally mediated IUGR. The Doppler information allowed us to deliver these twins at what seemed like the best time under the conditions. However, one can never be sure.

References

1 Sebire NJ, Snijders RJ, Hughes K, et al. The hidden mortality of monochorionic twin pregnancies. Br J Obstet Gynaecol 1997; 104(10): 1203–7.

2 Souka AP, Heath V, Flink S, et al. Cervical length at 23 weeks in twins in predicting spontaneous preterm delivery. Obstet Gynecol 1999; 94: 450–4.

3 Heath VC, Southall TR, Souka AP, et al. Cervical length at 23 weeks of gestation: prediction of spontaneous preterm delivery. Ultrasound Obstet Gynecol 1998; 12: 312–7.

4 Monteagudo A, Timor-Tritsch IE (eds). Ultrasound and Multifetal Pregnancy. New York: Parthenon; 1998.

5 Sperling L, Kiil C, Larsen LU, et al. How to identify twins at low risk of spontaneous preterm delivery. Ultrasound Obstet Gynecol 2005; 26: 138–1444.

6 Quintero RA, Dickinson JE, Morales WJ et al. Stage-based treatment of twin-twin transfusion syndrome. Am J Obstet Gynecol 2003; 188: 1333–40.

13 Advanced maternal age

Recent emphasis on noninvasive diagnosis has evolved over a time when the average age of pregnant patients has increased appreciably. For example, in 1985, 5.6% of patients who were pregnant were 35 years of age or older [1]. This rose in year 2002 to about 12.5% and recently it has been estimated that the figure now approaches 20% in the United States.

Up until the last decade it was common practice to offer, if not strongly encourage, all patients of advanced maternal age (AMA) to have an amniocentesis. However, the invasive route gave way to a practice of performing a triple biochemistry screen in some patients of AMA and to move to an amniocentesis if the risk were above a preset threshold for Down syndrome (usually 1 in 280).

Now, based in part on a patient-driven initiative, more noninvasive methods are available. The goal is to give patients the most accurate information available with which to make an informed decision regarding invasive sampling.

First, since the concept is to weigh the risks of invasive procedures against a given patient's risk of having a fetus with Down syndrome or trisomy 18, it is important to touch upon the known risks of two procedures, chorionic villus sampling (CVS) and amniocentesis.

Chorionic villus sampling

This first trimester procedure can be performed either transabdominally, using a needle guided under ultrasound direction into the placenta, or transcervically, using a catheter directed under ultrasound guidance into the placenta. Anterior placentas are easier to approach transabdominally while posterior placentas lend themselves to the transcervical route.

Spontaneous loss rates in apparently normal pregnancies are about 15% at 5–6 menstrual weeks, about 2% at 11 weeks, and slightly less than 1% at 16 weeks. Raw loss rates after CVS have varied between 1.6 and 3.4% in experienced centers in the United States [2]. We quote a procedure-related risk of between 1 and 1.5% for CVS.

There is no doubt that the more needle insertions that are required to obtain an adequate sample, the greater is the risk of the procedure, and the greater the experience of the operator, the less the need for multiple needle insertions. One investigator [3] noted that his loss rate dropped by 50% after he had more than 200 cases under his belt.

Based on a paper that emerged in 1992 [4], a question arose regarding a link between CVS and transverse limb defects. However, it was clear later that the problem had to do with how early the procedure was performed, and data from a large registry involving over 200,000 patients showed an incidence of transverse limb reduction defects, when the procedure was performed after 9 weeks, to be about 6 per 10,000, which is the prevalence of this abnormality in the overall population [5].

Amniocentesis

The labeling of a woman of 35 years of age as being AMA stemmed from the concept that her age-related risk for Down syndrome was approximately the same as the risk of amniocentesis (1 in 270). Actually, the risk figure that is most commonly used is 1 in 200. Although this figure was derived many years ago, most contemporary data seem to validate this estimate. Nevertheless, many feel that this figure is too high.

The only randomized trial [6] in the literature comes from Denmark in which half of 4606 patients were randomized, after a normal ultrasound examination, to have an amniocentesis. The fetal loss rate up until 24 weeks of gestation in the amniocentesis group was 1.7% and in the control group was 0.7%, giving a procedure-related risk of 1%. The results were surprising, but the study has stood up to heavy scrutiny because the numbers were reasonable,

Obstetric Ultrasound: Artistry in Practice. John C. Hobbins. Published 2008 Blackwell Publishing. ISBN 978-1-4051-5815-2.

the operators were very experienced, and the procedures were all performed under ultrasound direction.

To evaluate the procedure-related loss rate from contemporary mid-trimester amniocentesis, Seeds [7] analyzed data from 29 studies, each including more than 1000 patients having mid-trimester amniocentesis. Although these were not randomized studies, five studies included control data. In the controlled studies the procedure-related loss rate appeared to be 0.6%. In the entire sample of 33,795 patients having amniocentesis, the raw loss rate was 2.1% and the procedure-related risk was calculated to be 0.7%.

Note: just before this manuscript was submitted to the publishers, a report emerged from the authors of the First and Second Trimester Evaluation of Risk (FASTER) trial suggesting a very low risk of amniocentesis (6 per 10,000) in 3096 patients having this procedure, compared with over 25,000 patients who did not (loss rate of 1% vs 0.94%). Interestingly, in another similar contemporary screening study involving 47,000 patients (SURUSS study) [8] the procedure-related risk of amniocentesis was reported to be 1% (1.8% vs 0.79% not having amniocentesis).

Since the FASTER trial data are completely out of sync with everything else in the literature, we will continue to quote the risk figure of amniocentesis of 1 in 200 (with the caveat that it may be less in some centers). If other information surfaces that validates the FASTER data, we will adjust our counseling appropriately. However, it could change the risk/benefit paradigm appreciably.

First trimester nuchal translucency investigation

In 1992, Nicolaides [9], a tireless investigator and major force in the field, reported that an enlarged fetal nuchal translucency (NT) was frequently noted to be associated with fetal chromosome abnormalities. This measurement was made behind the fetal neck and represented a diameter that was measured from the inner margin of the membrane to the inner margin of the underlying tissue (Figure 13.1a–13.1c) In a later prospective study [10] involving 96,127 patients, he and his group used a risk calculation that involved the patient's age, the crown–rump length of the fetus, and the size of the NT itself. The detection rate for trisomy 21 was 77% at a screen positive rate of 5%. This exceeded the sensitivity of other diagnostic tests for fetal aneuploidy.

The first study from the United States resulted in data that conflicted with the above results. However, virtually every other prospective study surfacing after the large prospective Nicolaides study, including the North American Maternal Serum Biochemistry and Fetal Nuchal Translucency Screening (BUN) [11] and the FASTER [12] trials, validated the original data. For example, the BUN

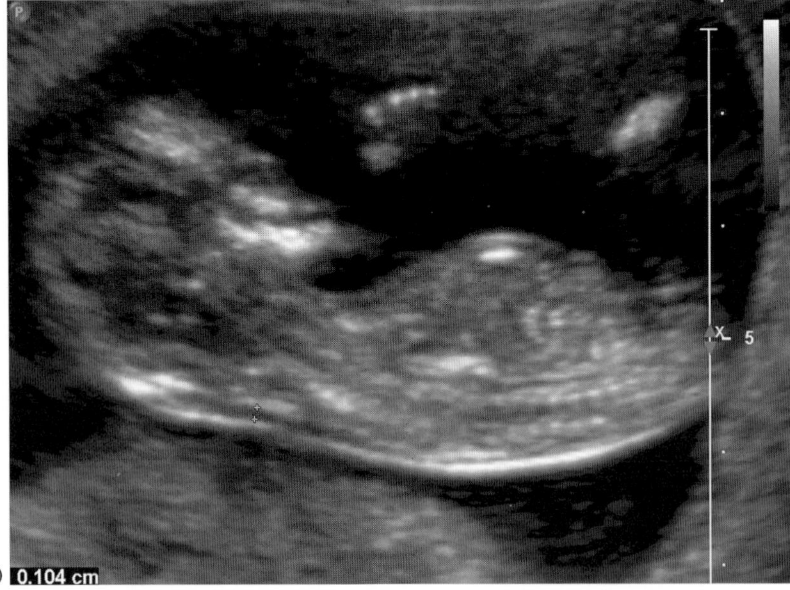

(a)

Fig 13.1 (a) Normal nuchal translucency (NT).

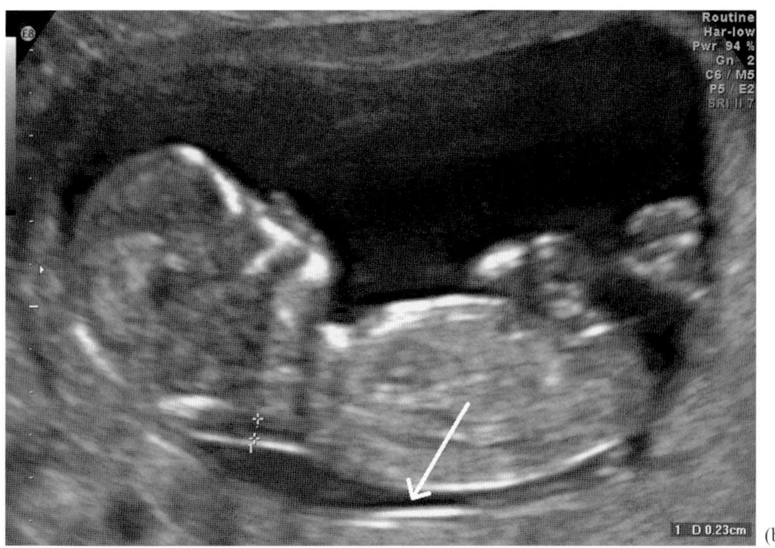

(b)

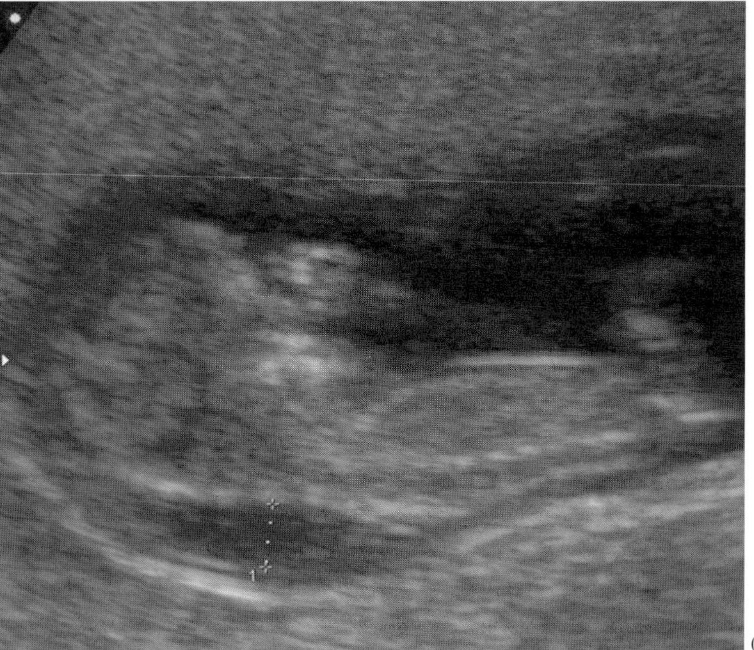

(c)

Fig 13.1 (continued) (b) Slightly enlarged NT and questionable nasal bone. Arrow points to amnion. (c) Very abnormal NT.

trial, involving 8514 patients had a sensitivity for NT alone of 69% at a 5% screen-positive rate, and the FASTER trial involving 35,000 patients had a similar detection rate. The effect of first trimester biochemistry in these two studies will be discussed below. However, despite the fact that NT alone has been shown to be a very reasonable way to screen for chromosome abnormalities in the first trimester, it is clear from quality-control studies that a carefully standardized method must be used by properly trained and experienced operators for optimal performance. The eight requirements are outlined in Table 13.1.

Two placental hormones, pregnancy-associated plasma protein-A (PAPP-A) and the beta subunit of human chorionic gonadotropin (beta hCG) have been found to be

Table 13.1 Fetal Medicine Foundation criteria for obtaining NT measurements.

- Fetal head, neck and upper thorax should occupy 75% of image area
- Fetus in mid-sagittal plan
- Measure at widest space
- Use only "+" calipers
- Calipers border black space
- Try to measure when perpendicular
- Head neither flexed nor extended
- Away from amnion

useful adjunctively in screening protocols involving NT. The former analyte is generally depressed and the latter analyte is usually elevated in Down syndrome (average of 0.39 and 1.83 MoM, respectively). Based on the data from the above studies, if used without NT, the sensitivity is about 62% at a 5% screen positive rate and, if used with NT, the sensitivity rises to 82% at a 5% screen positive rate.

This would mean that one could more than halve a patient's risk for Down syndrome with NT alone and derive a first trimester numerical risk that would be less than a patient's age-related risk in the majority of cases. Also, most commonly, one could take this risk well below the risk of invasive sampling, either by CVS or amniocentesis.

Second trimester biochemistry

For many years, the common method for screening patients for aneuploidy was a triple screen. This consisted of maternal serum alpha-fetoprotein (MSAFP), hCG, and estriol, which has a sensitivity (according to BUN data) of 67% at a 5% screen-positive rate. Recently, another placental product, inhibin-A, has been added to the mix to make the test a "quad" screen. According to the FASTER trial data, this combination yields a sensitivity of 83% at a 5% screen positive rate.

The fetal nasal bone

Cicero [13] first published a study in which she and her colleagues explored the possibility that first trimester fetuses with Down syndrome might have small nasal bones, an observation Langdon Down made in infants in 1866. The group found that 73% of first trimester fetuses with this condition had absent nasal bones, compared with only 0.5% in the normal fetal population (Figures 13.2a and 13.2b). With expanded data the sensitivity leveled off at 67% [14]. When added to NT and first trimester biochemistry (the "combined test"), the sensitivity for Down syndrome rose to 97% at a screen positive rate of 5%.

Although the FASTER trial data did not show a similar correlation with the nasal bone, all other studies in the literature have.

Two new markers that put into play color and pulse wave Doppler involve flow through the tricuspid valve and the ductus venosus. Falcon et al. [15] have found that 74% of Down syndrome fetuses will have tricuspid regurgitation, compared with 7% of chromosomally normal fetuses. In our experience, it is common for second trimester fetuses to have a small amount of tricuspid regurgitation. However, the above studies were done predominantly in the first trimester and the authors required that the regurgitant jet have a velocity of at least 60 cm/s before being considered positive.

Back in 1996, Matias [16] reported on a strong association between the finding of absent or reverse flow in the ductus venosus during atrial contraction and Down syndrome. They found that 91% of Down syndrome fetuses had this in the first trimester, compared with 3% of normal controls. Although others have not found this strong an association, there is no doubt that this can be a useful marker for Down syndrome as well as for cardiac anomalies.

Nicolaides has conceptualized a type of contingency screening program that would involve NT as a first line test and assessment of tricuspid regurgitation, ductus venosus, and nasal bone (which require more experience) as a second-tier endeavor in those with an abnormal NT.

The efficiency of various first and second trimester diagnostic combinations

In this small section, I will attempt to sort out the various diagnostic options available to the AMA patient or any pregnant patient for that matter. The confusion stems from the disparate designs of the studies to date and the inconsistent labeling of the various diagnostic packages, which seem to read out like a Chinese restaurant menu—one from column A, one from column B, etc.

First, a ground rule: when dealing with the efficacy of the test, instead of the words "false positive," I will use the term "screen positive." To many, false-positive means that the test says the fetus has something he/she does not

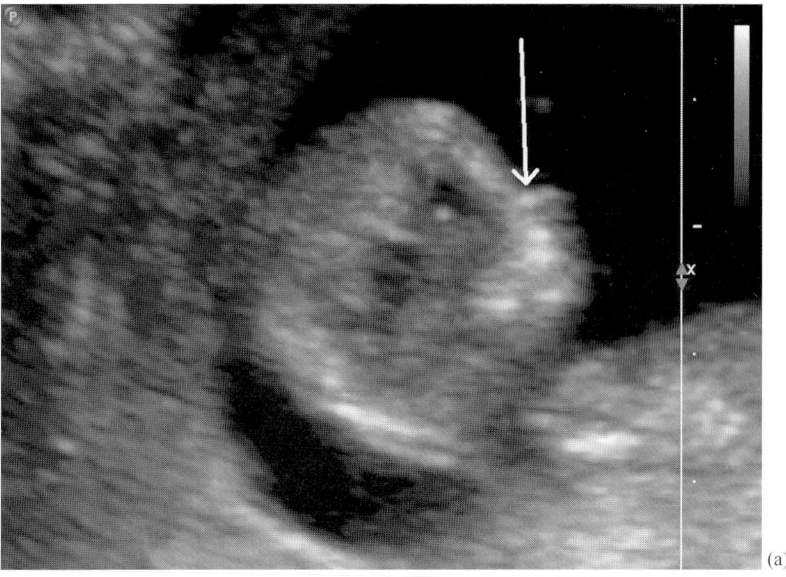

(a)

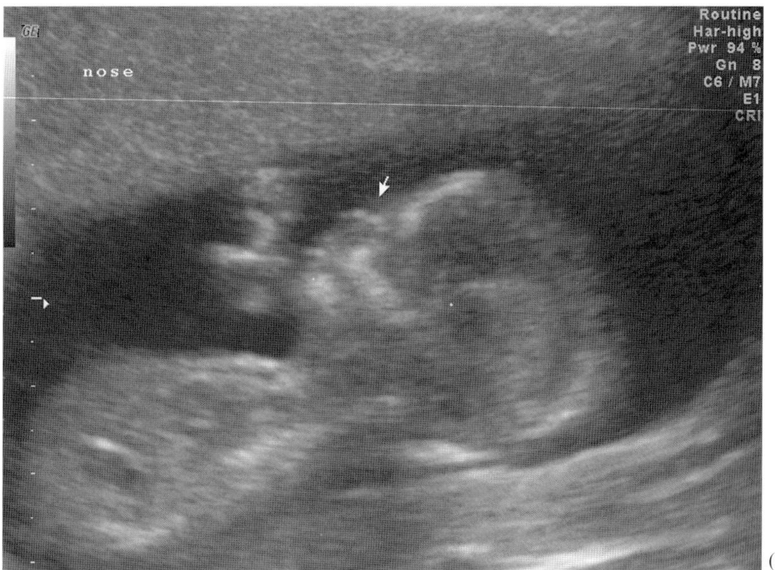

(b)

Fig 13.2 (a) Normal nasal bone. (b) The arrow points to skin interface, not bone.

really have. A screening test is not a diagnostic test, and "screen positive" simply means that the risk of something is elevated.

This may seem like an obvious distinction, but we have had many patients decline to have the above screening tests because "it is wrong most of the time" and, sadly, this phrase often came from their providers.

Here are the options as of this writing. For the sake of comparison, I am using a risk of Down syndrome of 1 in 270 and, with one exception; we'll deal with a screen positive rate of 5%.

1 *First trimester NT (based on CRL and maternal age).* This yields a sensitivity of 83% at a 5% screen positive rate (Nicolaides).

2 *"Combined" test.* This combination folds in first trimester biochemistry (HCG and PAPP-A) with NT, CRL, and maternal age. This has a sensitivity of 82% at a screen positive rate of 5% (Malone and D'Alton).
3 *"Sequential" test.* Here, the patient has the above combined test and is apprized of this first trimester result. Then later she has a quad screen as a separate diagnostic test. The drawbacks are that two answers are confusing and, although the sensitivity is excellent (96%), the screen positive rate is too high (14%), because the patient's age is used twice as a pretest (posterior) risk. This was the protocol used in the BUN study.
4 *"Integrated" test.* This test amalgamates the combined test results with the second trimester biochemistry, which results in only one answer being given to the patient after all the data are in. This was the design of the FASTER trial. The downside is that the first trimester results are withheld from the patient—something that initially was ethical to do in the FASTER trial, but may be questionable now that the study results have been published. As indicated above, the sensitivity of this approach is 96% at a 5% screen positive rate.
5 *"Stepwise" program.* This is the method that I feel has the greatest staying power, but, as yet, it does not have a commonly accepted name. Many of those that have begun to employ this method have used the label "Contingency Screen," with the idea that if the first trimester result is below a certain cut-off point, there would be little reason to pursue second trimester testing. On the other hand, if the risk is above a certain threshold, then the chance that second trimester testing would lower the risk below that of invasive testing is negligible. Of course, this would have cost saving implications. The results from the combined test are given to the patient, but the first trimester screen positive rate is not set at 5%, but at, let's say, 1.5% (which is about the risk of CVS). Then the second trimester biochemistry is added to the algorithm, which is set to have a total screen positive rate of 5% (1.5% plus 3.5%). This gives an excellent sensitivity while allowing the patient access to the first trimester results, followed by the "final answer" in the second trimester. The sensitivity of this approach is 95% at a total screen positive rate of 5% (modeling from FASTER trial data).

The algorithm given in Figure 13.3 is for screening for fetal chromosomal abnormalities.

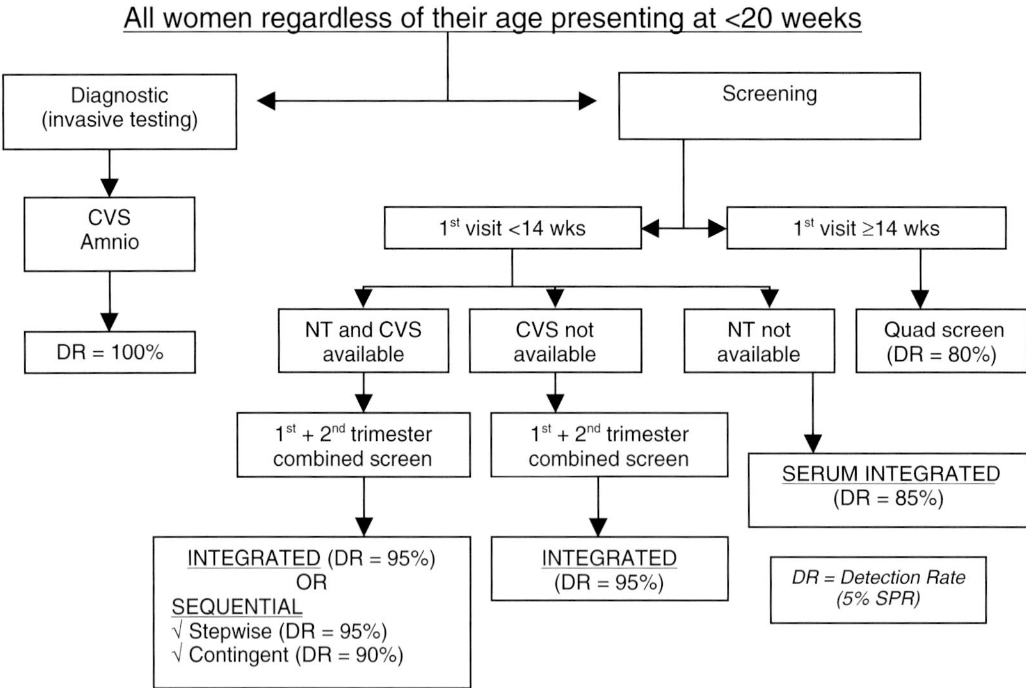

Fig 13.3 All women regardless of their age presenting at <20 weeks. (Adapted from Vintzileos AM [18], with permission from Lippincott Williams and Wilkins.)

Although ultrasound plays only one role in this comprehensive screening process, I have included discussion of the above methods because the ultrasound measurement of NT comprises an extremely important facet of these methods and everyone participating in NT screening needs to be aware of the nuances in the interpretation of the data. Most importantly, with an excellent sensitivity, patients can now be apprized of their individual risk for trisomy 21 and trisomy 18 so that they can make well-informed decisions as to whether or not to have further testing.

Follow-up of euploid fetuses with increased NT

If invasive testing proves the fetus with a large NT to have normal chromosomes, he/she is not quite out of the woods. A recent review by Souka [17], involving her data and those from other groups, has put the risk of anomalies in these patients into proper perspective. If the NT is between the 95th and the 99th percentile, the chance of an abnormal karyotype is 3.7%, and the risk of a major fetal anomaly is 2.5%. On the other hand, the chances of these fetuses being alive and well are still over 93%. These results can be contrasted with those from fetuses with very large NTs of greater than 6.5 mm, where the risk of major anomaly rises to greater than 50% and the chances of being alive and well after birth are only 15%. We have found Souka's table (Table 13.2) to be very useful in counseling patients according to the size of the NT.

The most common anomalies related to increased NTs are diaphragmatic hernia, exomphalos, body stalk abnormality, skeletal defects, and various anomaly syndromes such as fetal akinesia, Noonan syndrome, Smith–Lemli–Opitz syndrome, and spinal muscular atrophy. Most of these affected fetuses have a cardiac abnormality. This should clue the investigator into where he/she should first start the diagnostic workup in these patients.

The anomalies least often associated with an increased NT are neural tube defects, renal abnormalities, holoprosencephaly, and gastroschisis.

The genetic sonogram

The genetic sonogram has emerged as another noninvasive way to further drop a patient's risk of having a fetus with Down syndrome, which can work adjunctively with all of the other methods mentioned thus far. It is a "souped up" second trimester ultrasound examination containing three components: standard biometry with the humerus added, a basic fetal anatomy survey, and a search for markers for Down syndrome. About 20% of fetuses with Down syndrome will have femur and/or humerus lengths that are 2 weeks less than dates, and about 20% of fetuses with this condition will have a major congenital abnormality, which, if present, generally involves the fetal cranium, heart, or renal system. The ultrasound signs of duodenal atresia, which occurs in about 12% of infants with Down syndrome, may not appear until the end of the second trimester.

Unfortunately, there is no standard procedure one follows when exploring "soft markers" for Down syndrome, although there is certainly information in the literature as to which are the best performers.

Nuchal skinfold thickness

In 1985, Benacerraf, a major contributor in prenatal diagnosis, noted that about 40% of fetuses with Down syndrome had a nuchal skinfold thickness (NSFT) that was 6 mm or greater [19]. As opposed to the NT measurement

Table 13.2 Relationship between NT thickness and prevalence of chromosomal defects, miscarriage, or fetal death and major fetal abnormalities.

Nuchal translucency	Chromosomal defects (%)	Fetal death (%)	Major fetal abnormalities (%)	Alive and well (%)
<95th percentile	0.2	1.3	1.6	97%
95–99th percentile	3.7	1.3	2.5	93%
3.5–4.4 mm	21.1	2.7	10.0	70%
4.5–5.4 mm	33.3	3.4	18.5	50%
5.5–6.4 mm	50.5	10.1	24.2	30%
>6.5 mm	64.5	19.0	46.2	15%

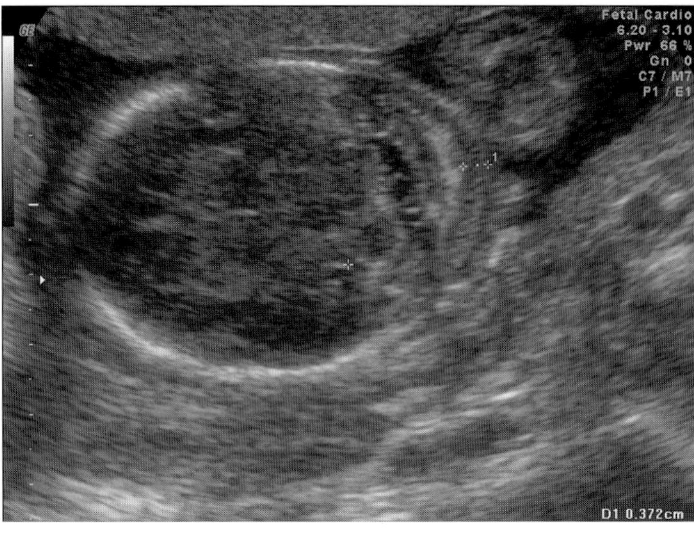

Fig 13.4 Nuchal skinfold thickness—normal.

in the first trimester, which is accomplished in the midsagittal plane, the NSFT is made from an angled cross-sectional view through the posterior fossa. Interestingly, there is little in the literature regarding standardization of this measurement, as there is for NT in the first trimester. This is surprising, since it is quite easy to overshoot on the measurement by freezing on a tangential image that is almost coronal in orientation, incorporating much of the inferior cerebellar vermis. Also, while the calipers should be placed precisely on the edge of the calvarium in the midline and the outer edge of the scalp, the former landmark is often shadowed by the calvarium itself. The apparent indentation (caused by an artifact) can cause the operator to overestimate the distance between the two calipers. This can be corrected by moving the transducer slightly off angle, thereby avoiding shadowing of the skull and at the same time exploiting the axial resolution of the transducer (Figure 13.4).

The reason to obsess over this measurement is that it is, by far, the best performer of all markers. Although Benacerraf initially reported a threshold diameter of 6 mm or more, in an eight-center study [20] we have shown that if one uses 5 mm between 16 and 18 weeks, and 6 mm between 18 and 20 weeks, the sensitivity rose by about 5% with little effect on the screen positive rate. A "positive" finding can increase a patient's risk for Down syndrome by 17-fold.

A variation on the nuchal thickening concept that is connected with a very high risk for aneuploidy in the first and second trimesters is the cystic hygroma (Figures 13.5 and 13.6). In the first trimester many chromosome abnormalities can be possibilities, while in the second trimester the greater proportion of these fetuses will have Turner syndrome. There is some controversy regarding whether a very large NT alone (Figure 13.1c) should be considered a cystic hygroma. Nevertheless, either one generally spells bad news for the fetus and parents.

The heart

At term, about 30% of infants with Down syndrome will have a cardiac defect, but it is clear that a higher percentage will have an interventricular septal defect in the second trimester, which will close over as pregnancy progresses. Also, many fetuses will have functional changes that should cue the wary observer to perform a marker search for Down syndrome. For example, in Down syndrome, even in the first trimester, there is right heart predominance, perhaps secondary to aortic narrowing, which can later be appreciated by a slight inequity in ventricular size, a deviation of the interatrial septum to the left (Figure 13.7), a slight outer ballooning of the atrium, and/or tricuspid regurgitation. By searching with color Doppler for these changes, DeVore [21] has improved the sensitivity of his genetic sonogram to well above 90%.

Echogenic intracardiac focus (EIF)

Bromley and Benacerraf [22] also were the first to report a relationship between echogenic foci in the fetal heart

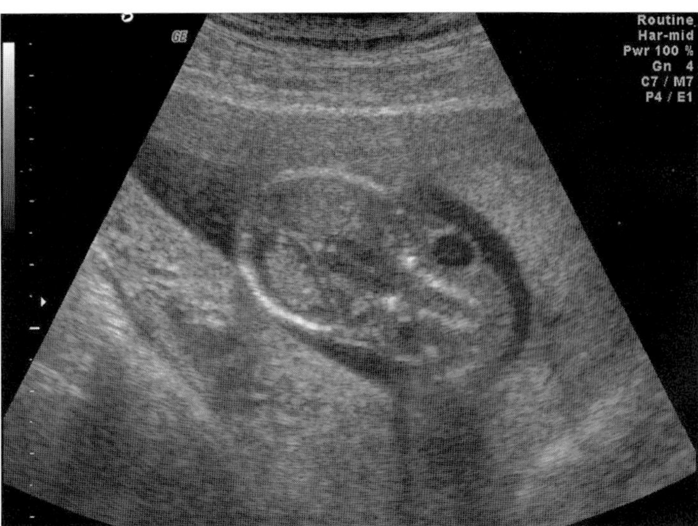

Fig 13.5 Smaller cystic hygromas in first trimester fetus.

and Down syndrome. Later studies have suggested that 15–26% of fetuses with Down syndrome will exhibit this finding, and a few studies have shown a somewhat increased likelihood for Down syndrome even if the finding is in isolation. However, other studies have not. An EIF is created by calcification of a papillary muscle within the ventricle (Figure 13.7), and its appearance is dependent upon the frequency of the transducer and the angle of insonation. Its presence even varies according to the population examined (one study shows a 15% incidence in Asian fetuses). Therefore, the whole EIF story has been difficult to interpret.

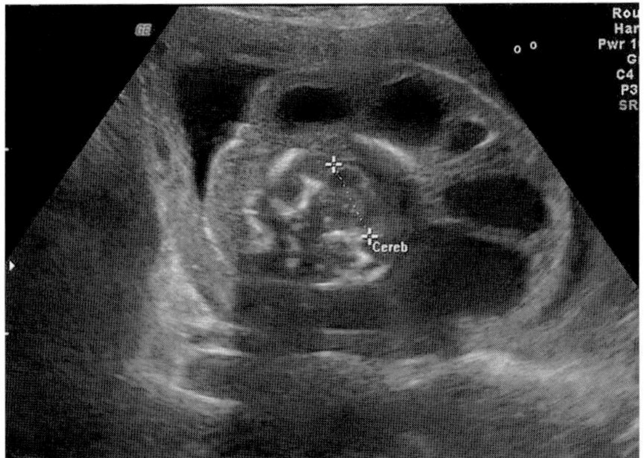

Fig 13.6 Large cystic hygromas in second trimester fetus with hydrops.

The most important question that arises pertains to its diagnostic impact, if it is isolated. Most single studies do not have the statistical clout to answer the question, and even meta-analyses are difficult to interpret because one wonders how diligently the investigators looked for other markers for Down syndrome; especially if the studies were conducted at a time when "isolated" simply meant there were no *obvious* fetal abnormalities. Also, many of the studies were done predominantly in patients having amniocenteses, where there was less incentive to do a thorough marker screen.

That said, one meta-analysis [23] involving 51,831 patients found a low sensitivity for EIF of 26%, in general, and 22%, if isolated. However, this caused the authors to state that the risk was increased fivefold for any patient with this finding.

Few studies have addressed the very patient who generates the greatest angst—a low-risk patient with an isolated EIF. Anderson et al. [24] followed 9167 women of age 34 or less. One hundred ninety three had in EIF and in 149 of these patients it was isolated. None of these patients had a fetus with Down syndrome.

As with every prenatal diagnostic method there are hawks and doves. The raw likelihood ratio from the above meta-analysis, without the necessary statistical embellishment, might give fuel to the hawks, who advocate "amniocentesis for all," and the low-risk study would favor the concept of not using an isolated EIF to adjust the risk for Down syndrome. To emphasize the need for sober thought on this subject, Caughey et al. [25] calculated that in those

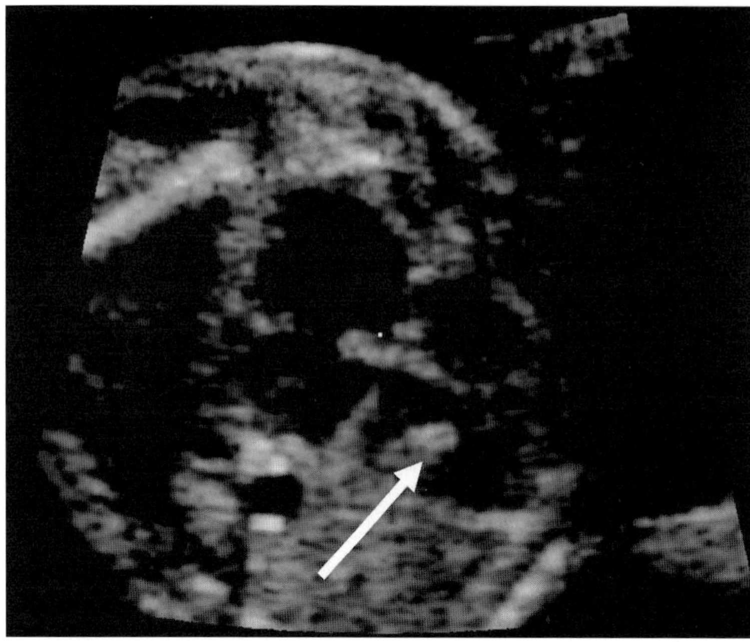

Fig 13.7 Echogenic focus in the left ventricle and levorotation in fetus with trisomy 21.

at low risk, 118,146 amniocenteses would be performed per year for an isolated EIF, and 244 fetuses would be lost, yielding 2.4 losses of normal fetuses for every Down syndrome fetus identified.

First, we will not label a little spot in the heart as being an EIF unless the intensity of the echogenicity is at least the same as adjacent bone. Second, we make very sure that the finding is isolated by performing a very thorough search for other markers or anomalies. If it is truly isolated, I neither raise nor lower a patient's risk for Down syndrome from her preultrasound risk. On the other hand, if this finding is clustered with another ultrasound marker(s), her risk for Down syndrome rises appreciably. Also, if the patient's prescan risk is high, then the finding of an EIF is hard to ignore.

Nasal bone

In the first trimester one simply decides whether or not a fetal nasal bone is visible. However, Bromley et al. [26] fine-tuned the concept in the second trimester. This group noted that if the nasal bone could be divided into the BPD measurement by 10 or more, 81% of Down syndrome fetuses would be screened in, with, unfortunately, a screen positive rate of 11%.

Other markers

The literature is replete with single studies with small numbers touting the benefit of various markers. In an attempt at thoroughness, I will list some of these below as second-tier markers:

1 *Frontal lobe length* [27] (Figure 13.8). This is measured from the back of the cavum to the front of the calvarium in the plane of the BPD (the diameter in millimeters is roughly the same as weeks of gestation up until 22 weeks; after this time the measurement is the same as the TCD). This measurement is usually smaller than expected in Down syndrome.

2 *Fetal ear length* [28] (Figure 13.9). The coronal measurement generally is less than 1 cm between 16 and 18 weeks in Down syndrome.

3 *Middle bone of the fifth digit* (Figure 13.10) [29]. This is sometimes absent in Down syndrome.

4 *Echogenic bowel* [30]. Mentioned in another chapter, this is one of the better markers for Down syndrome, especially since it has a low prevalence in the normal population.

5 *Iliac angle* [31]. Based on the observation of a higher rate of hip dysplasia in Down syndrome infants, a positive finding would constitute an iliac angle of greater than 90° (Figure 13.11). I have found this to be a very difficult

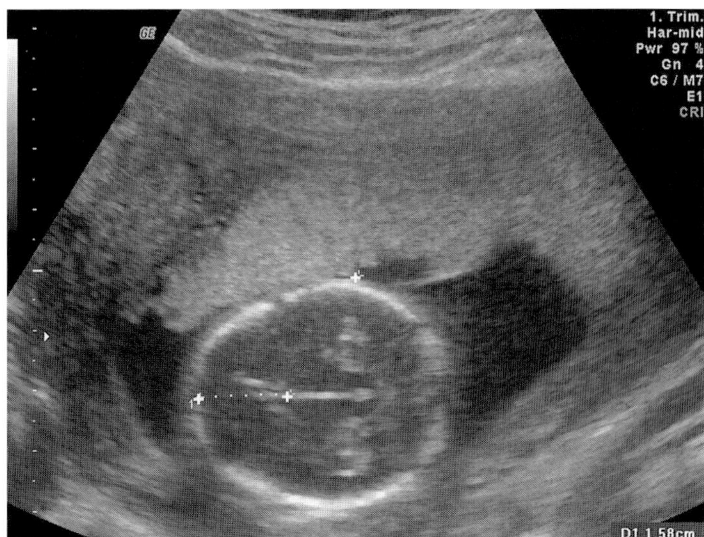

Fig 13.8 Indirect frontal lobe measurement at 15 weeks.

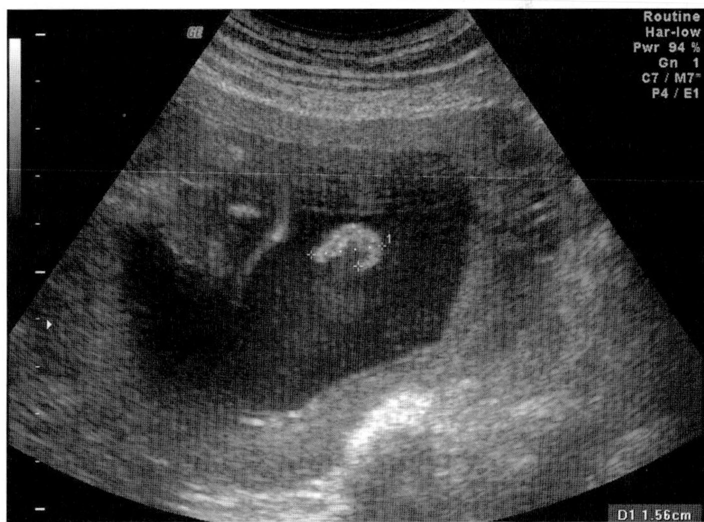

Fig 13.9 Ear 2D.

marker to standardize, because it is dependent upon fetal position and the height at which the cross-section is taken.

6 *Sandal gap*. Forget it.

7 *Bilateral pyelectasis* [32]. Although examination of the fetal kidneys is part of the basic fetal survey, I will include this as part of a marker search for Down syndrome. Up to 4.5% of fetuses will have enlarged renal pelves, defined as an A/P diameter of 4 mm or more before the twentieth week of gestation. In our eight-center study [20], we found that 20% of fetuses with Down syndrome had modest pyelectasis. However, a question confronting clinicians, seemingly every day, is what to do about the finding if it is isolated? Even older data [33], generated when "isolated" might not have had the same meaning as it would today, suggest that the risk is less than 1 in 300 if other signs of Down syndrome are excluded. Another factor to be considered is the "a priori" risk according to maternal age or postscreening results. Someone at age 40 with pyelectasis will generate more concern than a 25-year-old or one with a quad screen risk of 1 in 2000. Data from single studies, and even pooled data, are difficult to interpret because of the small numbers of affected fetuses in the studies. For example, in a recent study by Coco and Jeanty [34] a seemingly formidable number of patients

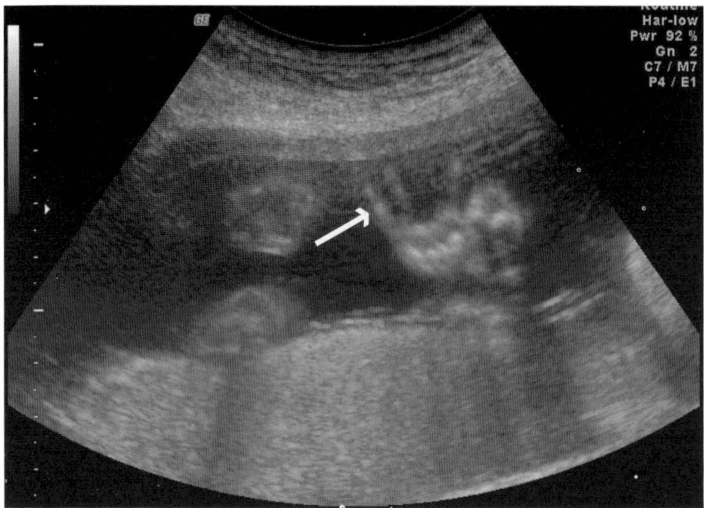

Fig 13.10 Arrow marks middle phalanx of fifth digit.

(12,672) were evaluated for ultrasound markers for Down syndrome in the second trimester. Three hundred sixty-six (2.9%) had renal pelves of equal to or greater than 4 mm. Eleven fetuses had Down syndrome and only one had isolated pyelectasis. The likelihood ratio for Down syndrome was 3.79, but the 95% confidence levels were 0.5–24.6, rendering that result meaningless. The authors concluded that isolated pyelectasis was not a good enough reason to recommend amniocentesis. Again, when pyelectasis is found in isolation, we neither drop nor elevate a patient's risk for Down syndrome from her preultrasound number.

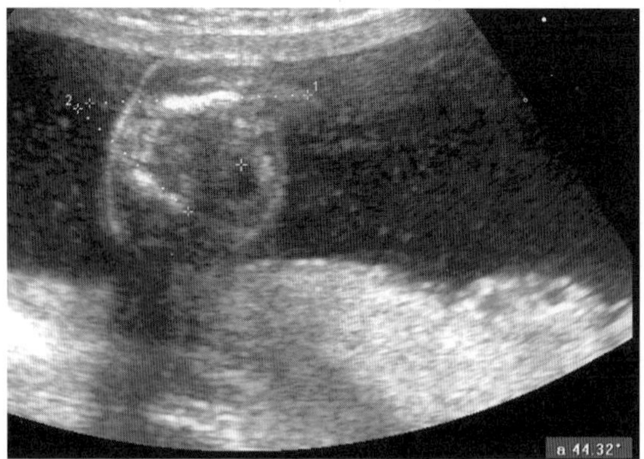

Fig 13.11 Iliac angle.

How to use the information provided by the genetic sonogram

The beauty of the genetic sonogram is that, if negative, it allows the clinician to diminish a given patient's risk by at least 50%. Some centers have enough experience to calculate their own sensitivities with regard to their screening performance. In our eight-center study [20] involving programs with substantial experience with genetic sonograms, the sensitivities among centers varied from 63.6 to 80%, with an average of about 72%.

Once sensitivity is ascertained, then a negative likelihood ratio can be calculated for each center by the formula 1− sensitivity/false positive rate. Then, using Bayes theorem, an adjusted risk can be estimated for a specific patient. For example, a woman of 36, having a prescan risk for Down syndrome of 1 in 220, will have a postscan risk of 1 in 660 after having a negative genetic sonogram in a center generating a negative likelihood ratio of 0.3 ($220 \times 0.3 = 660$). Theoretically, this calculation is legitimate for all patients, no matter whether their prescan risk comes from age alone or from any other testing method.

Many busy centers whose sonographers/sonologists have substantial experience with genetic sonograms may not have the wherewithal to gather outcome data on every patient passing through their program. Therefore, under these circumstances, a precise detection rate cannot be calculated for these centers. However, those not having their own sensitivity figure should be able to drop a given patient's risk by at least 50% by employing a conservative cushion (using average sensitivity figures from similar centers) to their calculations.

FASTER trial data have shown that, in a cohort of over 8000 patients having a genetic sonogram [35], the 3 fetuses with Down syndrome not screened in by the integrated test were picked up by the genetic sonogram. This brought the sensitivity of noninvasive testing in that group up to 100%.

The goal of all noninvasive testing is to avoid the need for unnecessary invasive procedures by creating a mismatch between risk for Down syndrome and risk of fetal loss from amniocentesis. Using 1974 to 1997 US figures and a procedure-related risk of 1 in 200, Egan [36] postulated that if every patient over 34 years of age having a reassuring biochemical screen were to forgo amniocentesis, 1971 normal fetuses would be saved per year from procedure-related loss. The same benefit could be attributed to the genetic sonogram.

That said, it is extremely important to honor our patient's wishes, and some may choose to have 100% assurance through amniocentesis. However, every patient needs to be fully informed regarding her options and the risks and benefits of each. Unfortunately, some patients are still being referred specifically for amniocentesis, armed only with a strong recommendation from their providers that they have one.

Trisomy 18

This devastating chromosome abnormality is more common in AMA patients. It is a condition that generally should not slip through unnoticed in any patient having first trimester screening, second trimester biochemistry, and a second trimester basic sonogram. Data from the BUN study [11] have shown that screening all patients with a first trimester "combined" method resulted in 91% sensitivity for trisomy 18 at a 2% screen positive rate. In those over 35 years of age there was 100% sensitivity at a 2.6% screen positive rate.

Using second trimester biochemistry alone many laboratories have been quoting 65% sensitivity for trisomy 18. However, for some strange reason the cut-off has been set at 1 in 100, which translates into a 0.5% screen positive rate. If the threshold were raised to 5%, the sensitivity would well exceed 90%.

Most importantly, this ultimately lethal abnormality is always associated with at least one fetal abnormality that can be identified on the standard ultrasound examination. Table 13.3 describes the abnormalities or markers commonly associated with trisomy 18.

Table 13.3 Ultrasound markers for trisomy 18.

- Choroid plexus cysts (40%)
- Cerebellar hypoplasia
- Large cisterna magna
- Strawberry-shaped calvarium
- Micrognathia
- Small ears
- Cardiac defects (~90%)
- Early intrauterine growth restriction with polyhydramnios
- Single umbilical artery
- Echogenic bowel
- Clubbed hands and feet
- Overlapping fingers
- Rocker bottom feet

The biggest problem with trisomy 18 screening is not missing one (which is difficult to do), but dealing with a patient's angst created by the finding of an isolated ultrasound marker or a second trimester biochemistry result that returns as "screen positive."

Choroid plexus cysts

Although the prevalence of choroid plexus cysts (CPCs) has been stated to be about 1% [37], this seems to be a major underestimation (Figure 13.12). However, because they have been found in up to 30% of fetuses with trisomy 18, they strike fear in the hearts of everyone whose fetus has them. Earlier studies suggested that occasionally CPCs could be "isolated" in this condition, but later studies have indicated that this is unlikely, if one clearly were to scrutinize thoroughly the fetus for signs of trisomy 18. Yeo et al. [38] have noted that fetuses with trisomy 18 have a minimum of four and a median of eight abnormalities on ultrasound evaluation. In 96% of these cases, clenched hands were noted, in 84% had cardiac abnormalities diagnosed in the second trimester.

When biochemistry is suggestive of trisomy 18, the hormone levels tend to be very low, especially the estriol, the latter also being associated with Smith–Lemli–Opitz syndrome and placental sulfatase deficiency. Nevertheless, if the search for all of the trisomy 18 markers and abnormalities noted in the table comes back clean, the chances of a fetus with CPCs or a positive biochemistry of having trisomy18 are close to zero, and certainly far less than the risk of amniocentesis.

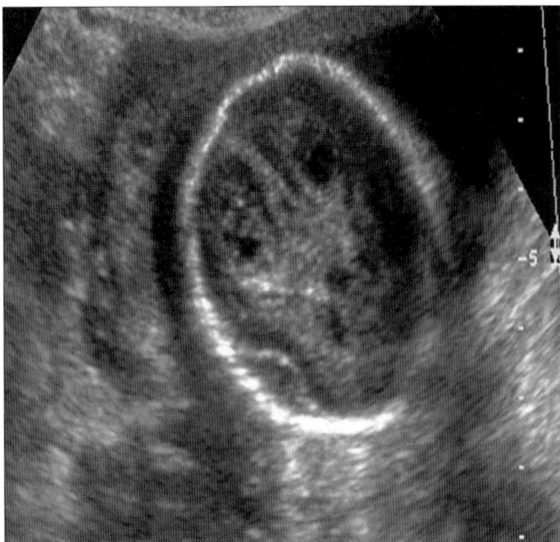

Fig 13.12 Choroid plexus cysts.

One last word about CPCs: some earlier reports have suggested a possible relationship between this finding and trisomy 21. Bromley et al. [39] did not find such an association, and the FASTER trial results further confirm the lack of a relationship between CPCs and trisomy 21.

References

1 National Center for Health Statistics. *Vital statistics of the United States, Natality, 1974–1993.* Hyattsville, MD: National Center for Health Statistics; 1977–1996.

2 Courtesy of Wapner RJ, Drexel University, Philadelphia, PA, USA.

3 Saura R, Gauthier B, Taine L, et al. Operator experience and fetal loss rate in transabdominal CVS. Prenat Diagn 1994; 14: 70–1.

4 Burton BK, Schulz CJ, Burd LI. Limb anomalies associated with chorionic villus sampling. Obstet Gynecol 1992; 79: 726–30.

5 Froster UG, Jackson L. Limb defects and chorionic villus sampling: results from an international registry. Lancet 1996; 347: 489–94.

6 Tabor A, Madesen M, Obel E, et al. Randomized controlled trial of genetic amniocentesis in 4606 low-risk women. Lancet 1986; 1: 1287–93.

7 Seeds JW. Diagnostic mid-trimester amniocentesis: how safe? Am J Obstet Gynecol 2004; 191: 608–16.

8 Wald NJ, Rodeck C, Hackshaw AR, et al. First and second trimester antenatal screening for Down's syndrome: the results in the Serum, Urine and Ultrasound Screening Study (SURUSS). Health Technol Assess 2003; 7: 1–77.

9 Nicolaides KH, Azar G, Byrne D, et al. Fetal nuchal translucency: ultrasound screening for chromosomal defects in first trimester of pregnancy. Br Med J 1992; 304: 867–9.

10 Snijders RJ, Nobel P, Sebire N, et al. UK multicentre project on assessment of risk of trisomy 21 by maternal age and fetal nuchal-translucency thickness at 10–14 weeks of gestation. Fetal Medicine Foundation First Trimester Screening Group. Lancet 1998; 352: 343–6.

11 Wapner R, Thom E, Simpson JL, et al. (for the First Trimester Maternal Serum Biochemistry and Fetal Nuchal Translucency Screening (BUN) Study Group). First-trimester screening for trisomies 21 and 18. N Engl J Med 2003; 349: 1405–13.

12 Malone FD, Wald NJ, Canick JA, et al. (for the First and Second Trimester Evaluation of Risk (FASTER Trial)). First- and Second-Trimester Evaluation of Risk (FASTER) trial: principal results of the NICHD multicenter Down syndrome screening study. Am J Obstet Gynecol 2003; 189: S56.

13 Cicero S, Curcio P, Papageorghiou A, et al. Absence of nasal bone in fetuses with trisomy 21 at 11–14 weeks of gestation: an observational study. Lancet 2001; 358: 1665–7.

14 Cicero S, Longo D, Rembouskos G, et al. Absent nasal bone at 11–14 weeks of gestation and chromosomal defects. Ultrasound Obstet Gynecol 2003; 22: 31–5.

15 Falcon O, Auer M, Gerovassili, et al. Screening for trisomy 21 by fetal tricuspid regurgitation, nuchal translucency and maternal serum free β-hCG and PAPP-A at 11 + 0 to 13 + 6 weeks. Ultrasound Obstet Gynecol 2006; 27: 151–5.

16 Matias A, Gomes C, Flack N, et al. Screening for chromosomal abnormalities at 10–14 weeks: the role of ductus venosus blood flow. Ultrasound Obstet Gynecol 1998; 12: 380–4.

17 Souka AP, Krampl E, Bakalis S, et al. Outcome of pregnancy in chromosomally normal fetuses with increased nuchal translucency in the first trimester. Ultrasound Obstet Gynecol 2001; 18: 9–17.

18 Vintzileos AM. Screening for fetal chromosomal abnormalities, No 77. ACOG Practice Bulletin 2007; 109: 217–27.

19 Benacerraf BR, Barss VA, Laboda LA. A sonographic sign for the detection in the second trimester of the fetus with Down's syndrome. Am J Obstet Gynecol 1985; 151: 1078–9.

20 Hobbins JC, Lezotte DC, Persutte WH, et al. An 8-center study to evaluate the utility of midterm genetic sonograms among high-risk pregnancies. J Ultrasound Med 2003; 22: 33–8.

21 DeVore GR. The role of fetal echocardiography in genetic sonography. Semin Perinatol 2003; 27: 160–72.

22 Bromley B, Lieberman E, Laboda L, et al. Echogenic intracardiac focus: a sonographic sign for fetal Down syndrome. Obstet Gynecol 1995; 86: 998–1001.

23 Sotiriadis A, Makrydimas G, Ioannidis JP. Diagnostic performance of intracardiac echogenic foci for Down syndrome: a meta-analysis. Obstet Gynecol 2003; 101: 1009–16.

24 Anderson N, Jyoti R. Relationship of isolated fetal intracardiac echogenic focus to trisomy 21 at the mid-trimester sonogram

in women younger than 35 years. Ultrasound Obstet Gynecol 2003; 21: 354–8.

25 Caughey AB, Lyell DJ, Filly RA, et al. The impact of the use of the isolated echogenic intracardiac focus as a screen for Down syndrome in women under the age of 35 years. Am J Obstet Gynecol 2001; 185: 1021–7.

26 Bromley B, Lieberman E, Shipp TD, et al. Fetal nose bone length: a marker for Down syndrome in the second trimester. J Ultrasound Med 2002; 21: 1387–94.

27 Persutte WH, Coury A, Hobbins JC. Correlation of fetal frontal lobe and transcerebellar diameter measurements: the utility of a new prenatal sonographic technique. Ultrasound Obstet Gynecol 1997; 10: 94–7.

28 Chitkara U, Lee L, Oehlert JW, et al. Fetal ear length measurement: a useful predictor of aneuploidy? Ultrasound Obstet Gynecol 2002; 19: 131–5.

29 Benacerraf BR, Sathanondh R, Frigoletto FD. Sonographic demonstration of hypoplasia of the middle phalanx of the first digit: a finding associated with Down syndrome. Am J Obstet Gynecol 1988; 159: 181–3.

30 Egan JFX. The genetic sonogram in second trimester Down syndrome screening. Clin Obstet Gynecol 2003; 46: 897–908.

31 Shipp TD, Bromley B, Lieberman E, et al. The iliac angle as a sonographic marker for Down syndrome in second-trimester fetuses. Obstet Gynecol 1997; 89: 446–50.

32 Benacerraf BR, Mandell J, Estroff JA, et al. Fetal pyelectasis: a possible association with Down syndrome. Obstet Gynecol 1990; 76: 58–60.

33 Corteville JE, Dicke JM, Crane JP. Fetal pyelectasis and Down syndrome: is genetic amniocentesis warranted? Obstet Gynecol 1992; 79: 770–2.

34 Coco C, Jeanty P, Jeanty C. An isolated echogenic heart focus is not an indication for amniocentesis in 12,672 unselected patients. J Ultrasound Med 2004; 23: 489–96.

35 Malone F, Nyberg DA, Vidaver J, et al. (for the FASTER Research Consortium). First And Second Trimester Evaluation of Risk (FASTER) trial: the role of second trimester genetic sonography. [abstract] Am J Obstet Gynecol 2004; 191: S3.

36 Egan JF, Benn P, Borgida AF, et al. Efficacy of screening for fetal Down syndrome n the United States, from 1974 to 1997. Obstet Gynecol 2000; 96: 979–85.

37 DeMasio K, Canterino J, Ananth C, et al. Isolated choroid plexus cyst in low-risk women less than 35 years old. Am J Obstet Gynecol 2003; 187: 1246–9.

38 Yeo L, Guzman ER, Ananth CV, et al. Prenatal detection of fetal trisomy 18 through abnormal sonographic features. J Ultrasound Med 2003; 22: 581–90.

39 Bromley B, Lieberman E, Benacerraf B. Choroid plexus cysts: not associated with Down syndrome. Ultrasound Obstet Gynecol 1996; 8: 232–5.

14 Diabetes

Pregestational diabetes complicates about 0.3–0.7% of all pregnancies. Gestational diabetes simply means that a patient's glucose intolerance has been diagnosed once pregnancy has started and 2% of all pregnant patients fall into this category. These individuals can further be divided into A1 diabetics, whose fasting glucoses are normal, and A2s, whose fasting values are not.

Fetuses and infants of diabetics can get into trouble in three ways, and the magnitude of the problems generally is proportional to the degree to which blood glucoses are out of control.

Fortunately, it is rare for fetuses to die today of maternal diabetes, as enhanced fetal surveillance employed in most pregnancies will prevent this. However, perinatal morbidity often is inevitable in poorly controlled diabetes.

Congenital anomalies occur in 10–16% of pregestational diabetic pregnancies, compared with about 2–3% in nondiabetics, and this is related to maternal glucose levels during organogenesis, which, in turn, are indirectly reflected in the glycosylated hemoglobin (HbA1c) levels. For example, if these levels are above 8.5 mg%, the anomaly rate is over 20%. Although one study [1] showed a rate of anomalies that was no different than the overall population if HbA1c levels are below 6, others have not. One large study [2] involving 145,196 deliveries in Dallas indicated that if gestational diabetics had normal fasting blood glucoses (A1s), their rate of congenital anomalies was 1.2% (essentially the same as that of the nondiabetics in the study of 1.5%). In those with elevated fasting glucoses (A2s), representing 10% of gestational diabetics, the prevalence for anomalies was 4.8%, and in pregestational diabetics the rate was 6.1%.

The point is that, while gestational diabetics maintaining normal glycemia were not at greater risk for fetal anomalies, those with abnormal fasting glucoses were at almost the same risk for anomalies as pregestational diabetics, probably because they really were pregestational diabetics waiting to be diagnosed.

The two fetal organ systems that are hit the hardest are the heart and the CNS. Cardiac anomalies complicate, on average, 27 per 1000 pregnancies versus 8 per 1000 in nondiabetics. Also, the rate of neural tube defects in diabetics is about 20 per 1000 versus 1 per 1000 in the overall population. Although the numbers are not as dramatic as the incidence of heart and spine anomalies, fetuses of diabetics are also at slightly greater risk for gastrointestinal and genital urinary abnormalities. The best-known anomaly to which diabetes is linked is caudal regression syndrome. This occurs in about 1 in 200 diabetic pregnancies and can involve many or only a few spinal segments.

Diabetes should be all about prevention of anomalies through strict diabetic control during organogenesis, and early detection of anomalies through staged ultrasound investigation is essential in the management of diabetes.

Cardiac anomalies

Hyett [3] noted that 40% of fetuses with cardiac defects had nuchal translucency (NT) measurements (covered in the segment on advanced maternal age) that were above the 95th percentile, and the larger the NT, the greater the chance of a cardiac anomaly. Therefore, diabetics should benefit from NT screening between 10/6 and 13/6 menstrual weeks. If NT is normal, this should drop the risk of cardiac anomalies by half, to about 1.5%, and if glucose control is reasonable by normal HbA1c and fasting glucose levels, the next logical ultrasound step would be a detailed second trimester examination. If the NT is large, then a transvaginal evaluation of the fetal heart can be attempted on the spot, and if the fetal heart is not easily accessible, this should be given another try at 14–16 weeks.

Obstetric Ultrasound: Artistry in Practice. John C. Hobbins. Published 2008 Blackwell Publishing. ISBN 978-1-4051-5815-2.

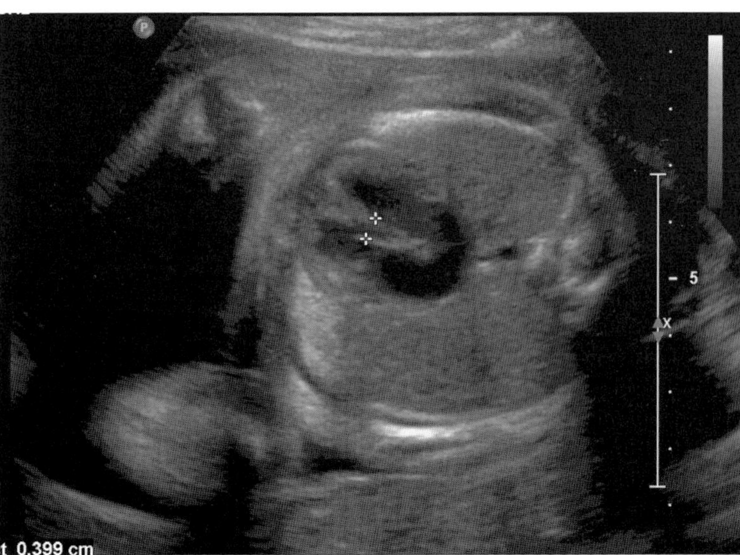

Fig 14.1 Measurement of IVS thickness.

Every diabetic should have a detailed anatomy survey after 16 weeks. Unfortunately, diabetes and obesity go hand in hand and, therefore, if the transabdominal route is chosen, then the later, the better (greater than 17 weeks) for the fetal survey, and a fetal echocardiogram would best be scheduled after 20 weeks.

One last examination of the fetal heart can be undertaken after 34 weeks to look for cardiac hypertrophy. In fetal hyperglycemia, glycogen can be overdeposited in the fetal cardiac muscle and liver, and growth of the fetal organs, in general, will be stimulated by the abundance of insulin being produced by the overworked fetal pancreas. This can result in some degree of cardiomyopathy in about 30% of fetuses/infants. If the problem is compounded by microvascular disease in the placenta, thus creating an increased after load, the resulting hypertrophic cardiomyopathy can on rare occasions become a very serious problem. This may have been the mechanism responsible for the many "unexplained" fetal deaths of yesteryear in diabetes.

Cardiac hypertrophy can be suspected if the interventricular septum, midway up the elongated triangle, measures more than 5 mm at any time in gestation (Figure 14.1). If it does, then with M-mode one can measure the thickness of the ventricular walls and, most importantly, can appreciate the size of the ventricular cavities. Hypertrophic subaortic stenosis can result from an overly thickened septum, and can be appreciated with M-mode or new 4D ultrasound techniques.

CNS anomalies

In the late first trimester anencephaly can be easily ruled out. Every diabetic should also have screening with MSAFP since mothers of 85% of fetuses with spina bifida will have elevations of this fetal protein. Nevertheless, the court of last resort is a detailed ultrasound evaluation of the fetal spine, since virtually 100% of open defects can be diagnosed by at least the eighteenth week of gestation, and most before the seventeenth week.

Macrosomia

The second major potential problem for fetuses of diabetics is macrosomia, which can result in birth injury and, indirectly, hypoglycemia in the newborn. About 20% of gestational diabetics and 25% of insulin-requiring diabetics deliver large-for-gestational-age (LGA) infants [4] and they run a threefold higher risk of having shoulder dystocia and, with it, the occasional brachial plexus injury. Although macrosomia results from accelerated fetal growth in later pregnancy, there is a recent study from Italy [5] to indicate that even the strictest of maternal glucose control did not prevent 17% of fetuses of pregestational diabetics from being LGA. In fact, the writing seemed to be on the wall at 20 weeks of gestation when the abdominal circumferences were already well above the mean for gestation in fetuses destined to be LGA at birth.

The take-home message is that if the abdominal circumference (AC) is within normal limits at the 18-week ultrasound examination, this does not completely preclude the fetus to be an LGA baby later, but the chances diminish appreciably. On the other hand, if the AC is large, tight glucose control may not be enough to prevent fetal macrosomia.

What is the best way to diagnose an LGA fetus in diabetes?

In the section on intrauterine growth restriction (IUGR), a pitch was made for using the AC alone because it incorporates the liver and subcutaneous fat in one swoop. Standard formulas for EFW tend to overestimate weight in large babies, but formulas fashioned specifically for large babies have added little to the predictive accuracy. One study showed that femur and AC performed as well in diabetes as more complicated formulas. While looking for the best formula to diagnose macrosomia at 37–41 weeks, Mongelli and Benzie [6] found that 5 of the 18 formulas tested would never yield a weight of above 4500 g, and 3 formulas yielded a 15% false positive rate for 4500 g.

As indicated in the segment on 3D, measurements of the fetal thigh and upper arm, by themselves, or folded in with other fetal measurements, do improve the accuracy of EFW, but are somewhat cumbersome to use.

Abramowicz [7] has reported on a clever concept based on the observation that corpulent fetuses have fat cheeks. He found that the cheek-to-cheek diameter correlated well with macrosomia and shoulder dystocia; especially if the measurement exceeded 7.9 cm. The measurement is made from a coronal slice through the face incorporating both cheeks. We have found this image to be difficult to capture in late pregnancy for a variety of reasons, but a coronal image can always be obtained to include one cheek in the same plane as the nasal width. By putting one caliper on a midpoint between the nostrils and the other on the outer margin of the cheek, half the cheek-to-cheek distance can be determined, and then multiplied by two (Figure 14.2).

Shoulder dystocia: can it be predicted?

Some statistics regarding shoulder dystocia should get our attention. It is obvious that the chances of shoulder dystocia are greater in macrosomia fetuses. Add diabetes to the mix and the risk escalates even more. In fact, fetuses of diabetics carry a three- to sevenfold greater chance of shoulder dystocia at every weight category. This is due to the predilection for body-to-head disproportion in this condition. Fetuses of diabetics tend to have the same-size heads as other fetuses, but under the influence of insulin, which is a growth stimulator, preferential treatment is given to the fetal chest, abdomen, and shoulder girth (versus the head). The conduct of labor is determined more by the size of the fetal head, which comes through first, and less upon what comes through the pelvis afterward, and, not surprisingly, the large shoulders occasionally get stuck, depending upon the size of the maternal pelvis.

Body-to-head disproportion can be assessed in a variety of ways. The often used HC/AC ratio represents a very indirect reflection of the relationship of the fetal head to shoulders, and variations of this method have been published. Elliott [8] was the first to describe a relationship between the abdomen and head as a way to predict shoulder dystocia. This was later refined by Cohen et al. [9] who compared the average abdominal diameter (AAD), taken at the standard plane for AC, with the biparietal diameter (BPD). If the AAD exceeded the BPD by more than 2.5 cm, the risk of shoulder dystocia was 33%. If this figure was less than 2.5, the risk of shoulder dystocia was zero.

Winn et al. [10] evaluated in utero many biometric variables in comparison with the bisacromial diameters of the neonate. The chest circumference correlated better with the size of the infant's shoulders than any other in utero biometric variable, with the exception of the fetal clavicle length, which correlated very well with the bisacromial diameter. Unfortunately, this bone is often difficult to image in late pregnancy. However, with 3D planar reconstruction this measurement could have promise.

Conway and Langer [11] have made a case for delivering the macrosomic fetus of a diabetic (greater than 4000 g) by elective cesarean section in order to obviate the possibility of birth trauma. I agree that at a time when more than 1 out of 4 women in the United States are delivered by cesarean section, we obviously have performed these operations for far less compelling reasons than avoiding birth injury. However, I think we can be far more selective in diabetics by assessing fetal body-to-head disproportion, estimating the size of the maternal pelvis, employing a 3D estimation of the EFW, and reviewing the past obstetrical history (previous successful vaginal deliveries of big babies), before automatically resorting to this type of invasive operation; especially when the decision often is based purely on standard 2D EFW formulas. Table 14.1 represents a diagnostic plan for diabetic management involving ultrasound.

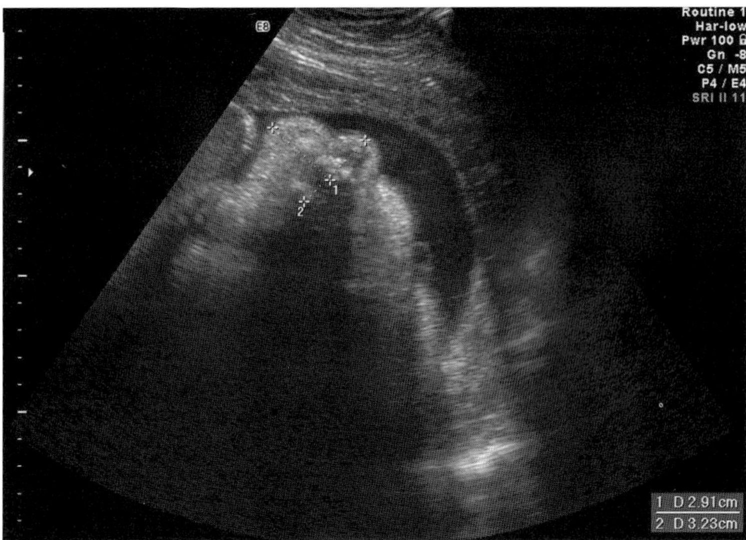

Fig 14.2 Cheek-to-cheek method in nonmacrosomic fetus. One doubles the hemidistance.

Table 14.1 Ultrasound diagnostic menu for diabetes.

Timing of ultrasound	Task and rationale
First trimester	
Early to 6–9 weeks	Date pregnancy and establish viability
10–13 weeks	Crown–rump length to confirm dates and assess size
Second trimester	
16–18 weeks	Anomaly scan with particular attention to posterior fossa, spine, heart, and limbs
20–24 weeks	Fetal echocardiogram; look for early macrosomia
Third trimester	
34–36 weeks	Fetal size and watch for body-to-head disproportion

A case in point

A 34-year-old woman in her first pregnancy was referred at 34 weeks because her uterus seemed large for dates. Her mother was a diabetic but she was not tested for glucose intolerance until 30 weeks, at which time she had a 1-hour glucose screen of 160 mg%. A full glucose tolerance test was positive, and her fasting sugar was 105 mg%. She was put on a standard diabetic diet, but she missed her next appointment.

Her fundal height was 38 cm when she showed up for her next visit at 36 weeks. The biometry was as follows: the BPD and HC were appropriate for 36 weeks, the AC at 38 weeks, and the long bones were compatible with 35 weeks. The EFW was 3700 g, well above the 90th percentile. The largest vertical pocket was 8 cm. Although no anomalies were noted, the interventricular septum measured 6.7 cm.

We chalked up the macrosomia, body-to-head disproportion, thick septum (and even ample cheeks) to her glucose intolerance, which existed from early on.

At 38 weeks, she went into labor. On admission the EFW was 3900 g, the (AAD)-BPD was 3.0 cm, and cheek-to-cheek diameter was 8.7 cm. She made sluggish progress in the active stage of labor, and we sectioned her rather than tempt fate later.

The baby weighed 4400 g, had some transient tachypnea, and some brief hypoglycemia in the nursery.

Comment

The last EFW was off by 500 g, which is not atypical in macrosomia. The body-to-head disproportion in a fetus, seemingly weighing 3900 g, was not enough to push toward a cesarian section on admission, but this was certainly concerning enough to interdict an instrument delivery had she progressed to full dilatation.

(Continued)

Why not perform a cesarean section empirically in a diabetic whose fetus weight was thought to be close to 4000 g? The controversy regarding elective cesarean section for large babies with or without diabetes will continue as long as there is no concrete evidence that either delivery route is superior. At the moment, I feel each case should be treated separately according to all of the available information. As indicated above, shoulder dystocia occurs most frequently when the head is not overly large, but the fetal trunk is; thus setting up potential disaster for a large baby passing through a small pelvis.

Multiparameter ultrasound examinations can certainly forewarn the clinician of trouble on the horizon.

References

1 Miller E, Hare JW, Cloherty JP, et al. Elevated maternal hemoglobin A1c in early pregnancy and major congenital anomalies and infants of diabetic mothers. N Engl J Med 1981; 304: 1331–4.

2 Sheffield JS, Butler-Koster EL, Casey BM, et al. Maternal diabetes mellitus and infant malformations. Obstet Gynecol 2002; 100: 925–30.

3 Hyett JA. Increased nuchal translucency in fetuses with a normal karyotype. Prenat Diagn 2002; 22: 864–8.

4 Gabbe SG, Mestman JH, Freeman RK, et al. Management and outcome of class A diabetes mellitus. Am J Obstet Gynecol 1977; 127: 465–9.

5 Greco P, Vimercati A, Scioscia M, et al. Timing of fetal growth acceleration in women with insulin-dependent diabetes. Fetal Diagn Ther 2003; 18: 437–41.

6 Mongelli M, Benzie R. Ultrasound diagnosis of fetal macrosomia: a comparison of weight prediction models using computer simulation. Ultrasound Obstet Gynecol 2005; 26: 500–3.

7 Abramowicz JS, Rana S, Abramowicz S. Fetal check-to-cheek diameter in the prediction of mode of delivery. Am J Obstet Gynecol 2005; 182: 1205–11.

8 Elliott JP, Garite TJ, Freeman RK, et al. Ultrasonic prediction of fetal macrosomia in diabetic patients. Obstet Gynecol 1982; 60: 159–62.

9 Cohen B, Penning S, Major C, et al. Sonographic prediction of shoulder dystocia in infants of diabetic mothers. Obstet Gynecol 1996; 88: 10–3.

10 Winn HN, Holcomb W, Shumway JB, et al. The neonatal bisacromial diameter: a prenatal sonographic evaluation. J Perinat Med 1997; 25: 484–7.

11 Conway DL, Langer O. Elective delivery of infants with macrosomia in diabetic women: reduce shoulder dystocia versus increased cesarean deliveries. Am J Obstet Gynecol 1998; 178: 922–5.

15 Preeclampsia

Preeclampsia complicates about 1 in 11 pregnancies, and it can represent a major threat to mother and fetus when it emerges. It is clear that the predisposition for this condition is in place even in the first trimester, many weeks before the clinical triad (hypertension, edema, and proteinuria) of preeclampsia appears. Today, it is uncommon for patients to progress into eclampsia, manifested by seizures, simply because today's emphasis on early detection and early delivery (the only cure) has averted this dreaded complication. However, preeclampsia, by itself, can result in substantial maternal and perinatal morbidity (maternal hemorrhage, IUGR, and prematurity).

As indicated in the section on the placenta, the current theory, backed by placental biopsy investigation, is that the trophoblast normally invades the decidual portion of the spiral arteries beginning by week 8, and this invasion is usually complete by the thirteenth week. After this time the second stage of spiral artery invasion kicks in, whereby the myometrial portion of the spiral arteries are similarly invaded by the trophoblast. This process is usually complete by 18–19 weeks, but occasionally the process is delayed until the twenty-second to twenty-fourth week in "late bloomers." In the overwhelming majority of preeclamptics this transformation does not occur in the spiral artery bed, and, from early on, there is increased resistance to flow into the intervillous space. Unfortunately, this can have a negative domino effect on the development of the fetal side of the placenta, which depends upon a free flow of oxygen-rich maternal blood into the intervillous space.

The method of choice to indirectly monitor the status of the spiral artery bed is to tap upstream information provided by uterine artery waveforms. When trophoblastic invasion has occurred, the end diastolic flow increases. If it has not, the end diastolic flow never rises and a diastolic notch is often present.

Although we have obtained waveforms from the uterine arteries transvaginally in the first trimester, the most common approach is to image transabdominally the iliac vessels in their longest axis alongside the uterus, and to search for the uterine artery as it crosses the external iliac artery. It should be sampled just below or just above the iliac artery (Figure 15.1), because the further away one is from this vessel, the greater the chance of straying into a cervical branch, which obviously will not reflect the resistance in the placental bed. Over 80% of the time both uterine artery waveforms are accessible, but, occasionally, either because the artery takes an aberrant course or is running at right angles to the plane of insonation, the signal is difficult to obtain. The trick is to approach the expected pathway of the uterine artery at an acute angle, and this should yield a waveform that is of suitable amplitude to measure (Figures 15.2a and 15.2b).

In general, the S/D ratio should not exceed 2.5, or the RI should not be above 55 in the second trimester.

Campbell, a pioneer and consistent leading light in obstetric sonography, was the first to explore the potential of uterine artery waveforms in predicting preeclampsia. Initially, he and his colleagues used a handheld continuous wave Doppler device to find the characteristic waveform at about 18 weeks. Although his initial results were encouraging with regard to its predictive ability for preeclampsia, others initially could not repeat his results. However, it became clear that the continuous wave Doppler did not allow an ability to pinpoint the sampling site (as with pulse wave Doppler), and, most importantly, a good 25% of patients who initially have abnormal Doppler's at 18 weeks do convert over to a normal waveform by 24 weeks. These late converters do not have the same predilection for preeclampsia as those whose waveforms remain abnormal at 24 weeks.

Ever since the method emerged there have been reams of data generated from many investigators, some of which have shown the method to be a reasonable predictor of preeclampsia, while others have not. These confusing results stemmed from inconsistency regarding when to test, the lack of a standard definition of "abnormal" (PI, RI,

Obstetric Ultrasound: Artistry in Practice. John C. Hobbins. Published 2008 Blackwell Publishing. ISBN 978-1-4051-5815-2.

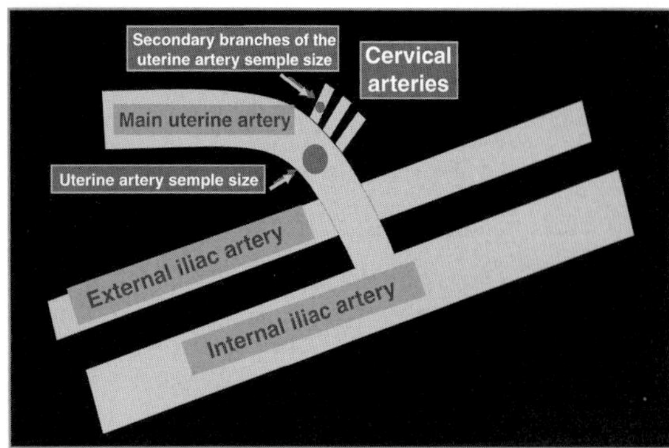

Fig 15.1 Sampling site for uterine artery waveform. Also one can sample just below external iliac artery.

or S/D ratio; bilateral or unilateral; the subjective nature of a notch, etc.), and the difficulty in making the clinical diagnosis of preeclampsia.

The largest difficulties in interpretation came from the high second trimester screen positive rate in unselected populations in whom there was a low prevalence of true preeclampsia. In a subgroup of low-risk patients enrolled in the FASTER trial, we found the incidence of true preeclampsia to be far lower than expected. This plays havoc with the positive predictive value, which in many studies was between 20 and 30%. On the other hand, in a high-risk population, the predictive accuracy of uterine artery waveform for preeclampsia and IUGR is between 60 and 95%.

I am inclined to look at the bright side of uterine artery investigation, and will start by citing an observation published in 1993. Bower and Campbell [1] screened an unselected group of patients (2058) with uterine artery Doppler evaluations at 18–20 weeks, and again at 24 weeks. Every woman delivering at less than 34 weeks because of preeclampsia had abnormal Dopplers at both stages of testing. Perhaps this is the most important point on which to focus because of its implications regarding the severity of the maternal disease and of its neonatal impact (IUGR, fetal distress, and prematurity). This relationship has been confirmed by the majority of other authors.

Also, it is now clear that abnormal spiral artery remodeling is associated with other pregnancy complications such as thrombophilia, chronic hypertension, and placentally mediated IUGR. For example, Donohoe [2] found a direct relationship between abnormal uterine artery waveform and the presence of anticardiolipins, and Frusca [3] noticed that the incidence of IUGR was 54% in chronic hypertensives with abnormal uterine arteries compared with an incidence of IUGR of 2% in hypertensives with normal uterine arteries. Last, Ferrazzi et al. [4] found that 93% of IUGR placentas from normotensive mothers had the same ischemic changes in the maternal vascular bed as those seen in 97% of IUGR placentas from hypertensive mothers. All of the above studies imply that, in addition to preeclampsia, the pathway to IUGR leads through the spiral arteries.

I particularly like a scoring system reported by Sekizuka et al. [5], which allows us to predict the chances of collective adverse outcome with second trimester uterine artery Dopplers. In a small study involving high-risk patients the authors awarded a point for a notch and a point for low end diastolic flow in each waveform. A score of 4 would indicate bilateral notches and high S/D ratios. There were 89 cases with adverse pregnancy outcome and those with scores of 1 and 2 had adverse outcome rates that were roughly similar to those with a score of 0, which was about 9%. However, this rate rose to 48% in those with a score of 3 and to 83% with a score of 4. Data from our institution also suggest little increased risk of adverse outcome in patients with scores of 0–2, but a huge jump in risk for scores of 3 and 4.

What is appealing is the ability to drop the risk of trouble to come for patients who, for example, had HELLP syndrome in a previous pregnancy or another recurring problem, to that of a low-risk patient.

One of the criticisms of uterine artery "screening," even in high-risk patients, is our inability to change the course of preeclampsia, despite our having been forewarned of it by abnormal uterine artery Dopplers. As indicated below, since there is now evidence that low-dose aspirin, initiated in the second trimester, seems to diminish the incidence of severe preeclampsia, there has been a push to move uterine artery Doppler investigation into the first trimester; a time when aspirin might have greater effect.

The uterine artery can be imaged transabdominally in the first trimester by either attempting to line up the iliacs longitudinally, or to use a cross-sectional tomogram at the level of the internal cervical os. It can also be assessed transvaginally.

The problem with early screening at 11–13 weeks is that many patients will be somewhat tardy in accomplishing their first phase of trophoblastic invasion, resulting in a 32–57% screen positive rate, according to some studies. However, a recent study by Nicolaides et al. [6] suggests that if uterine artery Dopplers are used selectively in conjunction with a new biochemical predictor of preeclampsia, plasma protein 13 (PP13), which is involved in spiral artery remodeling, the sensitivity for severe preeclampsia would be 90% at a 10% screen positive

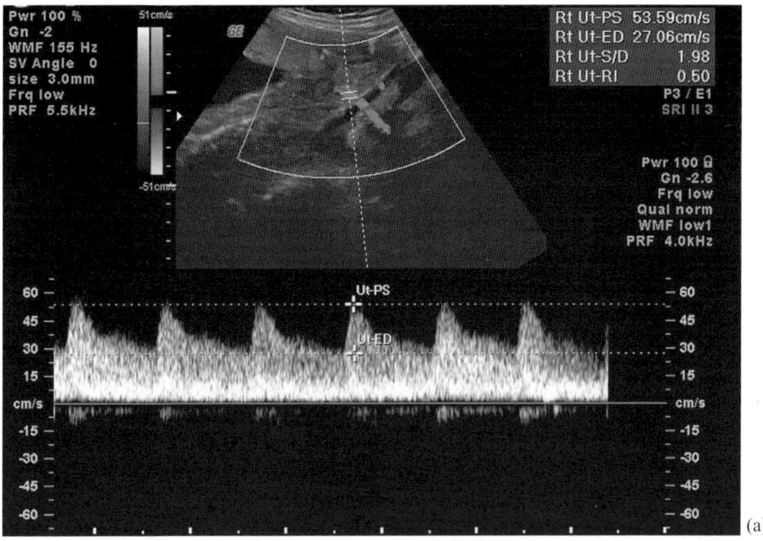

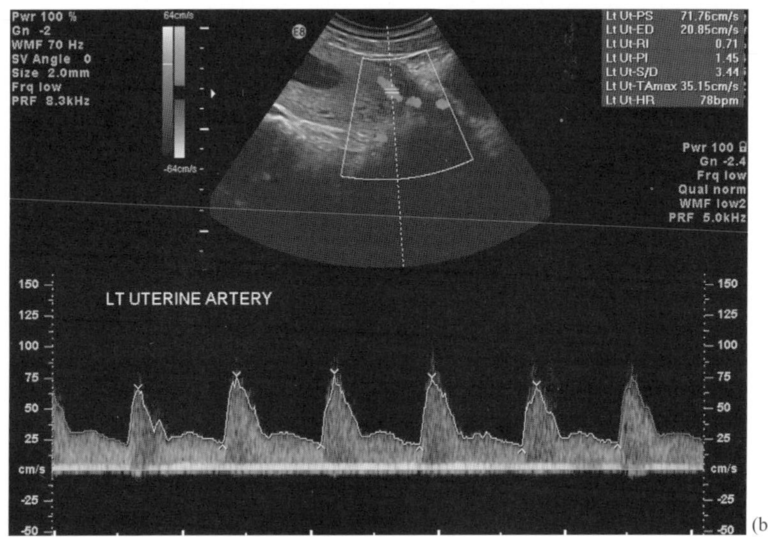

Fig 15.2 (a) Normal uterine artery waveform. (b) Mildly abnormal uterine artery.

rate. The concept would be to employ a contingency approach by doing Dopplers only in the 14% with low PP13 values between 11 and 13 weeks.

Regarding the prevention of preeclampsia, at first glance the results in the literature might seem to be conflicting. For example, an NIH sponsored study [7] involving high-risk patients did not bear out the efficacy of low-dose aspirin in preventing preeclampsia. However, a meta-analysis by Coomarasamy [8], involving 14 studies and a total of 12,416 patients, showed that giving aspirin resulted in a statistically significant drop in perinatal death (OR = 0.79), preeclampsia (OR = 0.86) and preterm birth (OR = 0.86), and an increase in infant weight of 215 g. These studies did not incorporate uterine artery waveforms in the mix. However, this had been done earlier by the same author in 2001 [9] in which he pooled data from five second trimester randomized clinical trials involving low-dose aspirin versus placebos in patients with abnormal uterine artery waveforms. A benefit was demonstrated by a decrease in severe preeclampsia (OR = 0.55).

Very recently, two small randomized trials have surfaced in which aspirin was started in the first trimester. Both studies have suggested the benefit of low-dose aspirin in decreasing the incidence of preeclampsia.

After sifting through the literature, here is my take on the utility of uterine artery investigation:

1 There is a very high screen positive rate in the first trimester.

2 It may be more useful when used selectively, and in conjunction with other first trimester predictors of preeclampsia such as PP13 and beta hCG.

3 Those patients who convert to a normal waveform by 18 weeks (after having abnormal waveforms in the first trimester) probably have the same chance of adverse outcome as those who started out with normal waveforms.

4 Although it is clear that "late bloomers" who wait to convert to normal by 24 weeks will have better outcomes than those who do not, they still may have a higher rate of IUGR than the background rate.

5 Uterine artery Dopplers are less useful in predicting preeclampsia, in general, than their ability to predict severe preeclampsia requiring delivery at less than 34 weeks.

6 There is evidence that low-dose aspirin can decrease adverse pregnancy outcome, and now there is a suspicion that beginning aspirin prophylaxis in the first trimester might afford even greater benefit in those with faulty spiral artery remodeling.

Thrombophilias

These inherited factors usually surface when patients with a history of pregnancy loss or venous thrombosis are worked up for a recurrent cause. It seems that every year a new factor emerges to worry us. However, patients who are heterozygous for one of these factors still run an excellent chance of an uneventful pregnancy despite their occasionally requiring anticoagulation. I am inserting this small section into this chapter on preeclampsia simply because patients possessing one of these thrombophilic factors are often referred to ultrasound laboratories for this reason alone. Hopefully, this will help to avoid being blindsided.

Pregnancy, being a hypercoagulable state, predisposes patients with any of the thrombophilic factors, collectively representing 15% of the population, to thromboembolism and a fivefold increase in stillbirth, abruption, IUGR, and preeclampsia. However, some are more potent troublemakers than others.

Anticardiolipin antibodies

Antiphospholipid antibody syndrome was a label placed on those patients with adverse pregnancy outcome who were noted, often after the fact, to have these antibodies in their blood. However, this has been overplayed, and only high levels of anticardiolipin antibody IgM and IgG are related to pregnancy loss or preeclampsia.

Factor V Leiden

This mutation is found in 5–10% of the Caucasian population and may be responsible for about 40% of thromboembolism in pregnant patients. It has been linked to stillbirth and severe preeclampsia.

Prothrombin gene mutation

This occurs in 2–3% of the Caucasian population, and increases the risk for clotting because it results in elevated levels of prothrombin. Like factor V Leiden, this has been associated with increased rates of stillbirth, abruption, severe preeclampsia, and IUGR.

Antithrombin deficiency

Despite this coagulopathy being a potent cause of thromboembolism and being associated with a fivefold increase in stillbirth, it is only weakly associated with other adverse pregnancy outcomes.

Protein S and protein C deficiencies

These deficiencies occur in only 0.2–0.5% of pregnant individuals and carry a 5–20% risk of thromboembolism. Slightly increased rates of stillbirth, preeclampsia, abruption, and IUGR have been reported.

Methylenetetrahydrofolate reductase (MTHFR) deficiency

This factor is involved in homocysteine metabolism and elevations of this substance can increase coagulability, can decrease folic acid levels (which in turn predispose fetuses to neural tube defects), and has been associated with increased rates of severe preeclampsia, stillbirth, and IUGR. The key to adverse pregnancy outcome is the actual level of homocysteine, and, fortunately, the majority of those heterozygous for MTHFR have normal homocysteine levels. Patients with this deficiency should be treated with folic acid, and some have advocated the use of supplemental vitamin B-12 and B-6. Heterozygotes generally have an excellent prognosis, if this is the only factor that is deficient.

The protocol du jour is to treat the above patients having any of these factors with heparin prophylaxis if they already have had a thrombotic event or second trimester loss, and to prescribe low-dose aspirin for the remainder.

Again, the reason I have devoted these few paragraphs to thrombophilias is that ultrasound will play an important diagnostic role in detecting early signs of IUGR and, although little information is available on this group of patients, uterine artery waveform analysis may offer an excellent way of predicting severe preeclampsia, or, better yet, excluding this complication of pregnancy early on.

Abnormal biochemistry

Screening with second trimester biochemistry has become almost universal and, as indicated earlier, elevations of AFP, hCG, and inhibin have been associated with preterm birth, preeclampsia, stillbirth, and abruption; the same unfortunate events that have been linked to thrombophilias. Now there is information to tie low PAPP-A in the first trimester with preterm birth, and the relationship may be independent of second trimester biochemistry. For example, one study shows a twofold increase of preterm birth for either elevated AFP or low PAPP-A, and a ninefold increase in preterm birth if both are abnormal.

Only a few small studies have surfaced combining uterine artery waveform analysis with combinations of second trimester biochemical markers. One study [10], using elevated MSAFT, hCG, and abnormal uterine arteries as variables, found a LP of 3.3 for preterm birth prior to 32 weeks and a LR of 3.9 for severe IUGR. Aquilina et al., also found a combination of increased inhibin-A and abnormal uterine arteries to be a very good predictor of preeclampsia requiring delivery prior to 37 weeks [11].

Table 15.1 Quad markers and adverse pregnancy outcomes.

Outcome	Marker	Odds Ratio
Spontaneous loss <24 weeks	AFP	7.8
Fetal death ≥24 weeks	Inhibin-A	3.7
Preterm birth ≤ 32 weeks	Inhibin-A	5.0
Preterm PROM	AFP	1.9
Preeclampsia	Inhibin-A	3.8
Gestational hypertension	Inhibin-A	2.7
Abruption	AFP	1.9
Previa at delivery	AFP	3.1
IUGR	Inhibin-A	3.0
Birthweight ≤ 5th percentile	Inhibin-A	2.3
– Delivery ≤ 37 weeks	Inhibin-A	8.0
– Delivery ≤ 32 weeks	Inhibin-A	18.6

Dugoff et al. published a table that links adverse pregnancy outcome with various components of first and second trimester biochemical screening [12].

References

1 Bower S, Schuchter K, Campbell S. Doppler ultrasound screening as part of routine antenatal scanning: prediction of pre-eclampsia and intrauterine growth retardation. BJOG 1993; 100: 989–94.

2 Donohoe S, Geary M, Kingdom JC, et al. Maternal cardiolipins, beta 2-glycoprotein-I and prothrombin antibody expression in high-risk pregnancies with bilateral abnormal uterine artery Doppler waveforms. Ultrasound Obstet Gynecol 1999; 13: 317–22.

3 Frusca T, Soregaroli M, Zanelli S, et al. Role of uterine artery Doppler investigation in pregnant women with chronic hypertension. Eur J Obstet Gynecol Reprod Biol 1998; 79: 47–50.

4 Ferrazzi E, Bulfamante G, Mezzopane R, et al. Uterine Doppler velocimetry and placental hypoxic-ischemic lesion in pregnancies with fetal intrauterine growth restriction. Placenta 1999; 20: 389–94.

5 Sekizuka N, Hasegawa I, Takakuwa K, et al. Scoring of uterine artery flow velocity waveform in the assessment of fetal growth restriction and/or pregnancy-induced hypertension. J Matern Fetal Invest 1997; 7: 197–200.

6 Nicolaides KH, Bindra R, Turan OM, et al. A novel approach to first-trimester screening for early pre-eclampsia combining serum PP-13 and Doppler ultrasound. Ultrasound Obstet Gynecol 2006; 27: 13–7.

7 Caritis S, Sibai B, Hauth J, et al. Low dose aspiring to prevent preeclampsia in women at high risk. NICH/HD Network of Maternal-Fetal Medicine Units. N Engl J Med 1998; 338: 701–5.

8 Coomarasamy A, Honest H, Papaioannau S, et al. Aspiring for prevention of preeclampsia in women with historical risk factors: a systematic review. Obstet Gynecol 2003; 101: 1319–32.

9 Coomarasamy A, Papaioannou S, Gee H, et al. Aspirin for prevention of preeclampsia in women with abnormal uterine artery Doppler: a meta-analysis. Obstet Gynecol 2001; 98: 861–6.

10 Alkazaleh F, Chaddha V, Viero S, et al. Second trimester prediction of severe placental complications in women with combined elevations in alpha-fetoprotein and human chorionic gonadotrophin. Am J Obstet Gynecol 2006; 194:821–7.

11 Aquilina J, Thompson O, Thilaganathan B, et al. Improved early prediction of pre-eclampsia by combining second-trimester maternal serum inhibin-A and uterine artery Doppler. Ultrasound Obstet Gynecol 2001; 17:477–84.

12 Dugoff L, Hobbins JS, Malone FD, et al. for the FASTER Trial Research Consortium. Quad Screen as a predictor of adverse pregnancy outcome. Obstet Gynecol 2005; 106:260–7.

16 Preterm labor

Preterm birth (PTB), defined as birth before 36 weeks, complicates 11.4% of pregnancies in the United States. Birth before 34 weeks occurs between 4 and 7% of the time. Interestingly, despite concentrated efforts to reduce the PTB rate, it has actually risen in the United States by 20% since 1981, probably as a result of the doubling of the incidence of twins and a 400% increase in higher order multiples. Perhaps the reason that we have not been successful in reducing this concerning trend is that PTB is not a result of only one factor on which to take aim, but on many factors, some of which make elusive targets.

Since most PTBs are preceded by labor, the simplistic idea is that the primary focus of therapy should be to stop contractions. However, every randomized clinical trial using various tocolytics in different ways has shown no effect on the rate of PTB except to delay delivery by 48 hours; long enough to get steroids on board.

The latest agent du jour to prevent PTB in those at historical risk is progesterone. In one recent study, this uterine quieting hormone was given early in pregnancy by weekly intramuscular injections and by daily suppositories in another. Both randomized trials demonstrated some effect in reducing PTB. Frankly, I was surprised that this type of modest hormone priming could override some powerful stimuli to end pregnancies. However, the results were compelling.

Various etiologic factors for PTB have been identified or contemplated, which include infection, silent abruption, uterine anomalies, multiple gestation, cervical conization, ruptured membranes, and cervical "incompetence." However, very often there is no obvious cause for the PTB.

One fact is clear. The cervix shortens in patients delivering early, and often the shortening is present by 20–24 weeks of gestation. So, although little progress has been made in preventing PTB, much progress has been accomplished in predicting PTB—mostly through ultrasound studies involving the cervix.

The cervix contains collagen for stability, and elastin for flexibility. The relationship between these two tissue components has much to do about how the cervix behaves, and these and other constituents of the cervix are influenced by exogenous factors such as the balance between estrogen and progesterone (which changes as labor approaches) or cytokines, elaborated secondary to an inflammatory process. Messages from these sources, either separately or together, will cause the cervix to soften, shorten, and, ultimately, to dilate.

Mid-trimester cervical length as a predictor of PTB

Many investigators have made contributions to our knowledge about the cervix and its relationship to PTB. However, Iams [1] was the first to put this link into proper perspective. He and others have constructed normative values for cervical length (CL) in pregnancy and noted that at 20–24 weeks the median CL is 3.5 cm and the 10th percentile is 2.5 cm. He found that a CL below this threshold was associated with a sixfold increase in PTB, compared with those above the median. It was also clear that cervical shortening occurs linearly as a continuum.

It should be pointed out, however, that the prevalence of PTB, defined in Iams' original study as occurring at <35 weeks, was 4.3% in the overall population and 17.3% in those with CLs below 2.5 cm. This means that more than 4 out of 5 women with short cervices did not deliver preterm.

Heath [2], using an endpoint of 32 weeks, below which the neonatal morbidity increases appreciably, found that 50% of patients delivering in this time frame had CLs at 20–24 weeks that were 1.5 cm or less. Interestingly, he and his colleagues found that in twins the CL at which 50% of patients delivered by 32 weeks was 2.5 cm.

Obstetric Ultrasound: Artistry in Practice. John C. Hobbins. Published 2008 Blackwell Publishing. ISBN 978-1-4051-5815-2.

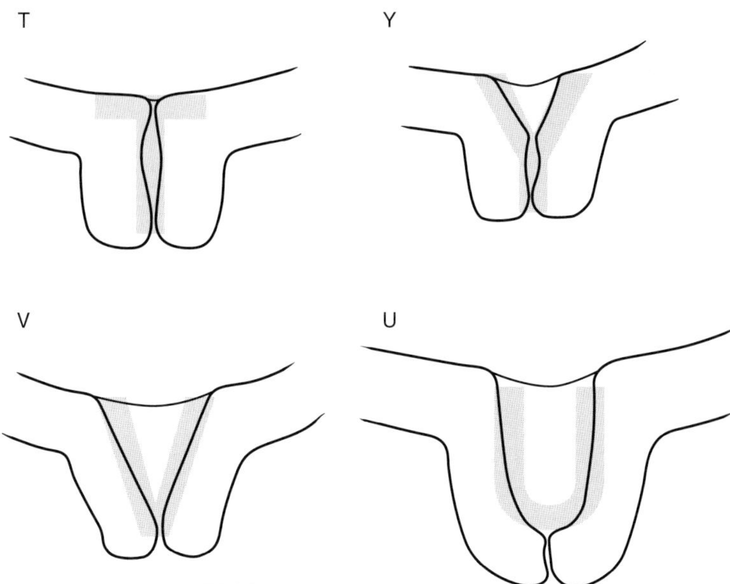

Fig 16.1 Cervical progression in preterm labor.

Zilianti [3] first noted that in most cases of PTB the cervical configuration follows a pattern described by the letters TYVU—"trust your vaginal ultrasound" (Figures 16.1 and 16.2). Basically, the cervix most often thins from the internal os outward by the creation of funneling or wedging, but occasionally the cervix does shorten without the accompaniment of funneling.

Examination of the cervix

The probe is inserted into the vagina in the standard fashion, which usually means the transducer makes contact with the cervix in the anterior fornix. For some reason, early critics of transvaginal ultrasound were worried about dragging bacteria from the vagina into the cervix or causing intracervical trauma in patients with placenta previa. This is not the case, because it is extremely unusual for the cervical canal to be lined up in such a way as to be within the pathway of the advancing transducer.

The best and most accurate method for CL evaluation is to advance the transducer until both the endocervix and exocervix are in the same plane with an intervening line, representing the cervical canal, all within the same image. Step 2 involves backing off until the image degrades a bit, and then gently advancing the transducer again until a crisp image returns (Figure 16.3). This maneuver will assure that the pressure of the transducer does not artificially lengthen the cervical canal. The cleanest endpoint is the endocervix. The exocervix can be elusive to nail down and, therefore, care should be taken to place the other caliper on the Y-shaped outer margin of the cervix (and not the vagina—represented by a robustly echogenic line).

Regarding funneling, many have attempted to measure the width and length of the funnel itself, but the only really important diameter involves what is left of the cervix—the CL, measured from the apex of the wedge to the exocervix. Also, all that matters diagnostically is whether funneling is present or absent.

With CL, more than one measurement should be accomplished and the shortest one should be recorded. While a straight cervical canal is often associated with a short cervix, the curved canal virtually always is associated with a long cervix. Also, a study from Japan [4] has suggested that the width of the canal, representing lush glandular surface, can be correlated with CL and preterm delivery (a thin-lined canal being less reassuring).

The transabdominal approach in most cases can give the observer a rough idea of CL, but it is fraught with problems of an overfilled bladder causing an erroneous impression of a long cervical canal. Also, there is diminished ability to precisely define the necessary landmarks, especially in obese patients. For low-risk patients this approach to the cervix should be adequate as part of the basic ultrasound examination, but in high-risk patients there is no substitute for the transvaginal approach. The translabial (or transperineal—TPU) approach avoids the

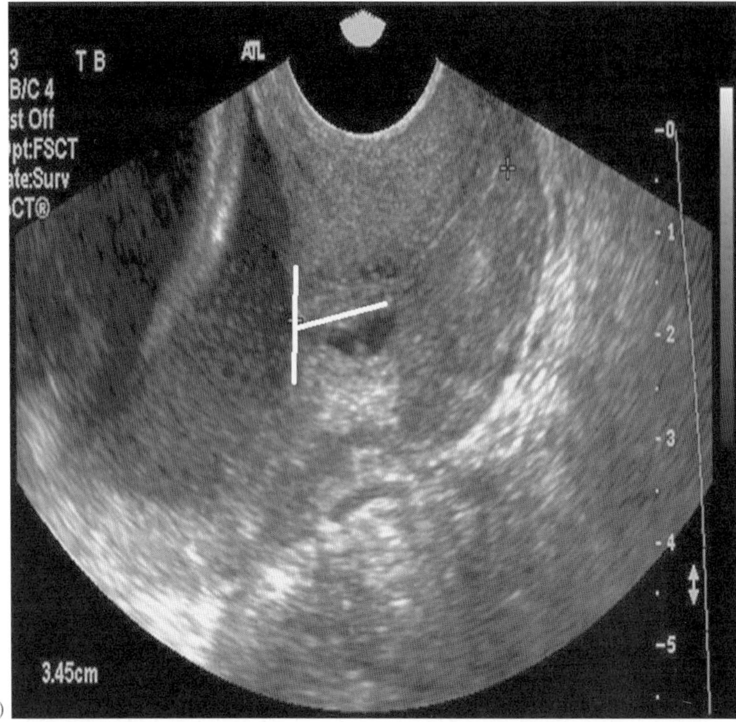

(a)

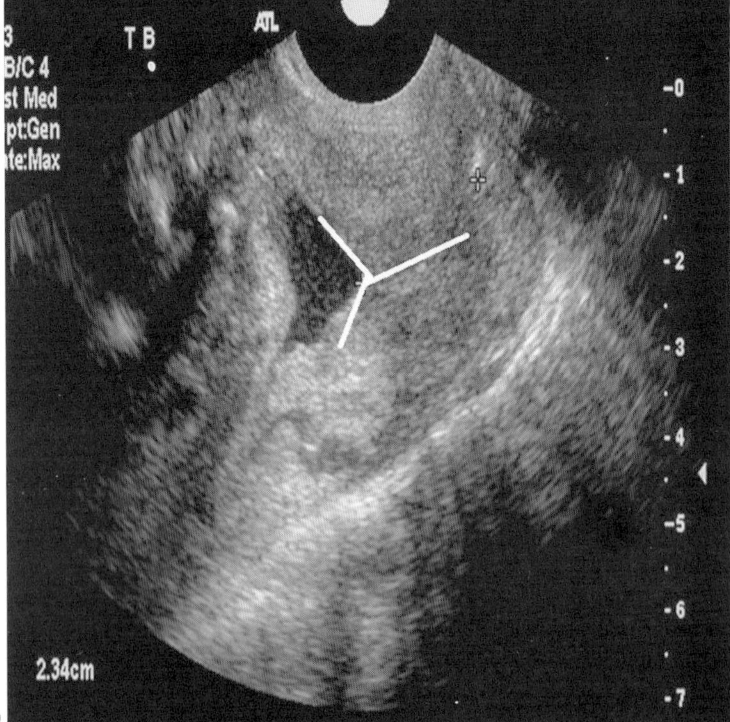

(b)

Fig 16.2 (a) T-shape: no funneling. (b) Y-like shape.

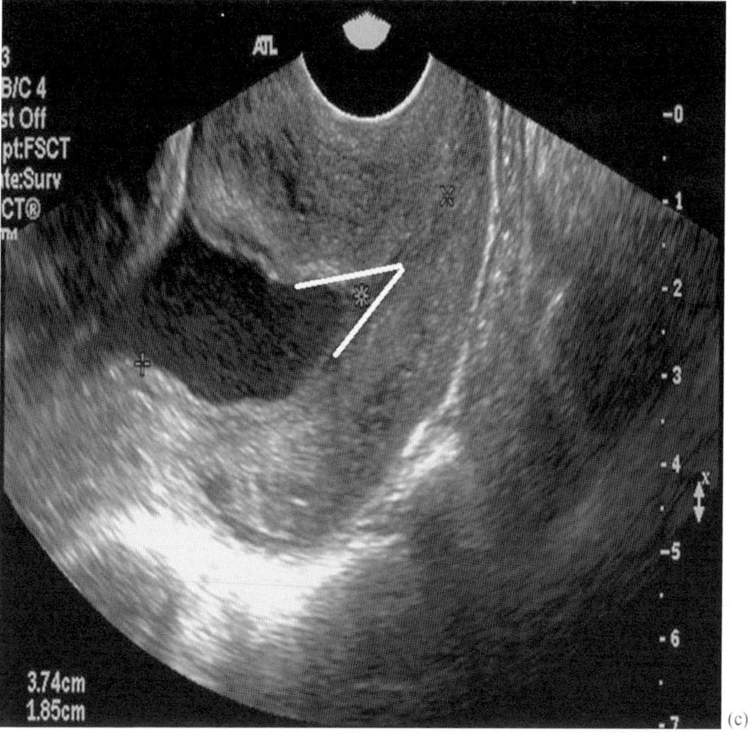

(c)

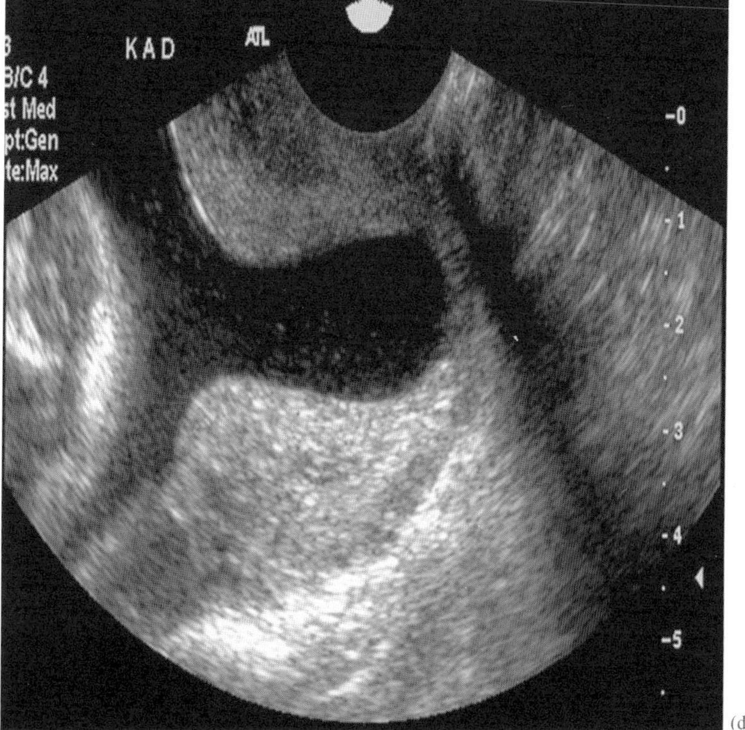

(d)

Fig 16.2 (continued) (c) V-shaped cervix. (d) U-shaped cervix.

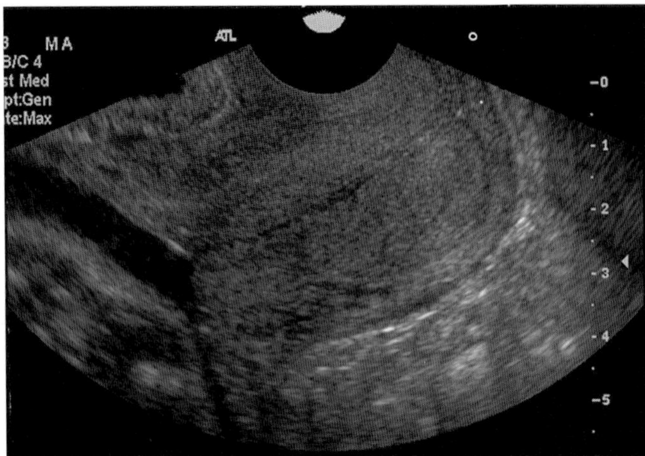

Fig 16.3 Normal cervix.

introduction of the probe into the vagina and, therefore, is less uncomfortable. It can be used as a substitute for the transvaginal approach, but, although I am a strong proponent of TPU in laboring patients, it is a poor substitute for transvaginal sonography in assessing CL, especially at 20–24 weeks.

The association between second trimester CL and PTL

The literature indicates that the shorter the cervix, the greater the chance of the patient delivering prior to term. However, the most important predictive ability of CL involves very early delivery, which is accompanied by high rates of perinatal mortality and morbidity. For example, Romero, one of today's real stars in perinatal medicine, and his group [5] have found the same relationship as Heath in very short cervices: a 50% rate of PTB at <32 weeks with a CL of 1.5 cm. However, only 8% of those who deliver at that time will have a CL of 1.5 cm. Therefore, the test is best used to adjust the relative risk of PTB in high-risk patients, but, as a screening test, especially in low-risk populations, it has questionable value. The high negative predictive value of a long cervix (>3.5 cm) at 20–24 weeks of gestation can be very reassuring, especially in those with a history of mid-trimester or early third trimester losses. On the other hand, a short cervix does not always portend gloom and doom for every woman who has one.

How important is funneling?

Some studies have attempted to correlate the presence of funneling by itself with PTB. However, the strongest correlation is with CL, which has to be shorter, in any case, in the presence of funneling. Nevertheless, Rust and other authors have found that the presence or absence of a funnel has an independent relationship with early birth, over and above that of a shortened CL. Althuisius [6] has suggested that there are different processes leading to labor and a TYVU continuum may not fit every situation because the cervix may thin out without a wedge, and effacement in early labor will give way to a short T-shaped cervix.

We simply have been measuring the length of the cervix and note the presence or absence of a funnel.

What is the meaning of a dynamic cervix?

The first time I saw the cervix shrink before my eyes, I thought I had consumed too many glasses of wine the night before. The cervix can wedge and unwedge in a matter of seconds, playing havoc with one's ability to measure the CL (Figures 16.4a–16.4c). One study [7] has shed some light on the meaning of this phenomenon. The authors monitored some patients' contractions while observing the cervix continuously for 10 minutes. Forty-eight percent of those who felt contractions (when the monitor said they had them) had a change in CL during the observation period, while only 9% of those who did not feel contractions had a dynamic change. In general, those with symptoms of PTL had the shortest CLs but often it took 5 minutes to attain the shortest measurement.

The cervix is not supposed to be "dynamic" and this finding represents a prelude to a state of permanent shortening. Yes, it is better to have a dynamic cervix that occasionally thins to 1 cm than to have a consistently short

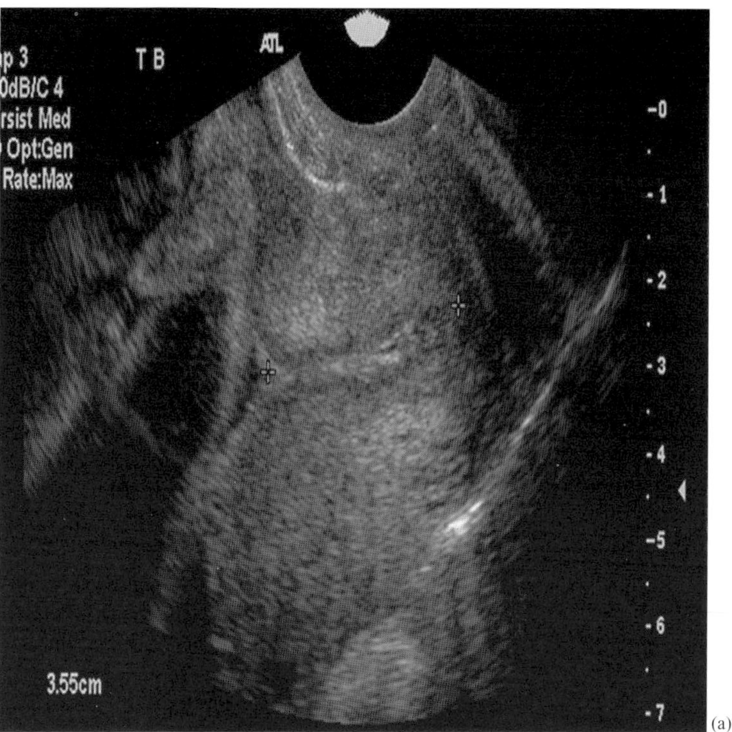

(a)

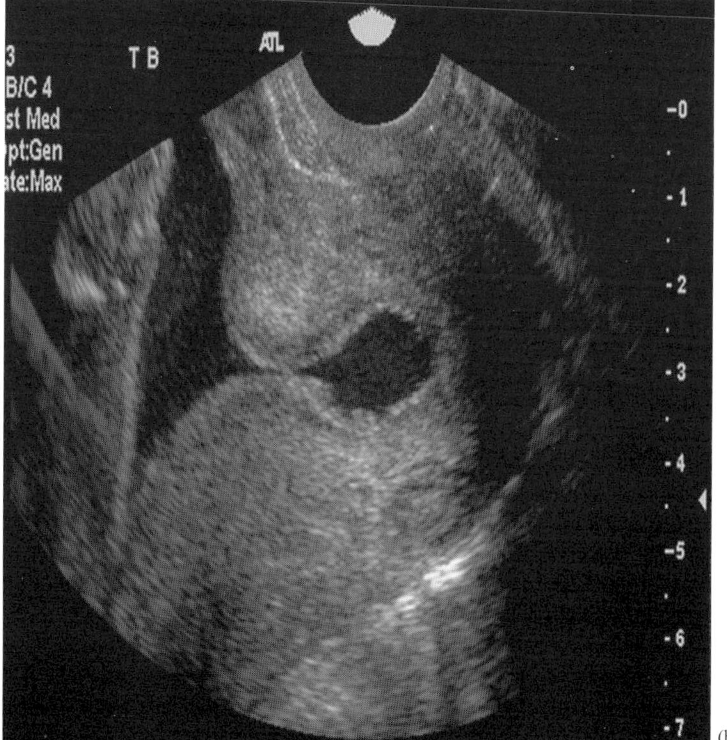

(b)

Fig 16.4 (a) Dynamic cervix sequence. Unexciting start. (b) 30 seconds later.

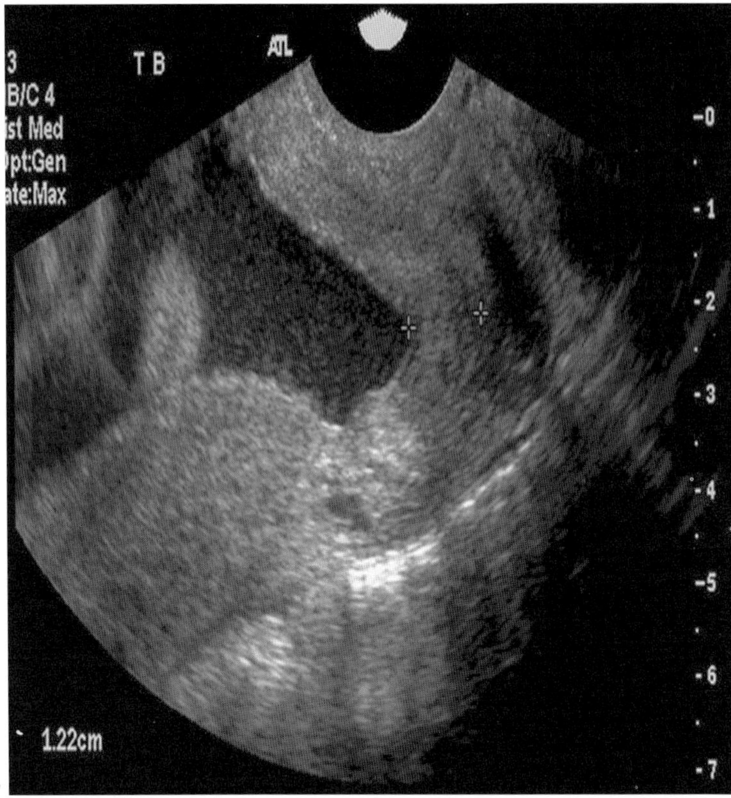

(c)

Fig 16.4 (continued) (c) Another 15 seconds later.

cervix, but, unfortunately, it suggests that the writing may be on the wall for an early delivery.

To quantify a dynamic cervix, use the shortest measurement as the final answer—not the largest or an average of all measurements.

Fundal pressure during transvaginal sonography

Guzman [8] reported that fundal pressure often created funneling and cervical shortening in patients who delivered early. He and others have used this technique to identify patients at risk for incompetent cervix. We have not found this method to be useful, and have had difficulty in quantifying the amount of pressure to, let's say, make the patient's eyes bulge. The continuous 10-minute study above found that fundal pressure did not shorten the cervix in any of the patients studied, and, therefore, did not have the same effect that documented strong contractions had on CL, the very clinical event that fundal pressure was supposed to mimic.

Why not measure CL very early in pregnancy?

One study did show a relationship between CL at 16 weeks and PTB, but others have found that CL has far better positive and negative predictive values when accomplished between 20 and 24 weeks.

Cervical insufficiency

The term "cervical incompetence" has been used for years to identify the patient who, by a history of having had a PTB preceded by silent, painless, and short labor, has been labeled as having a cervix that is mechanically incapable of containing the pregnancy. Today, the word "retardation," originally responsible for the "R" in IUGR, now has been replaced by the term "restriction." Similarly, the label "incompetence," applied to the cervix, is being phased out in favor of "insufficiency" because nobody wishes to be, or to have any body part that is, "incompetent." Whatever name is used, this has to be one of the most tenuous diagnoses ever made, because there are so many reasons to have mid-pregnancy loss and/or short cervices other than from pure cervical insufficiency.

We know that intrauterine infection will cause the myometrium to become irritable and the cervix to soften and shorten. Often in PTL, organisms enter the cervix and ascend within the uterine cavity to a place outside the membranes where they settle in. Here they produce phospholipases that cleave off arachidonic acid from the membranes, which, in turn, is involved in the production of prostaglandins. These trigger the uterus to contract and, undoubtedly, the cervix to shorten. At the same time cytokines, elaborated in the presence of infection, may also have an independent effect on the uterus and cervix, as well as on the fetal brain.

Labor becomes Mother Nature's way of protecting the mother and fetus against further intrauterine harm. Unfortunately, often these events evolve without any signs or symptoms of infection, with the only sign of trouble being a short cervix.

One early study [9] showed that as many as 51% of those patients admitted with preterm labor (PTL) had positive amniotic fluid cultures, and in another large study [10] involving 400 patients admitted in PTL between 22 and 35 weeks, it was noted that 26% of those whose CLs were less than 1.5 cm had positive amniotic fluid cultures. Hassan et al. [11] have found that as many as 9% of asymptomatic patients with short cervices, and a seemingly clear diagnosis of cervical insufficiency, have bacteria in the amniotic cavity. Actually, this observation could represent an underestimation of the problem because not all subchorionic infections capable of inducing labor will have advanced to the point where the bacteria have gained entry into the amniotic cavity.

Also, there are other theories that put the cart before the horse. For example, one thought is that if the cervix shortens substantially, the distance between the bacteria in the vagina and the membranes diminishes, predisposing the patient to intrauterine infection, and then labor.

Even if infection is not the culprit, there are many other reasons for asymptomatic patients to have short cervices, which include a change in the hormonal status prior to spontaneous labor, overdistention of the uterus (as in twins), or silent abruption (one study suggests this). These will not be cured by a stitch in the cervix. Also, it is clear that trying to prolong a pregnancy that is already infected is a bad idea, in view of the recent information regarding the effect of intrauterine infection on the fetal brain (periventricular leukomalacia and, later, cerebral palsy) and the lack of effectiveness of antibiotics in this clinical setting.

There are two types of patients prone to PTL who have inherently short cervices: teenagers, and those who have had cervical conizations (but not cryosurgery) [12]. We have found that the average CL in teenagers in our Young Mothers Program is significantly shorter than those in older pregnant women. Also, studies have indicated that CL, on average, is shorter in those who have had tissue removed from the exocervix through colonization (a logical "slam dunk"). Both groups of patients also have higher rates of PTB. However, even short cervices in these patients do not always translate into early delivery. For this reason, *serial* transvaginal ultrasound examinations are far more informative than the initial CL.

Back to cervical insufficiency. There probably *is* such an entity, but it constitutes a far smaller proportion of PTL than can be accounted for by the amount of cerclages being performed in the USA.

Is there a place for cerclage in cervical insufficiency?

It is interesting that so many prophylactic 13-week cerclages are still being performed in high-risk patients with a history of silent second trimester loss, cervical surgery, or previous cerclages, since randomized trials [13,14] and a systematic review [15] published more than a decade ago showed no benefit from this practice. When CL was added to the clinical backdrop, a meta-analysis [16] published in 2003 of more recent studies has shown no benefit from cerclage in patients with short cervices noted in the second trimester.

A study by Althuisius and colleagues [17] provided a new wrinkle. In one randomized trial, they took patients with historical predispositions toward cervical insufficiency and performed early cerclage in roughly one-third of them. The others were followed with serial ultrasound examinations until 24 weeks of gestation, and if the CL dipped below 2.5 cm, the patients were randomized either to watchful waiting or to cerclage. The lowest PTB rate was in those whose cervices never shortened below 2.5 cm. The next best outcomes were in those with second trimester cerclages, which outperformed early cerclages. The worst outcomes were in those with progressively short cervices and no cerclage. The authors' conclusion was that early elective cerclage in high-risk patients was of questionable benefit, when compared with a protocol of serial ultrasound evaluations of CL. They also concluded that the few patients whose cervices shortened prior to 24 weeks might benefit from a cerclage. Interestingly, a 2005 meta-analysis which included these and other data from Althusius, showed benefit of cerclage in some patients with short CL (as opposed to other pooled data published earlier) [18].

A study from Japan [19] speaks for the benefit of cerclage in the late second trimester in a select group of patients, but the data pointed against doing cerclages in those with evidence of intracervical infection. Interleukin-8 (IL-8) is an inflammatory cytokine that the authors evaluated in the cervical mucus of 16,000 patients in a 5-year study. Two hundred and fifty-six patients (1.5%) had cervices at 20–24 weeks that were <2.5 cm. One hundred and sixty-five patients had cerclage procedures, and the remaining 81 patients were simply observed.

There was no difference overall in the rate of PTB between the cerclage and the no cerclage groups. However, the negative IL-8 patients with cerclages had a lower rate of PTB than the control group. The group that fared the worst consisted of those who had a positive IL-8 and cerclage. The study indicated that there may be a place for cerclage in a select group of patients with short CLs and no evidence of intracervical or intrauterine infection. However, the results also indicated that it is clearly a bad idea to perform cerclage in patients with any sign of infection.

So, to summarize, many studies show no benefit from cerclage in high-risk patients with or without short cervices, while the two studies from the Netherlands do suggest benefit in some patients who have progressively shortening cervices. The differences could be due to dissimilar study designs and types of patients enrolled. Certainly, if cerclage is being contemplated, the Japanese study shows that every attempt should be made to rule out intrauterine infection beforehand.

Rescue cerclage

Some patients have already passed through the stage of cervical shortening and have reached a point where the cervix is dilated to 4–6 cm with membranes protruding. Two trials have addressed the efficacy of cerclage in these patients. Olatunbosun et al. [20] studied women at 22–24 weeks with advanced cervical dilatation (equal to or greater than 4 cm). Twenty patients obtained a cerclage and the rest were observed on bed rest. The cerclage group delivered, on average, 1 month later than the bed rest group. The numbers were small and the study was not randomized.

In one of the above studies from the Netherlands [17], a cohort of 23 women was found to have advanced cervical dilatation with membranes below the external os at 21–23 weeks. Thirteen had cerclages and ten had bed rest. The cerclage group's pregnancies lasted 30 days longer on average than the bed rest patients, although one patient did rupture membranes during the procedure.

I am passing this information on simply to indicate that the door should not necessarily be completely closed for cerclage, even in patients with this very guarded clinical scenario.

Salient points regarding CL at 20–24 weeks

1 The measurement must be scrupulously performed under a standardized protocol.
2 Studies do not demonstrate the efficacy of screening with CL in a low-risk population.
3 Funneling will increase the likelihood of PTB as an independent predictor, but it is no better a clinical performer than CL alone.
4 A dynamic cervix is probably a forerunner of permanent shortening and may require a longer examination time to detect it.
5 Empiric early cerclage is not a useful option in patients at risk for cervical insufficiency.
6 Some highly selected patients, representing a very small percentage of those with short CLs in the second trimester, may benefit from cerclage.
7 Any patient with a short CL should be worked up for intrauterine or intracervical infection. I think that the rare patient who might benefit from a cerclage should have a preprocedure amniocentesis and fluid culture, particularly looking for ureaplasma. The ability to do a cervical IL-8 may negate the need to sample amniotic fluid.

Use of CL in patients with preterm contractions

PTL is responsible for the bulk of admissions to the antepartum service of most large hospitals, where PTB is the second most common cause of perinatal mortality and morbidity. Although more than 80% of patients with preterm contractions are not in PTL, we overreact to these patients for fear of turning someone loose who will return soon after, fully dilated and ready to deliver. It does not matter that even in the hospital there seems to be no effective treatment to keep fetuses in the uterus for more than about 48 hours. However, we are sensitized to this unhappy ending and wind up hospitalizing these patients for many unnecessary days away from their families.

Now, there are ways to sort out those patients at risk for delivery from those who are not, and this involves a simple transvaginal evaluation of CL.

Surprisingly, there is a paucity of studies with adequate numbers to address this dilemma, but what is out there makes a very strong case for performing CL measurements on admission in all patients entering with preterm contractions. One study [21] involved 216 women presenting with a regular painful contractions between 24 and 36 weeks. Forty-three patients had a CL of <1.5 cm and 16 (37%) delivered within 7 days. However, only 1 of the 132 women with CL of >1.5 cm delivered within 7 days.

A study from Germany [22] yielded almost identical results. Interestingly, receiver operator curve (ROC) analysis indicated a CL threshold of 1.5 cm to be the best predictor of early delivery in patients with preterm contractions. Forty-seven percent of patients with cervices <1.5 cm delivered within 7 days and only 1.8% of patients with CL >1.5 cm delivered within 7 days.

A similar study from Greece [23] showed that if the CL exceeded 3 cm, 100% of these patients delivered after 34 weeks.

These three studies strongly endorse the concept of using CL to carefully select out those patients needing special attention and to allow the other patients, representing the majority of those with preterm contractions, to be left alone. Presently, patients admitted with preterm contractions are kept in the hospital for many days or weeks, long after their contractions peter out. Here they are treated to bad institutional food and exposed to our hospitals' own special brands of pathogens. In addition, while the total cost of health care is skyrocketing, these unhappy campers are occupying beds at a cost of up to $1800 per day.

A long cervix should allow us to safely discharge these patients to home, where they will be far more content.

Where does fetal fibronectin fit in?

Fetal fibronectin is an extracellular protein that is responsible for fastening the fetal membranes to the decidua. Normally, it can be found in the cervix and vagina up until 22 weeks of gestation, but can return in threshold amounts (>50 ng/ml) later if there is disruption of the decidua /membrane interface. When found in the vagina after 22 weeks it is a reasonable predictor of PTL.

A collaborative study [24] involving 215 patients, admitted with preterm contractions, was undertaken in Chile and Detroit. CL was assessed, as well as vaginal fetal fibronectin. Twenty percent delivered before 35 weeks and CL outperformed fetal fibronectin as a predictor of this event. However, the two tests together formed a very powerful diagnostic combination. If both were positive, 81.3% delivered before 35 weeks. If both were negative, only 2.2% delivered within a week of the examination and none delivered at less than 32 weeks. After sifting through the data, I noticed that if the CL was greater than 3 cm, fetal fibronectin added little to the negative predictive value. Therefore, a simple CL alone would suffice in those with long cervices, and fetal fibronectin would only be required in the 40% of cases where the CL was <3 cm.

Algorithm for threatened PTL:

1 History
 (a) Are the dates accurate? Determined through early documentation with ultrasound or compelling information about the patient's menstrual dating or time of conception.
 (b) Previous history of PTL?
 (c) On tocolytics now or in the past?
 (d) Any history compatible with rupture of membranes in this pregnancy?
2 Transabdominal ultrasound
 (a) Assess amniotic fluid volume.
 (b) Obtain biometric estimation of gestational age (AUA).
 (c) On occasion, look for epiphyseal centers (see section on ultrasound and labor and delivery).
 (d) Repeat the full fetal survey—especially if done earlier in pregnancy.
 If the history and/or ultrasound confirm the patient's dates, then move to the next step.
3 Transvaginal ultrasound
 (a) Do CL measurement
  (1) If CL is greater than 3 cm, simply observe patient and send her home when contractions abate.
  (2) If CL is 1.5–3 cm, send off fetal fibronectin.
  (3) If fibronectin is positive, admit as long as contractions persist.
  (4) If fibronectin is negative, discharge.
  (5) If CL is less than 1.5 cm, admit.

Premature rupture of the membranes (PROM)

While 40% of PTB is contributed by PTL, about 35% results from PROM. Like PTL, there are many causes of PROM, but infection plays an even greater role here. The membranes, which provide the barrier to ascending infection, can rupture as a result of weakening, secondary to bacterial infiltration. A less common cause of PROM is hour-glassing through the incompletely closed cervix, where the event becomes an accident waiting to happen. Placental abruption has been linked to PROM. An extramembranous clot will cause the membranes to tent away from their source of nutrition, the decidua. This renders them more vulnerable to rupture. Romero, a leading light in understanding preterm labor, has noted through placental bed biopsies that patients with PROM often have a deficiency in spiral artery remodeling, which speaks for a long-term process being responsible for the PROM. This finding also adds another diagnostic modality, uterine artery waveform, as a potential predictor of PROM.

In a study from Philadelphia, Odibo et al. [25] found that in 321 high-risk patients a short cervix (defined as a CL <2.5 cm) between 14 and 24 weeks was more predictive of very early PROM than it was of very early PTL. Specifically, short cervices were associated with a 10-fold increase in the risk for PROM, and a 4-fold increase for PTL at <32 weeks. Unfortunately, although this allows the clinician to identify those at highest risk for PROM, we still do not have a reliable way to prevent it.

Oligohydramnios is the rule after PROM, and this can easily be assessed by transabdominal ultrasound. Occasionally, the presenting part of the fetus will settle down into the pelvis to produce a ball valve effect with the cervix. Although this can stop the leakage briefly, virtually always there is a dramatic decrease in amniotic fluid volume.

As indicated in the segment on oligohydramnios, transvaginal ultrasound can be used to identify the presence or absence of membranes coursing over the endocervix. If they are there, then the rupture could only represent the "high leak", something I think is very rare. Even then, the protective function of the membranes should still be intact at the endocervix.

Also, as mentioned earlier [26], it is possible to tell if the patient will be going into labor, sooner rather than later, by CL measurements on admission. If the CL is <2 cm, the average latent period is about 10 hours, while if the CL is <2 cm, the average time until labor begins is 50 hours.

In prolonged rupture of membranes, pulmonary hypoplasia is a devastating consequence, and 2D methods can give a rough approximation of fetal lung size, while 3D methods (covered in the 3D section) can do it more precisely.

Last, over and above the obvious problems awaiting any infant being delivered very early from prematurity alone is the additive potential threat of superimposed intrauterine infection in pregnancies complicated by PROM. As suggested earlier, the presence of chorioamnionitis in PROM should trump any reason to keep the fetus in utero. For this reason, most protocols for PROM call for induction of labor in patients with PROM >33 weeks because of the potential for infection (whether or not there is evidence for it). However, there are ways to indirectly assess the presence of intrauterine infection in patients with PROM.

The degree of oligohydramnios has been correlated with both the length of the latent period and the presence of chorioamnionitis. In many cases, after the initial loss of fluid, the uterine cavity will seem "dry," and will stay that way over time. These patients are at higher risk of infection and have very short latent periods, compared with those patients who retain residual amounts of amniotic fluid (1–2 cm single vertical pocket).

Another method of surveillance in hospitalized patients involves the use of the biophysical profile (BPP). Under the influence of intrauterine infection, the fetus usually moves and breathes less and has a smooth heart rate pattern. These observations were put into proper perspective by Vintzileos and his colleagues in 1985 [27], when they first found that BPP correlated with clinical infection in patients with PROM. Since then there have been 10 studies addressing this relationship. Seven showed the BPP to be a reasonable predictor of infection, while three studies did not. In the latter negative studies the protocols called for sampling intervals of between 48 and 72 hours, compared with 24-hour intervals in the studies showing a positive relationship.

Although no investigator recently has been enticed to continue this research, most of the available data suggest that low BPP scores will precede clinical evidence of chorioamnionitis early enough to properly alert providers to its presence in a majority of cases, with the caveat that it must be employed at least once a day. Vintzileos also has shown that, for some reason, fetal behavior is not affected when mycoplasma is the primary organism involved.

Some years ago, when this type of testing was in vogue at Yale, we found that infection had its most powerful effect on fetal breathing, which would be virtually absent in patients with PROM before clinical signs of amnionitis emerged or labor ensued.

In summary, patients with a history of previous PROM, cerclage, PTB, and now, I will wager, abnormal uterine artery waveforms, are at high risk for PROM. These individuals should benefit from a CL determination at 20–24 weeks of gestation. At this time, depending upon the length of the cervix, these individuals' risk could be elevated or, better yet, diminished. Later, in patients presenting with a history of vaginal leakage of fluid and an equivocal clinical examination, a transvaginal ultrasound examination can be useful in assessing the status of the membranes over the cervix, and in estimating, through CL, when labor is most likely to begin (if the membranes *are* ruptured). For example, if patients are <34 weeks and the CL is >2.0 cm, there is a high likelihood that they will not go into labor within 1 week. These patients could benefit from daily BPPs, with heavy emphasis on the presence or absence of fetal breathing.

If the CL is <2.0 cm, one should expect delivery imminently, but, with a 50-hour average latency period there should be enough time to get steroids on board to discourage the development of intraventricular hemorrhage, if the patient is <32 weeks (an ACOG recommendation).

References

1 Iams JD, Goldenberg RL, Meis PJ, et al. The length of the cervix and the risk of spontaneous premature delivery. National Institute of Child Health and Human Development Maternal fetal medicine Unit Network. N Engl J Med 1996; 334: 567–72.

2 Heath VC, Southall TR, Souka AP, et al. Cervical length at 23 weeks of gestation: prediction of spontaneous preterm delivery. Ultrasound Obstet Gynecol 1998; 12: 312–7.

3 Zilianti M, Azuaga A, Calderon F, et al. Monitoring the effacement of the uterine cervix by transperineal sonography: a new perspective. J Ultrasound Med 1995; 14: 719–24.

4 Yoshimatsu K, Sekiya T, Ishihara K, et al. Detection of the cervical gland area in threatened preterm labor using transvaginal sonography in assessment of cervical maturation and the outcome of pregnancy. Gynecol Obstet Invest 2002; 53: 149–56.

5 Hassan SS, Romero R, Berry SM, et al. Patients with an ultrasonographic cervical length of < or = 1.5 mm have nearly a 50% risk of early spontaneous preterm delivery. Am J Obstet Gynecol 2000; 182: 1458–67.

6 Althuisius S, Dekker G. Controversies regarding cervical incompetence, short cervix, and the need for cerclage. Clin Perinatol 2004; 31: 695–720.

7 Kurtzman JT, Jenkins SM, Brewster WR. Dynamic cervical change during real-time ultrasound: prospective characterization and comparison in patients with and without symptoms of preterm labor. Ultrasound Obstet Gynecol 2004; 23: 574–8.

8 Guzman ER, Vintzileos AM, McLean DA, et al. The natural history of a positive response to transfundal pressure in women at risk for cervical incompetence. Am J Obstet Gynecol 1997; 176: 634–8.

9 Romero R, Gonzalez R, Sepulveda W, et al. Infection and labor. VIII. Microbial invasion of the amniotic cavity in patients with suspected cervical incompetence: prevalence and clinical significance. Am J Obstet Gynecol 1992; 167: 1086–91.

10 Gomez R, Romero R, Nien JK, et al. A short cervix in women with preterm labor and intact membranes: a risk factor for microbial invasion of the amniotic cavity. Am J Obstet Gynecol 2005; 192: 678–89.

11 Hassan S, Romero R, Hendler I, et al. A Sonographic short cervix as the only clinical manifestation of intra-amniotic infection. J Perinat Med 2006; 34: 13–9.

12 Crane JM, Delaney T, Hutchens D. Transvaginal ultrasonography in the prediction of preterm birth after treatment for cervical intraepithelial neoplasia. Obstet Gynecol 2006; 107: 37–44.

13 Rush RW, Isaacs S, McPherson K, et al. A randomized control trial of cervical cerclage in women at high risk of spontaneous preterm delivery. Br J Obstet Gynaecol 1984; 91: 724–30.

14 Lazar P, Gueguen S, Dreyfus J, et al. Multicentred control trial of cervical cerclage in women at moderate risk for preterm delivery. Br J Obstet Gynaecol 1984; 91: 731–5.

15 Final multicentre report of Medical Research Council/Royal College of Obstetricians and Gynaecologists randomized trial of cervical cerclage. MRC/RCOG Working Party on Cervical Cerclage. Br J Obstet Gynaecol 1993; 100: 516–23.

16 Drakeley A, Roberts D, Alfirevic Z. Cervical cerclage for prevention of preterm delivery: meta-analysis of randomized trials. Am J Obstet Gynecol 2003; 102: 621–7.

17 Althuisius SM, Dekker GA, Hummel P, et al. Final results of the Cervical Incompetence prevention Randomized Cerclage Trial (CIPRACT): therapeutic cerclage with bed rest versus bed rest alone. Am J Obstet Gynecol 2001; 185: 1106–12.

18 Berghella V, Odibo AD, To MS, et al. Cerclage for short cervix on ultrasound: meta-analysis of trials using individual patient-level data. Obstet Gynecol 2005; 106: 181–9.

19 Sakai M, Shiozaki A, Tabata M, et al. Evaluation of effectiveness of prophylactic cerclage of a short cervix according to interleukin-8 and cervical mucus. Am J Obstet Gynecol 2006; 194: 14–9.

20 Olatunbosun OA, al-Nuaim L, Turnell RW. Emergency cerclage compared with bed rest for advanced cervical dilation in pregnancy. Int Surg 1995; 80: 170–4.

21 Tsoi E, Akmal S, Rane S, et al. Ultrasound assessment of cervical length in threatened preterm labor. Ultrasound Obstet Gynecol 2003; 21: 552–5.

22 Fuchs IB, Henrich WO, Osthues K, et al. Sonographic cervical length in singleton pregnancies with intact membranes presenting with threatened preterm labor. Ultrasound Obstet Gynecol 2004; 24: 554–7.

23 Daskalakis G, Thomakos N, Hatziioannou L, et al. Cervical assessment in women with threatened preterm labor. J Matern Fetal Neonatal Med 2005; 17: 309–12.

24 Gomez R, Romero R, Medina L, et al. Cervicovaginal fibronectin improves the prediction of preterm delivery based on sonographic cervical length in patients with preterm uterine contractions and intact membranes. Am J Obstet Gynecol 2005; 92: 350–9.

25 Odibo AO, Talucci M, Berghella V. Prediction of preterm premature rupture of membranes by transvaginal ultrasound features and risk factors in a high-risk population. Ultrasound Obstet Gynecol 2002; 20: 245–51.

26 Gire C, Fabbianelli P, Nicaise C, et al. Ultrasonographic evaluation of cervical length in pregnancies complicated by preterm premature rupture of membranes. Ultrasound Obstet Gynecol 2002; 19: 565–9.

27 Vintzileos AM, Campbell WA, Nochimson DJ, et al. The fetal biophysical profile in patients with premature rupture of the membranes — an early predictor of fetal infection. Am J Obstet Gynecol 1985; 152: 510–6.

17 Rh disease (erythroblastosis fetalis)

This condition is now uncommon due to the common practice of giving anti-immunoglobulin after delivery and once during pregnancy. This injection will tie up fetal red blood cells before the mother can recognize their presence to later mount an antibody response.

If the mother is Rh negative and has a partner who is Rh positive, she runs a 50% chance, if the partner is heterozygous (Dd) for the Rh factor, of having a fetus who is Rh positive. If the father of the baby is one of the 15% who is homozygous for the Rh factor (DD), she runs 100% chance of the fetus being Rh positive. If the father is heterozygous for the Rh factor (or for Kell), it has been a part of many protocols to perform amniocenteses to obtain fluid for fetal typing in seemingly sensitized pregnancies in order to weed out the 50% of fetuses who are negative for these factors. In these pregnancies no further testing would be required. Today, in some laboratories fetal DNA can be separated out of maternal blood, allowing fetal typing without the need for invasive measures.

When the patient is sensitized (producing antibodies against Rh positive cells), the IgG antibody gets across the placenta and can indirectly cause breakdown of the fetal red cells, sometimes rendering the fetus anemic.

Kell sensitization often occurs from a blood transfusion given to the mother. A Kell negative mother, mating with a Kell positive partner, can produce a Kell positive fetus whose red blood cells are vulnerable to maternal antibody via the same basic mechanism as in Rh disease.

Unfortunately, Kell can kill quickly after an initial unexciting, almost dormant, early stage of pregnancy. Because of this, the wary physician should be ever vigilant when managing a Kell sensitized pregnancy.

In the "old days" the diagnostic method of choice in following Rh and Kell sensitized pregnancies was to monitor antibody titers and to perform serial amniocenteses if the titer exceeded a certain threshold (usually 1:16). The fluid then would be evaluated by optical density characteristics for indirect bilirubin—a product of fetal red blood cell breakdown. Using a curve originally developed in New Zealand by Liley, and initially implemented by many around the world, including Queenan and Frigoletto in the USA, if the optical density difference (ΔOD) at 450 nm was elevated, then intrauterine transfusions would be initiated if the fetus were too premature to be delivered at that point.

Today, ultrasound has revolutionized the diagnosis and therapy of this condition. First, when fetuses with erythroblastosis fetalis are engaged in the removal of their own red blood cells, the spleen, which can be quite large in this condition, gets put into play in two ways: (1) by breaking down the fetal red blood cells and removing them from the circulation and (2) by acting as another organ to produce new red cells, since the bone marrow cannot keep up with the rate of destruction. Also, the liver is enlarged in the process because it also becomes involved in extramedullary hematopoiesis. Last, the fetal heart can be challenged by severe fetal anemia (sometimes simplistically alluded to as high output failure), and hydrops eventually ensues.

The spleen can be identified just behind the stomach on cross-sectional views and can be measured in two planes or quantified with a trackball as a perimeter (Figure 17.1). Splenomegaly is one of the earlier signs of increased splenic activity and, indirectly of the severity of the fetal condition.

The liver size can be quantified by liver length measurements made from the dome of the diaphragm to the tip of the liver (Figure 17.2).

Cardiac failure can be suspected by the presence of ascites (Figure 17.3). However, long before the ascites is noted in the fetal abdomen (always indicating a fetus that has a hematocrit of below 15), there is often the appearance of echogenic bowel. Fluid between the bowel loopswill

Obstetric Ultrasound: Artistry in Practice. John C. Hobbins. Published 2008 Blackwell Publishing. ISBN 978-1-4051-5815-2.

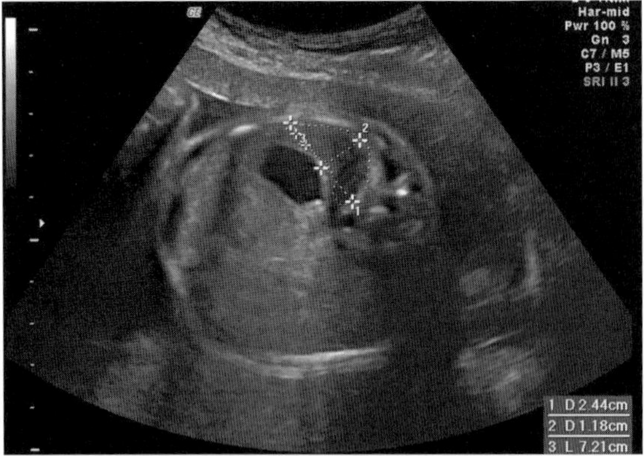

Fig 17.1 Fetal spleen.

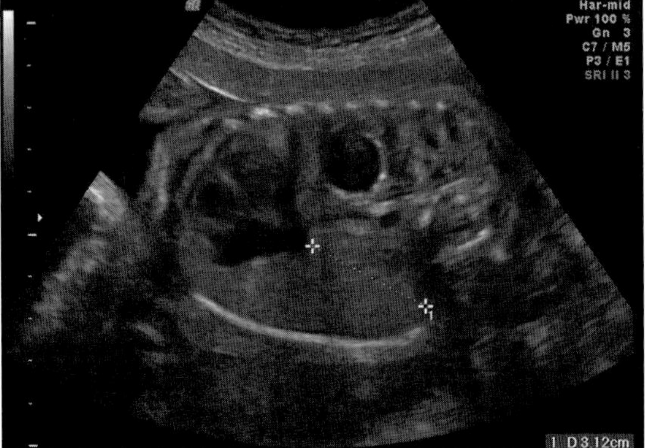

Fig 17.2 Liver length (but tangential cut).

cause a mismatch in acoustic impedance between it and the bowel wall, causing the bowel to appear bright.

The above are all indirect reflections of fetal anemia and its aftermath, and are probably worth pursuing. However, the most precise way to evaluate fetal anemia is to analyze Doppler waveforms from the middle cerebral artery (MCA). When the fetus is anemic, the oxygen content (but not the PO_2) is low, and the fetus will virtually always start autoregulating to spare his/her brain. As opposed to IUGR, this time we are interested in the peak velocity in the MCA and not so much the amount of end diastolic flow. Peak velocities are generally sky high in fetal anemia because cardiac output is increased, the viscosity of the blood is low, and, therefore, the table is set for blood to shoot up through this vessel to protect the cerebral cortex.

Years ago Campbell suggested looking at the MCA in Rh disease, but Mari [1] was the one who put the process in place through creative investigation. He developed a peak velocity curve that is used in most high-risk centers around the world. In short, if the fetus is severely anemic, the peak velocity in the MCA is always above 1.5 MoM. The false positive rate is between 12 and 18%. However, because it is almost unheard of for fetuses to be severely anemic when peak velocities are below 1.5 MoM, thousands of unnecessary amniocenteses and risky cord sampling procedures have been averted over the last few years.

Now that I have touted the method, it is important to emphasize that the technique must be very carefully performed. Since obtaining a simple ratio is not the goal here, the angle of insonation with the MCA must be as close to zero as possible, and angle correction must occur before the peak velocities are recorded (Figure 17.4). Any angle of $>30°$ will yield worthless information. Fortunately, most fetuses spend their time in an occipital transverse position, and the pathway of the MCA lends itself to an ideal setup for this type of waveform analysis. We prefer to sample just above the circle of Willis. Three measurements should be made, and the cleanest waveform chosen. The curve into which this measurement is plotted is in the appendix.

Prospective study has indicated this to be an excellent excluder of fetal anemia resulting from Rh disease, Kell sensitization, and parvovirus (which can cause severe fetal anemia). Amniocentesis now is rarely needed, but if the peak velocity of the MCA is >1.5 MoM, one should go right to cord sampling, poised to do an intrauterine transfusion if the fetus is proven to be anemic.

Although there has been accumulating anecdotal experience of a concerning tendency for a high rate of false positives of MCA peak velocities after 33 weeks (enough to cause some clinicians to use amniotic fluid preferentially at this time in gestation), in a cursory poll of clinicians with the greatest experience with MCA investigation, I have found only one false negative case (an infant with severe anemia after a reassuring MCA peak velocity). Mari indicates that he has had none. Until new information emerges, I will be suspicious of a high MCA peak velocity after 33 weeks and, depending upon the clinical backdrop, I will either move to an amniocentesis (also with assessment of fetal pulmonic maturity), or will consider delivery. However, if the MCA waveform is reassuring, I will continue to believe it.

Algorithm for management of Rh and Kell sensitization

Historical criteria

1 High risk: those whose fetuses or infants required transfusions in previous pregnancies.

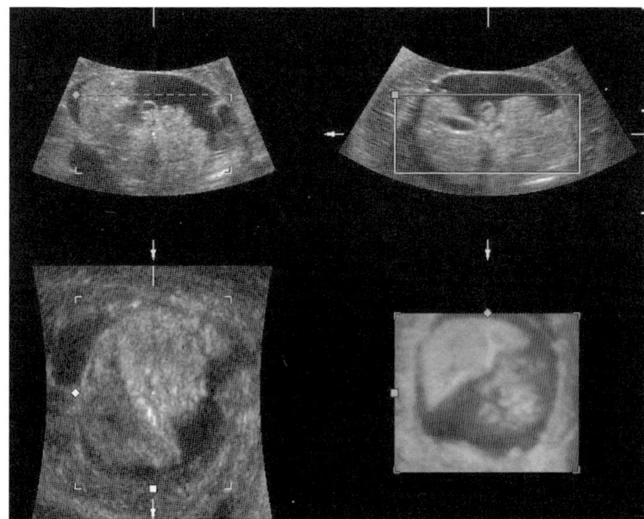

Fig 17.3 Ascites.

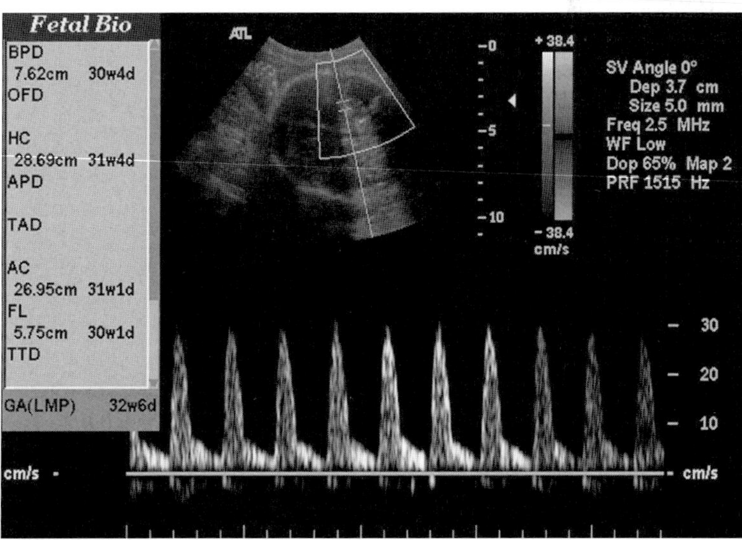

Fig 17.4 Normal peak velocity in MCA.

2 Lower risk: those who had low titers in a previous pregnancy or developed a titer in the current pregnancy.

An attempt should be made to test the zygosity of the father of the baby. If he is heterozygous for D, then there is a 50% chance that the fetus will be unaffected. If he is homozygous, the chances of the fetus being D positive, and, therefore, susceptible to erythroblastosis are 100%.

Protocol for those at historical high risk

1 Start MCA waveforms at 18–20 weeks and continue every 2 weeks if the peak velocity is below 1.5 MoM.
2 If MCA is above 1.5 MoM, then consider cord sampling and possible intrauterine transfusion.
3 If the slope is not steep and MCA peak velocities hover around the 1.5 MoM, then use the presence or absence of splenomegaly or preascites to determine

whether to do cord sampling and the intrauterine transfusion.

4 If the fetal hematocrit is below 30 mg%, transfuse and repeat transfusion in 2 weeks if less than 34 weeks' gestation.

Protocol for those at historical low risk

1 Start monthly titers; if anti-D titer is above 1:16, go to MCA waveforms every 2 weeks.

2 If MCA peak velocity is above 1.5 MoM, and the slope is steep, do cord sampling and possible intrauterine transfusion.

3 If MCA peak velocity is borderline or just above 1.5 MoM, and the slope is not steep, consider amniocentesis for delta OD assessment (since there is up to an 18% false positive rate with MCA peak velocities). If the delta OD is not reassuring, go to cord sampling and possible intrauterine transfusion.

4 Repeat transfusion in 2 weeks.

In all transfusions, use the last intrauterine hematocrit, the patient's gestational age, and MCA peak velocities to decide whether and/or when to transfuse again. Delivery time is based on clinical judgment. Because of the complications of intrauterine transfusion, we rarely transfuse after 32 weeks and would rather deliver the fetus at this time.

Kell sensitization warrants the same management plan, but with a much lower threshold to transfuse and/or deliver the patient early. Weiner and Manogura recently published a review of the management of fetal hemolytic disease [3].

References

1 Queenan JT, Tomai TP, Ural SH, King JC. Deviation in amniotic fluid optical density at a wavelength of 450 nm in Rh-immunized pregnancies from 14 to 40 weeks' gestation: a proposal for clinical management. Am J Obstet Gynecol 1993; 168:1370–76.

2 Mari G, Deter RL, Carpenter RL. Noninvasive diagnosis by Doppler ultrasonography of fetal anemia due to maternal red-cell alloimmunization. Collaborative Group for Doppler Assessment of the Blood Velocity in Anemic Fetuses. J Ultrasound Med 2005; 24: 1599–624.

3 Weiner CP, Manogura AC. Maternal alloimmunization and fetal hemolytic disease. In: Clinical Obstetrics: The Fetus and Mother. Reece EA, Hobbins JC (eds). Malden, MA: Blackwell Publishing, 2007.

18 3D and 4D ultrasound

There is no doubt that 3D ultrasound is useful in obstetrics and that 4D ultrasound has an emotional impact on everyone in the room when it is employed. The obvious questions to be asked, however, are how much does it really add to the diagnostic process, and when is it essential in making the diagnosis? In a review article published by Goncalves et al. [1], the authors found 706 papers in the world literature dealing with 3D and 4D ultrasound. Not surprisingly, about 20% were case reports, and fewer than 20% represented clinical studies, most of which did not answer the above questions. However, a few did, and some will be folded into this overview.

Although some of this information was covered in the chapter on the fetal heart, I will start with the mechanics of 3D and 4D. In standard 3D, the operator lines up an area of interest and either uses a 2D starting point that is longitudinal (the fetal profile) or cross-sectional (the four-chamber view of the heart). Then the mechanical array is activated to sweep through an arc, the size and speed of which are predetermined by the operator. The information is immediately displayed in three planes. The A plane represents the original starting point and will also provide the image with the best resolution. The B plane is an orthogonal slice taken at right angles across the A plane in the north–south axis. The C plane represents a tomogram at 90° from the B plane in the east–west axis. The point where the three planes converge is marked with a single spot. The fourth image, placed in the lower right-hand corner of the four-image display, is a surface rendered version of the view initiated from a separate trigger line. After acquisition, the line or spot can be moved by rotation through the x, y, and z axes, allowing the operator to view the four newly created images simultaneously. The good news is that with this type of planar reconstruction one can get views that are often impossible to obtain with standard 2D imagery. The bad news is that the resolution is generally inferior in the B and C planes because lateral and azimuthal resolution are being put into play during the initial acquisition.

Figures 18.1a and 18.1b show how the four standard images are displayed when the same second trimester fetus is investigated using two different acquisition approaches.

Volumes of 3D data can be stored for later manipulation and even transported to remote sites.

The images can be rendered, after the fact, to concentrate on dense tissue, such as bone, through maximum intensity mode, or on soft tissue in the surface rendering mode.

4D is technically a misnomer since there really is no fourth dimension. It refers to 3D in a real-time format. To accomplish this feat, the mechanical array sweeps repetitively through a field, obtaining, currently, at least 6 volumes per second. Since the information is being constantly refreshed, a 3D real-time image will be created. The screen will contain two images, a 2D slice through the area of interest, and the other, a surface rendered image from the plane of the line described above.

The disadvantage is that the image may suffer somewhat from the amount of voxels (3D pixels) making up the picture. The obvious advantage is that one can get remarkable surface rendered views of the fetus in motion (Figure 18.2).

It is likely that by the time this book is published further advances such as convex matrix arrays, involving 8000 separate elements, allowing machines to create 20 or more volumes per second, will be offered by many manufacturers. This will greatly enhance the 4D investigation of the fetal heart.

As indicated above, much already has been written about the brand new 3D and 4D technology, and some of it has the understandable flavor of bias from individuals naturally caught up in the wonder of the technology. I am no different, and am emotionally hooked on the technology to a point where I will engage in hand-to-hand combat with anyone about to take it away. However, I will try to tap my inner objectivity while describing how it offers distinct advantages in some fetal conditions.

Obstetric Ultrasound: Artistry in Practice. John C. Hobbins. Published 2008 Blackwell Publishing. ISBN 978-1-4051-5815-2.

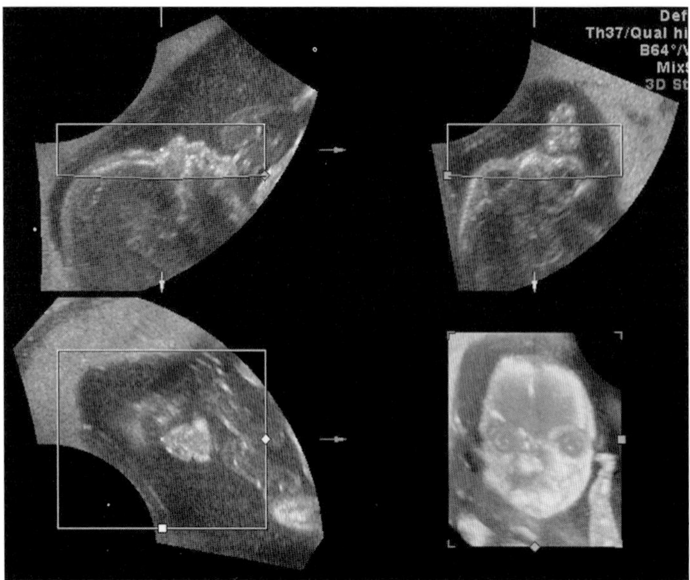

(a)

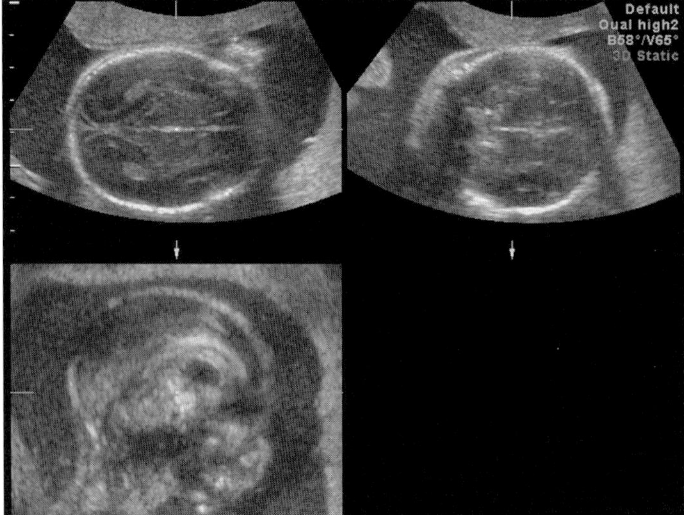

(b)

Fig 18.1 (a) Profile as starting point. (b) Cross-section through plane just above BPD as a starting point.

The face

Cleft lip can be diagnosed with 2D alone, but the clinical impact is dependent upon the extent to which the palate is involved. This is where 3D offers a superior edge. A cleft can involve the alveolar ridge, portions of the hard palate, and/or soft palate. By viewing sequential coronal slices through the face with "thick cuts" in maximum intensity mode, one can generally appreciate the size of the palatal defect. This can be done in the reverse format, as described by Campbell, or in a "flipped" cross-section, as first described to me by Platt and later published by Goncalves and Platt separately (Chapter 6, section "Fetal face"). For this indication, I would rate the worth of 3D as almost essential.

By giving a more graphic picture of a facial defect with 3D, parents can be more adequately prepared for their

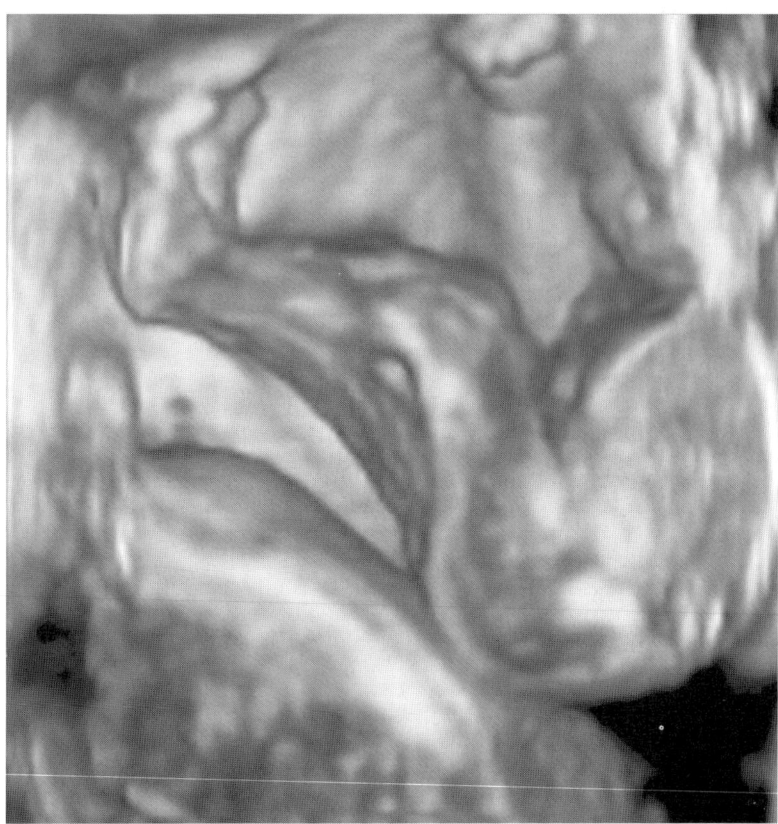

Fig 18.2 A 4D view of limbs in one twin.

babies' appearance at birth, while being counseled that this is the "before" portion of a scenario that has a very different "after" result postsurgery. We have also found 3D pictures to be quite useful in demonstrating to our colleagues in Pediatric Surgery the nature of the defect they will be dealing with after birth.

As Goncalves has indicated in his review, 7 studies have shown 3D to provide useful additional information in fetal lip abnormalities, while in four studies no additional benefit was accrued from 3D.

Intracranial abnormalities

Agenesis of the corpus callosum is a diagnosis that can only be suspected with standard abdominal 2D ultrasound when the fetus is in a vertex presentation. Under these circumstances only axial views of the brain can be obtained. Unfortunately, one needs coronal and/or mid-sagittal views in order to make the definitive diagnosis, and this can only be accomplished with 2D by directing the ultrasound beam through the anterior or posterior fontanelles—a job that can be done best transvaginally in fetuses in a vertex position. However, with 3D planar reconstruction both coronal and mid-sagittal views can be evaluated transabdominally. However, as indicated above, one is forced to employ inferior lateral resolution.

Wang et al. [2] noted an ability to image midline intracranial structures 78% of the time with 3D, compared with only 3% of the time with 2D alone.

The same benefit of 3D can be put into play when evaluating a fetus with partial agenesis of the cerebellar vermis. This also allows the investigator to view the size of the brainstem; something that may reflect the extent of neurological compromise in vermal dysgenesis (Chapter 6).

In spina bifida 3D is extremely useful, but not essential, in pinpointing the location and extent of the spinal defect, through first labeling the spinal bodies using an orthogonal plane to identify the twelfth rib, and then swinging the fetus around in the y-axis to locate the exact position of the defect (Chapter 8).

One study showed an ability to pinpoint the upper level of spinal defects to within one segment of the actual level in eight of nine fetuses, compared with six of the nine fetuses with 2D.

We have found 3D to be invaluable in identifying and quantifying the number of hemivertebra in an affected fetus and to discern the degree of angulation of the spine (Chapter 8).

Also, many skeletal dysplasias involving the limbs can be sorted out with greater ease with surface rendering and 3D planar reconstruction.

The fetal heart

This has been covered in more detail in the segment devoted to the fetal heart, but there is no doubt that, through planar reconstruction, and using STIC (spatial temporal image correlation) technology, a full panel of ideal views of the heart can be obtained, and events within each cardiac cycle can now be thoroughly analyzed. Newer techniques of reversing the color format through "inversion" methods allow all vessels leading into or immediately leaving the heart to be captured and rotated to the examiner's delight (Plate 18.1).

As indicated earlier, it is mainly the job of the initial observer to determine if there simply is something abnormal about the fetal heart. Fine-tuning by someone with special expertise is necessary on some of the more complicated cardiac abnormalities, and this is where all of the newer 3D and 4D technologies can be extremely helpful. However, the standard 2D technology should be sufficient in the first line evaluation of the fetal heart.

3D to increase the efficiency of ultrasound examinations

Benacerraf [3] recently has put forth the idea of using 3D to increase the efficiency of, and throughput for, the basic ultrasound examination. Four or five 3D volume acquisitions are made through the fetus, which will enable off-site evaluation of every aspect of the basic examination through planar reconstruction. This can be done as the patient is being scanned or can be interpreted later on. She and her group have found that the whole diagnostic examination can be condensed into 7.5 minutes versus 19.6 minutes required for the standard examination. She calculated that for 50 patients, the total time-saving with 3D was between 10.3 and 10.8 hours [4]. This has opened up an interesting and controversial debate, because this "conveyor belt" approach, while being more cost-effective, might leave the patient out of the loop by obviating any provider/patient contact, thereby generating unnecessary anxiety until the final interpretation is available.

An attractive spin-off of the above theme is the ability to send volumes through the Internet for interpretation by consultants.

As with any new technology, the risks and benefits need to be soberly examined. To me, the interplay between the health-care professional and the patient (and family) should be an integral part of the examination, and I would hate to see this devalued. Also, an inability to render a diagnosis on the spot would represent a move in the wrong direction from what is currently available in many centers. However, in many high-volume operations and/or situations where large populations need low-cost screening, various modifications of the above method might be implemented effectively.

3D and fetal organ size

Often the difference between life and death for a fetus is dependent upon lung function, which, in turn, is indirectly reflected by the size of the fetal lungs.

A variety of 2D attempts have been made to assess fetal lung size, which include thoracic circumference to abdominal circumference ratio, fetal lung length, lung diameter along the same axis of the interventricular septum, and the thoracic circumference to cardiac parameter relationship (the latter two being accomplished in the plane of the four-chamber view of the heart). However, results from these studies have been inconsistent when predicting neonatal lung function after birth.

With the emergence of 3D many investigators have jumped into the fore with various techniques and formulas for quantifying lung volume. These methods basically have taken three forms: (1) 3D multiplanar techniques requiring the operator to trace around cross-sections of the lungs at different levels within the chest. (2) A method that involves tracing around the lung bases in addition to measuring the height of the right lung. These three measurements are put into a formula that assumes the lungs to be the geometric pyramid. (3) A new method, entitled virtual organ computerized aided analysis (VOCAL), which, although

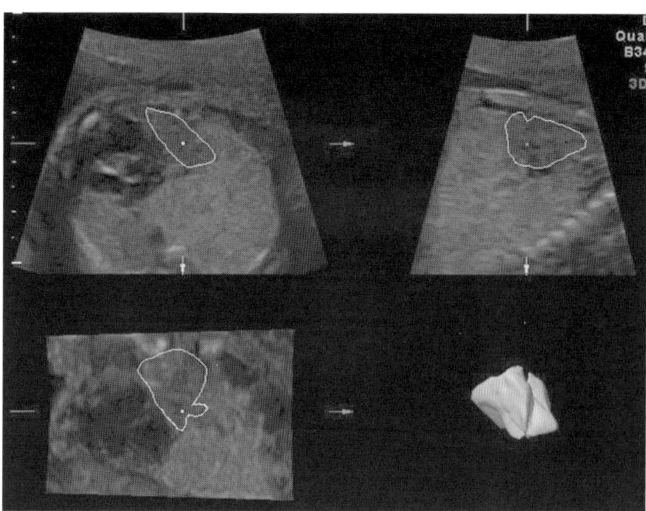

Fig 18.3 VOCAL depiction and quantification of normal lung on the same side as a CAMl.

somewhat cumbersome, allows the investigator to deal with organs that have irregular contours (Figure 18.3). In any case, the few studies available suggest these methods to be comparable to MRI in predicting fetal lung volume [5–7], but more studies are necessary to establish their worth in predicting neonatal pulmonary hypoplasia in prolonged oligohydramnios or diaphragmatic hernias.

Estimated fetal weight (EFW)

Recent attempts have been made to fold 3D measurements into formulas to improve the accuracy of EFW. Following the idea of Jeanty in 1985 [8], some investigators have added thigh volumes and, later, upper arm volumes to other biometric variables in their formulas for EFW, or as stand-alone measurements to accomplish this aim. Rather than review all of these methods, we will cut to the conclusion: limb volume improves the accuracy of EFW.

The latest, and perhaps greatest, method has been recently published by Lee et al. [9]. Their formula involves the use of fractional limb volume (based on length of the diaphysis and perimeter measurements around the "cylinder"), as well as the AC. In 100 fetuses, it was found that the 3D model was superior to 2D methods. In 66% the EFW was within 5% of the true weight with the 3D formula, compared with only 20% falling within 5% of the actual weight with 2D.

As indicated in the section on biometry and IUGR, this represents a distinct improvement in the predictive accuracy of ultrasound, but it does require extra effort and more fancy equipment.

3D, 4D, and maternal–fetal bonding

Years ago, Stuart Campbell [10] reported that mothers seeing an ultrasound image of their fetuses smoked fewer cigarettes and consumed fewer alcoholic beverages than mothers who were not shown images of their fetuses during the ultrasound examinations. The conclusion was that this altered behavior as a result of enhanced bonding.

With the advent of 3D and 4D, it became clear that the new technology could have an even greater effect on maternal attachment. However, the challenge involved how to test objectively for this behavior. The group in San Diego [11] has been involved with 3D from its inception, and last year they reported some soft findings suggesting a benefit of 4D in bonding. Eighty-two percent of those having 3D were able to get a better mental image of their fetuses, compared with 39% with 2D alone. Also, the 3D group was more prone to share their fetal pictures with others than those having 2D.

Unfortunately, bonding is difficult to nail down. An Italian group [12] randomized 100 patients to 2D or 3D and found no difference in the numbers of mothers with positive responses to the examination. They used a tool often cited in the psychology literature, maternal automated attachment scale (MAAS), to study bonding and found that in a small cohort of the above patients (46) there were no differences between patients having 2D alone and those in whom 3D was added. The study slowed down the bonding bandwagon.

The last study to surface emanates from Australia. Sedgmen et al. [13] randomized 68 patients to have 2D or 3D examinations at 12 and 18 weeks of gestation. Not all in this study had both. The participants were given two sets of questionnaires (one prescan and the other postscan), which allowed MAAS and maternal perception tools to be folded into the analysis, as well as in the evaluation of maternal behavior. The results indicated that having an ultrasound, in general, enhanced attachment, with the greater benefit stemming from the first trimester examination. The ultrasound exposure also resulted in a decrease in the number of alcoholic beverages consumed per week. The surprising part (to some) was that there were no differences in any of the categories between 2D and 3D methods.

In a companion editorial, Campbell [14] pointed out that 4D might well have had a more dramatic effect on women in the study than 3D alone, had it been used, and he even suggested that the quality of the 3D fetal image the authors used in their publication might not enhance any woman's ability to bond.

While many providers have latched onto the concept of maternal attachment as a reason to add 4D to every examination (and some have even used this rationale to justify nonmedical 3D and 4D activities), there are at least as many naysayers who cite a lack of evidence of its merit, and even question its safety in this setting. Although this will be discussed in a segment below on keepsake videos, I think that a minute or two of "warm and fuzzy" 4D ultrasound, offered gratis, at the end of each indicated ultrasound examination, will do wonders for maternal attachment and for patient, family, and operator enjoyment. If done routinely, it just might put the "keepsake industry" out of business.

References

1 Goncalves L, Lee W, Espinosa J, et al. Three- and 4-dimensional ultrasound in obstetric practice: does it help? J Ultrasound Med 2005; 24: 1599–624.

2 Wang PH, Ying TH, Wang PC, et al. Obstetrical three-dimensional ultrasound in the visualization of the intracranial midline in corpus callosum of fetuses in cephalic presentation. Prenat Diagn 2000; 20: 518–20.

3 Benacerraf BR, Shipp TD, Bromley B. Improving the efficiency of gynecologic sonography with 3-dimensional volumes: a pilot study. J Ultrasound Med 2006; 25: 165–71.

4 Benacerraf BR, Shipp TD, Bromley B. How sonographic tomography will change the face of fetal ultrasound: a pilot study. J Ultrasound Med 2005: 24: 371–8.

5 Ruano R, Joubin L, Sonigo P, et al. Fetal lung volume estimated by 3-dimensional ultrasonography and magnetic resonance imaging in cases with isolated congenital diaphragmatic hernia. J Ultrasound Med 2004; 23: 353–8.

6 Kalache KD, Espinoza J, Chaiworapongsa T, et al. Three-dimensional ultrasound fetal lung volume measurement: a systematic study comparing the multiplanar method with the rotational (VOCAL) technique. Ultrasound Obstet Gynecol 2003; 21: 111–8.

7 Moeglin D, Talmant C, Dyme M, et al. Fetal lung volumetry using two- and three-dimensional ultrasound. Ultrasound Obstet Gynecol 2005; 25: 119–27.

8 Jeanty P, Romero R, Hobbins JC. Fetal limb volume: a new parameter to assess fetal growth and nutrition. J Ultrasound Med 1985; 4: 273–82.

9 Lee W, Deter R, Ebersole JD, et al. Birth weight prediction by three-dimensional ultrasonography: fractional limb volume. J Ultrasound Med 2001; 20: 1283–92.

10 Campbell S, Reading AE, Cox DN, et al. Ultrasound scanning in pregnancy: the short term psychological effects of early real time scans. J Psychosom Obstet Gynaecol 1982; 1: 57–61.

11 Ji EK, Pretorius DH, Newton R, et al. Effects of ultrasound on maternal-fetal bonding: a comparison of two- and three-dimensional imaging. Ultrasound Obstet Gynecol 2005; 25: 473–7.

12 Rustico MA, Mastromatteo C, Grigio M, et al. Two-dimensional vs. two- plus four-dimensional ultrasound in pregnancy and the effect on maternal emotional status: a randomized study. Ultrasound Obstet Gynecol 2005; 25: 468–72.

13 Sedgmen B, McMahon C, Cairns D, et al. The impact of two-dimensional versus three-dimensional ultrasound exposure on maternal-fetal attachment and maternal health behavior in pregnancy. Ultrasound Obstet Gynecol 2006; 27: 245–51.

14 Campbell S. 4D and prenatal bonding: still more questions than answers. Ultrasound Obstet Gynecol 2006; 27: 243–4.

19 The safety of ultrasound

About twice a week, we are asked about the safety of ultrasound. Either the patient or her partner is concerned about the effect of this type of energy on their fetus. Often providers cannot generate specific answers to these questions other than to state, "there is no evidence that it is unsafe." This will satisfy some readers of childbirth magazines in which the wonders of ginger and St. John's wort are extolled and the dangers of ultrasound are "exposed." However, others push further for more concrete evidence. Although the above-condensed statement is true, I am covering the subject in a little more detail to help in responding to those who want (and should have) more.

First, a few words about ultrasound physics. Electrical energy is converted to mechanical energy in the form of sound waves by intermittently pulsing current across elements in the transducer made of a piezoelectric material. This results in pulses of ultrasound that are extremely short in length and, because they need time to pass through tissue and return to the same element that sent them out, the time interval between pulses is quite long. This means that the time spent emitting, compared with the time spent "listening" (the duty cycle) is analogous to about 1 part "on" to 1000 parts "off".

The "gain" function on the keyboard deals only with returning sound waves, which are amplified in an effort to counter the normal dissipation of sound in tissue. However, the "output" or "power" function represents a way to muscle in more energy on the front end by increasing the intensity of the ultrasound.

The intensity produced by the elements in the transducer is measured at the apex of the pulse wave as "peak pulse intensity," and the average intensity over time is referred to as the "spatial peak temporal average (SPTA)." For example, if the peak pulse intensity, captured at the ideal focal distance from the transducer, is 10 W/cm^2, then, based on a duty cycle of 1 to 1000, the above figure is divided by 1000 to yield an SPTA at the center of interest of 10 mW/cm^2.

There are two known pathways through which ultrasound can have a biological effect at very high intensities:

1 Through cavitation, which is dependent upon the peak pulse intensity and is likely a one-cycle event.

2 Through a rise in tissue temperature, which is related more to average intensities over time (an SPTA effect).

Sonographers/sonologists can monitor peak pulse intensities by referring to the mechanical index (MI), displayed now on every ultrasound monitor. Average intensities are displayed on some machines as a thermal index (TI). This occasionally is broken down into the TI in bone and the TI in soft tissue. The goal should be to use the lowest power (intensity) required to get images of acceptable quality. This ALARA principle of keeping power "as low as is reasonably achievable" (to get an adequate image) should be the motto of everyone using ultrasound. Unfortunately, my impression is that not only do many users not understand what the ALARA principle means, but they are unaware that MI and TI generally should not exceed 1.0, unless there are special circumstances where you need it (generally related to obesity).

Within the AIUM is a watchdog group, the AIUM Bioeffects Committee, which is composed of sober scientists who undertake an ongoing review of the literature on the bioeffects of ultrasound. Many years ago, the committee issued a statement, which I will paraphrase. It indicated that there was no independently confirmed evidence of bioeffect in clinical practice or in an experimental setting when ultrasound was delivered at diagnostic power levels (below SPTAs of 100 mW/cm^2). Since then, the committee has revamped the wording somewhat, but the bottom line is still the same. The addition of the words "independently confirmed" indicates that a few in vitro experiments have shown bioeffect at diagnostic dosage, but other investigators have been unable to reproduce the results of these studies.

Two types of clinical studies have shown differences between infants exposed to ultrasound in utero and

Obstetric Ultrasound: Artistry in Practice. John C. Hobbins. Published 2008 Blackwell Publishing. ISBN 978-1-4051-5815-2.

controls. In an investigation from Norway [1], representing a spin-off of randomized trials to evaluate the efficacy of routine ultrasound, it was noted that there was a higher rate of left handedness in children exposed to ultrasound in utero, more specifically, males, in whom the chances of being left handed was 5% greater than in the overall population. The authors suggested that this might represent evidence of an effect of ultrasound on neuronal migration. Perhaps this idea should not be shared with the lefties out there who have been told by their parents that being one of the 15% lucky enough to be left handed puts them in the same category as some of the most creative individuals in history.

It is of interest that in these Norwegian randomized trials [2] many other endpoints were evaluated, all of which showed no difference in any outcome variable between ultrasound exposed infants and controls, and the above finding should not be a surprise statistically when so many dependent variables were tested.

The only other clinical study showing a difference between those exposed to ultrasound versus controls emanated from Australia [3]. One group of patients had serial Dopplers to determine if using umbilical cord waveforms enhanced perinatal outcome. The group having ultrasound had, on average, infants that weighed 25 g less than controls. Many of the patients in this study had multiple Doppler examinations and, although peak pulse intensities are not increased with Doppler, the SPTAs are appreciably higher because the pulses must be longer in order to appreciate a change in frequency. This results in a change in the duty cycle with more time "on" and less time "off." The point here is that if this small difference in infant weight is of any significance, it may be due to the fetuses in the study being exposed to higher average intensities repetitively over time; something that is not applicable to most clinical situations, especially where only 2D and 3D are used.

The authors [4] recently followed up 2714 children involved in the above study up until 8 years of age to see if there was still a difference in their size and their ability to meet various milestones. They then found no difference after one year in physical size between those exposed to repetitive Doppler ultrasounds in utero and those who were not after 1 year. Also, there were no differences in groups regarding speech, language, behavior, and neurological development.

Just before this manuscript was submitted for publication, a study [5] appeared which I am including for completeness. Obviously, it has not yet been explored by other investigators. It involved exposing pregnant mice to diagnostic dosages of ultrasound for variable amounts of time. Some of the offspring having lengthy exposure to ultrasound had up to 10% reduction in brain cells.

This study got the attention of the lay press and sparked questions about whether ultrasound might be interfering with neuronal migration. However, scientists and clinicians pointed out that the experiment in no way mimicked a standard ultrasound examination in the human. In this study, the animals were exposed to continuous ultrasound for up to 50 hours and the size of the animals required that the distance between the transducer and the fetuses be reduced to a point where there was little dissipation of ultrasound intensities. Last, none of the animals had any reduction in brain cells until the continuous exposure had exceeded 30 minutes, a situation that was not analogous to a typical clinical examination, where the transducer is rarely kept in the same area for more than a few seconds at a time. Nevertheless, the wide dissemination of the results of this study did mobilize the medical community to comment again about the prudent use of ultrasound.

It is important to point out that there is no compelling in vitro, fetal animal or human clinical investigation that has shown a bioeffect of ultrasound used at diagnostic dosage.

Does this mean that there is proof that it is incontrovertibly safe? No, and that is why we should use it prudently, as indicated by the AIUM and the FDA [6–8].

References

1 Salvesen KA, Vatten LJ, Eik-Nes SH, et al. Routine ultrasonography in utero and subsequent handedness and neurological development. BMJ 1993; 307: 159–64.

2 Salvesen KA, Eik-Nes SH. Ultrasound during pregnancy and subsequent childhood non-right handedness: a meta-analysis. Ultrasound Obstet Gynecol 1999; 13: 241–6.

3 Newnham JP, Evans SF, Michael CA, et al. Effects of frequent ultrasound during pregnancy: a randomized controlled trial. Lancet 1993; 342: 887–91.

4 Newnham JP, Doherty DA, Kendall GE, et al. Effects of repeated prenatal ultrasound examinations on childhood outcome up to 8 years of age: follow-up of a randomized controlled trial. Lancet 2004; 364: 2038–44.

5 Ang ES Jr, Gluncic V, Duque A, et al. Prenatal exposure to ultrasound waves impacts neuronal migration in mice. Proc Natl Acad Sci USA 2006; 103: 12903–10.

6 AIUM Practice Guidelines for the Performance of an Antepartum Obstetric Ultrasound Examination. Laurel, MD: American Institute of Ultrasound in Medicine; 2007; 1–13.

7 AIUM Official Statement: Prudent Use and Clinical Safety. Laurel, MD: American Institute of Ultrasound in Medicine; Approved March 19, 2007.

8 AIUM Official Statement: Limited Obstetrical Ultrasound. Laurel, MD: American Institute of Ultrasound in Medicine; Approved October 7, 1997.

20 The biophysical profile (BPP)

In 1980, Manning and Platt [1] fashioned a method for fetal surveillance in high-risk pregnancies that combine fetal heart rate monitoring with various ultrasound derived variables. Modeled after the Apgar score, 2 points were awarded in each of the five categories for reassuring results and no points for a nonreassuring result. A total score of 8 or 10 was indicative of a fetus that was not in trouble and a score of 6 or less was cause for some concern.

Each of the five categories represented a separate mini-evaluation of fetal behavior or function.

Fetal heart rate monitoring

The nonstress test (NST) involves monitoring the fetal heart rate over a 20-minute period. It involves the ability of the hypothalamus and the medulla to maintain a variable, rather than a smooth, baseline and to increase the heart rate when fetal movement occurs. This represents a sophisticated function of the brain that puts into play higher centers. Newer techniques with computerization, used more commonly in Europe, can quantify subtle changes in baseline beat-to-beat variability, but the classic NST interpretation depends upon the fetal heart rate to rise by 15 beats per minute over a 15-second time period, at least twice during the 20-minute observation period. If it does, 2 points are given, and if one or none are seen during this time, no points are awarded. Hypoxia, or really acidemia, will cause the heart rate to smooth out due to its effect on the CNS.

Fetal breathing

After 30 weeks of gestation, the fetus will spend about 30% of his/her time making breathing motions through action generated in the ventral surface of the fourth ventricle. Prolonged hypoxia and/or acidemia will blunt this activity. Fetuses having at least one episode of 30 seconds of fetal breathing during an observation period of up to 20 minutes will get two points, with no points going to those who do not.

Fetal movement

The fetal cortex generates the messages for the fetus to move his/her arms, legs, and trunk, and profound hypoxia and acidemia will stop this from happening. Two points go to the fetus who has at least three trunk movements during this observation period. Anything less than that results in zero points.

Fetal tone

Fetal tone, which is dependent upon an intact cortex and subcortex, is the last to go in a sequence of events ending in severe fetal compromise. Basically, the assessment of tone is predicated on the fetus' ability to flex and extend his/her hands or limbs. One episode of extension with a return to flexion during the examination period should suffice to garner two points. Although, in the original description flexion and extension of the spine was required, this is something most clinicians have abandoned as a requisite. Actually, fetal tone is the least useful variable since, by the time tone is lost, all of the other categories will have had scores of zero (unless the fetus has a primary neuromuscular disorder).

Amniotic fluid assessment

As indicated in the chapter on amniotic fluid, the original definition of oligohydramnios by Platt and Manning was the absence of a pocket of fluid of at least 1 cm in any vertical plane. This requirement has been loosened to one

Obstetric Ultrasound: Artistry in Practice. John C. Hobbins. Published 2008 Blackwell Publishing. ISBN 978-1-4051-5815-2.

2-cm pocket, for which two points are awarded, and below which no points are given. Some centers have converted over from the vertical pocket definition to an AFI of <6 cm (for a score of zero).

The amniotic fluid category relates only indirectly to the fetal brain, which, under the influence of hypoxia, will be "spared," resulting in blood being shunted away from the kidneys. This results in less urine production and, ultimately, oligohydramnios. The oligohydramnios seen in postterm pregnancy may represent an exception to the brain sparing concept. Here there is evidence to suggest that there may be a direct effect on the kidneys, rather than a stealing mechanism employed by the brain.

How the BPP relates to fetal behavior

The fetal brain develops in a very predictable order with the brainstem, medullary, and subcortical areas developing first, and the cortical areas and hypothalamus being refined last. Under the influence of progressive hypoxia, the characteristic behavior patterns linked to these portions of the brain are lost in reverse order from their appearance in the developmental time line. For example, the NST becomes nonreactive and the respirations are lost at roughly the same level of partial pressure of oxygen (PO_2) in the fetal blood. However, fetal movement slows and stops at a lower PO_2. The last to be affected is fetal tone, which from my standpoint is superfluous, since by the time tone is lost, so are all of the other variables.

Before discussing the data on the efficacy of the BPP, it is important to touch upon the concept of fetal sleep states and their effect on fetal behavior—specifically on fetal heart rate, respirations, and movement.

Although many investigators have contributed to our knowledge of fetal behavior, John Patrick was the one who used ultrasound continuously for many hours to correlate fetal heart rate changes with fetal respirations and movement in an effort to correlate these outward manifestations with fetal sleep states [2].

There are four fetal sleep states, 1F through 4F. Sleep state 1F represents quiet sleep, during which time the fetus moves little, breathes infrequently, and has a heart rate that is generally devoid of significant accelerations. Toward term the fetus spends about 25–30% of the time in sleep state 1F.

State 2F represents a period of active rapid eye movement sleep during which time the fetus actively moves, breathes, has increased beat-to-beat variability of the heart rate, and displays heart rate accelerations. This occupies about 60–70% of the fetus's time in late pregnancy.

Both 3F, representing "quiet awake sleep," and 4F, or "active awake sleep," comprise only 3% of the fetus's activity and are not worth further mention.

The BPP is affected by the two major sleep states. For example, NSTs are often nonreactive during quiet sleep and respirations and movement are normally depressed during this time. This is why one often has to be patient while performing a BPP. Patrick found that quiet sleep usually does not last more than 20 minutes (this is why the testing length of 20 minutes was initially chosen), but an occasional mellow, yet normal, fetus can frustrate the observer for more than 40 minutes. The trick is to monitor the fetus's heart rate first and the minute it is clear that the fetus is in active sleep (2F), by the demonstration of increased variability, to then move to the ultrasound portion of the test.

It is important to mention that factors other than hypoxia will affect the variables in the BPP. For example, various drugs such as narcotics, tranquilizers, alcohol, and cigarettes will depress fetal heart rate variability, respirations, and movement, while maternal hyperglycemia will increase fetal movement and respirations. In fact, if we see a large-for-dates fetus who seems to be breathing throughout the entire observation window (and throw in body-to-head disproportion, a large bladder, and generous amniotic fluid), we will explore, or re-explore, that mother's glucose tolerance.

A word about the use of acoustic or vibratory stimulators. Many of my colleagues, whom I respect, are enamored of this type of stimulation to shorten the length of BPPs in fetuses engaged in prolonged quiet sleep. However, I am philosophically opposed to this. The acoustic stimulator is essentially an artificial larynx that generates mixed frequency sound at rather high intensities. If you want to see an adult display a Morrow reflex, just walk behind some unsuspecting person and "buzz" him/her with this gadget. The vibratory method is a somewhat kinder, gentler approach, but this can create fetal hyperactivity for *many* minutes. I never have been impatient enough to use one.

The efficacy of the BPP

The NST, by itself, is a very reasonable excluder of fetal jeopardy. In large studies, the perinatal mortality rate in patients with reactive NSTs is 3–5 per 1000, while perinatal morbidity is 22% in nonreactive NSTs versus 5% in reactive NSTs. The false positive rate is quite high, ranging from 44 to 90% for a nonreactive NST [3]. If the test is continued for 80 minutes, the negative predictive and positive predictive values rise appreciably. However, with such a high false positive rate it makes sense to move to a test with more variables not only to save fetuses from unnecessary intervention, but to save time.

One of the most interesting studies came from Vintzileos, a prolific investigator, and colleagues [4] who correlated BPP findings with umbilical cord pH at birth, which backs up the "gradual hypoxia" concept. Breathing was lost at a pH of <7.20, while all movement and tone were gone at a pH of <7.10.

Manning found that the four ultrasound components of the BPP performed as well as the NST portion of the test, suggesting that maybe the time-consuming fetal heart rate monitoring portion of the BPP could be deleted.

The "modified BPP" also came into being as a pragmatic substitute for the full BPP. It consists of an NST and an evaluation of amniotic fluid. The NST assesses the fetus for acute hypoxia, and the amniotic fluid speaks for the chorionicity of a problem. Miller et al. [5] found a false positive rate of 60% with this test, but a 0.08% false negative rate (with regard to perinatal death).

My problem, as indicated in the chapter on amniotic fluid, is that the precise diagnosis of oligohydramnios is elusive, and, if it is isolated in a preterm baby, there is no evidence in the recent literature to mandate delivering these normal babies into newborn special care units where they will stay for many days.

Last, I have been caught up with the use of Doppler in IUGR, and how it makes physiologic sense in monitoring fetal well being, to a point where I had almost written off the BPP as a useful adjunctive tool in this condition. However, Baschat [6] has convinced me with his longitudinal IUGR studies that the BPP brings another modality (the fetal CNS) to the diagnostic table that has independent value.

References

1 Manning FA, Platt LD, Sipos L. Antepartum fetal evaluation: development of a fetal biophysical profile. Am J Obstet Gynecol 1980; 136: 787–95.

2 Patrick J, Carmichael L, Chess L, et al. Accelerations of the human fetal heart rate at 38 to 40 weeks' gestational age. Am J Obstet Gynecol 1984; 148: 35–41.

3 Hanley ML, Vintzileos AM. Antepartum and intrapartum surveillance of fetal well-being. In: Reece EA, Hobbins JC (eds.), *Medicine of the Fetus and Mother*, 2nd ed. Philadelphia, PA: Lippincott-Raven Publishers, 1999.

4 Vintzileos AM, Fleming AD, Scorza WE, et al. Relationship between fetal biophysical activities and umbilical cord blood gas values. Am J Obstet Gynecol 1991; 165: 707–13.

5 Miller DA, Rabello YA, Paul RH. The modified biophysical: antepartum testing in the 1990's. Am J Obstet Gynecol 1996; 174: 812–7.

6 Baschat AA, Galan HL, Bhide A, et al. Doppler and biophysical assessment in growth restricted fetuses: distribution of results. Ultrasound Obstet Gynecol 2006; 27: 41–7.

21 Ultrasound on the labor and delivery floor

Ultrasound is an indispensable tool on the labor and delivery floor. In most hospitals, the machine that is found on most delivery suites is a hand-me-down from another service, scavenged when a newer model has rendered the one eventually relegated to the labor floor obsolete. Frankly, beggars cannot be choosers, and the common clinical questions that need answering in the laboring patient do not require overly sophisticated equipment. In fact, portability may be a more important feature than image quality. On our labor and delivery floor we wheel these machines in and out of birthing rooms at least 15 times per day.

In this chapter, I have chosen only a few of many conditions encountered on most labor and delivery floors where ultrasound can provide an invaluable service to the managing clinician.

Fetal presentation and position

Most clinicians pride themselves on their ability to use their hands in determining fetal presentation and position. However, occasionally even very experienced physicians and nurse midwives are surprised to find that the fetus they initially thought to be in the vertex presentation wound up being a breech, after many hours of labor. Most often, this surprise happens in obese patients where in some cases it is almost impossible to tell which fetal pole is in the pelvis. The simplest 30-second transabdominal ultrasound examination will identify the exact location of the head, heart, and breech.

Similarly, although fetal presentation is much easier to assess with a digital examination, it is not unusual to be completely fooled regarding the position of the head. There is not a clinician out there who has not put forceps on a fetal head, thinking that the position was a left occiput anterior (LOA), only to realize that the head actually had been in the right occiput posterior (ROP) position when the fetus came out of the pelvis, staring straight up at the mortified operator.

This setup for maternal trauma is usually the result of difficulty in distinguishing on digital examination the anterior fontanelle from the posterior fontanelle (a "V" from a "Y"); especially when there is a significant caput, which we have quantified on occasion with transperineal ultrasound to be 3- to 4-cm thick.

Again, a simple transabdominal ultrasound scan will tell the caregiver where the fetal eyes are located, as well as about the rotation of the head, so that an ROP should not be mistaken for an LOA.

Placental position

This subject has been covered in Chapter 2, but the importance of knowing the position of the placenta needs to be particularly underscored in this segment on the use of ultrasound in the laboring patient. Fortunately, it is relatively rare for a clinician to put his/her finger through a previa or low-lying placenta, but performing a limited transabdominal ultrasound on every patient on admission would alert the clinician to the possibility of an undiagnosed placenta previa. Also, a malpresentation, a lower segment fibroid, or oligo- or polyhydramnios could be identified. In addition, we have found that identifying the location of the fetal heart (especially in an obese patient) helps in the placement of the fetal heart rate monitor.

Obstetric Ultrasound: Artistry in Practice. John C. Hobbins. Published 2008 Blackwell Publishing. ISBN 978-1-4051-5815-2.

Vaginal birth after cesarean section

As indicated earlier, the cesarean section rate has skyrocketed in recent years to 29% in the USA at last count. As the primary cesarean section rate rises, so does the repeat cesarean section rate, since many patients and their providers are unwilling to try for a vaginal birth after cesarean section (VBAC). However, a recent study shows that over 75% of attempted VBACs will succeed and the risk of uterine rapture is low. Macones et al. [1] reviewed 4 years worth of data from 11 centers in the United States and found that the uterine rupture rate in VBACs was about 1%. In those who had a successful vaginal birth prior to the VBAC, the uterine rupture rate is closer to 0.5%.

Recent attention has been directed to identifying patients with cesarean scars who are at greater risk of uterine rupture. Two studies that have shed important light on this subject have focused on the width of the uterine wall in the vicinity of the uterine scar. In a study from Japan [2] the authors evaluated the lower uterine segment wall thickness just under the bladder flap in patients about to have attempted VBACs. They found that if the thinnest diameter was 2 mm or less, there was a 30% risk of uterine rupture. Conversely, if the diameter exceeded 2.9 mm, no uterine ruptures occurred.

In another study [3] involving 642 patients, the same technique was used to assess the wall thickness before attempted VBAC. The unique wrinkle in this study is that the ultrasound examinations were undertaken by a single practitioner. The results indicated that the critical cut-off point for uterine rupture was a wall thickness of 3.5 mm, below which there was a 20-fold greater risk for uterine rupture and above which there was a 99% negative predictive value for uterine rupture. If the wall thickness was between 1.6 and 2.5 mm, a scar defect ultimately was found in 16% of these patients. Later, they used the 3.5 mm cut-off in a prospective trial in which managing physicians were given the uterine wall information and, although those with thin measurements were sectioned more frequently, the overall uterine rupture rate decreased appreciably.

Some investigators have suggested that the transvaginal route is more precise in measuring uterine wall thickness at the level of the old scar. However, we have found it sometimes difficult to get to the area in question through the vaginal route when there is enough urine in the bladder to identify the appropriate region and to outline the upper margin of the uterine wall.

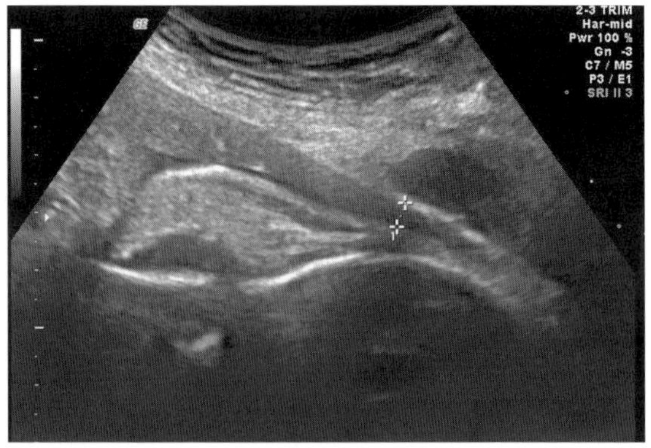

Fig 21.1 Uterine wall thickness. Measurement is made in area of old scar.

Others had invoked various scoring systems based on the past obstetrical history, the ripeness of the cervix, estimated fetal size, etc., in an effort to predict success of an attempted VBAC, in addition to the chances of uterine rupture. The above uterine wall technique could be used alone or in conjunction with these clinical guidelines.

The transabdominal method involves focusing on the lower uterine segment underneath the bladder flap (with some urine in the bladder) in the mid-sagittal plane and magnifying the image so that the anterior wall and bladder in the area of the cesarean scar occupy about one-third of the screen. The transducer is moved sagittally back and forth at the same level until the thinnest segment of the uterine wall is visualized. The clear space is measured with the calipers resting on the outer borders of myometrium (Figure 21.1).

Use of ultrasound in the patient having a cesarean section

"Be prepared" should be the credo of the clinician about to do a cesarean section, since sometimes there are structures between the patient's skin and the uterine cavity that can present difficulties, when traversed. For example, the placenta and pelvic varicosities can bleed copiously when the pathway to the fetus goes through them. The problem is compounded if the patient has a placenta accreta. By being forewarned, the clinician will know the diameter of the placenta to be traversed, and what approach to use in expeditiously extracting the fetus. On occasion, we have tailor-made an incision (often vertical) to avoid the placenta in patients in whom a tubal ligation (to follow) will prevent further pregnancies, or to shade one side or the

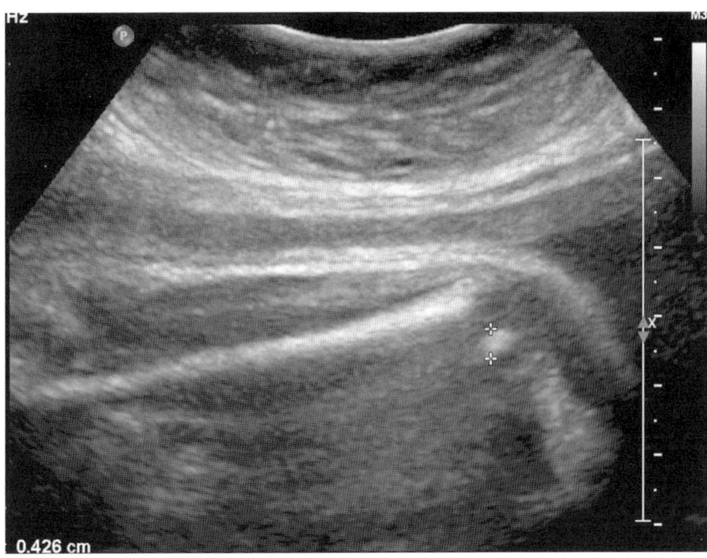

Fig 21.2 DFE measurement.

other when doing a transverse incision. This can be done in the operating room immediately before prepping the patient, or by applying the transducer (in a sterile sleeve) to the uterus, once the abdomen has been entered.

Certainly, the cord insertion should be located in the unlucky situation where the insertion site is along the prospective pathway of the scalpel—a rare potential disaster.

Last, in morbidly obese patients, one always wonders what type of incision to use. Since the low transverse skin incision is prone to infection, because it rarely sees the light of day in the postpartum period, many have advocated the paramedian approach where the incision is made above the major portion of the panniculus.

I have found that with ultrasound one can easily find the shortest distance between the skin and the uterus in these patients, and, with a magic marker, one can map out on the abdomen an approach that will allow the most direct access to the uterine cavity and also will avoid going through the skin twice—something I did many years ago by going through the folded-over pannus. This "he did what?" story circulated around the delivery floor far longer than I think it deserved.

The use of ossification centers in predicting gestational age and maturity

The distal femoral epiphysis (DFE) is rarely seen with ultrasound before 33 weeks, when it appears as a thin disk-like collection of echoes. By 36 weeks, it becomes a thick echogenic spot, which is seen just below the end of the ossified shaft of the femur. Using the axial resolution, one can precisely measure the thickness of this epiphyseal center in the north/south axis (Figure 21.2).

The proximal tibial epiphysis (PTE) is rarely seen before 36 weeks, when it appears as an echogenic dot at the proximal end of the tibial shaft (Figure 21.3). The last long bone epiphysis to appear in utero is the proximal humeral epiphysis, which rarely shows up before 37 weeks.

These observations can be used to advantage in unregistered patients entering the labor and delivery suite with little or no documentation of dating. Not infrequently the average ultrasound age is discordant with the patient's dates and often in the late or no care patients, there are no reliable dates. When the fetus is smaller than expected, the epiphyseal centers can help in deciding whether to stop labor, if the fetus appears to be premature, or even to induce labor if the fetus is growth restricted.

Let's take a typical scenario occurring at least once every few days on a busy labor and delivery service. The patient enters in preterm labor with a history of being 37 weeks by menstrual dates alone. The average ultrasound age is determined to be 33 weeks, but a thick DFE is seen and a PTE is visualized. The fetus most likely is mature and perhaps growth restricted. This would also suggest the patient's dates to be correct, and there would be no need to stop her labor.

On the other hand, if the DFE is absent, or appears as only a thin echogenic wisp, it is likely that the patient's

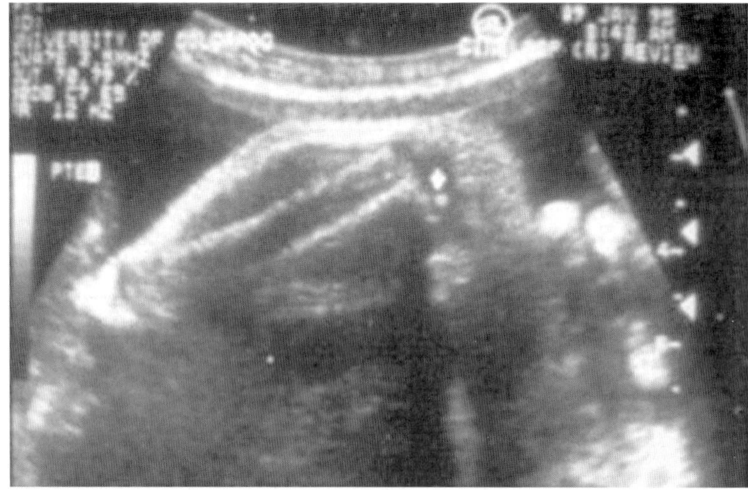

Fig 21.3 Proximal tibial epiphysis.

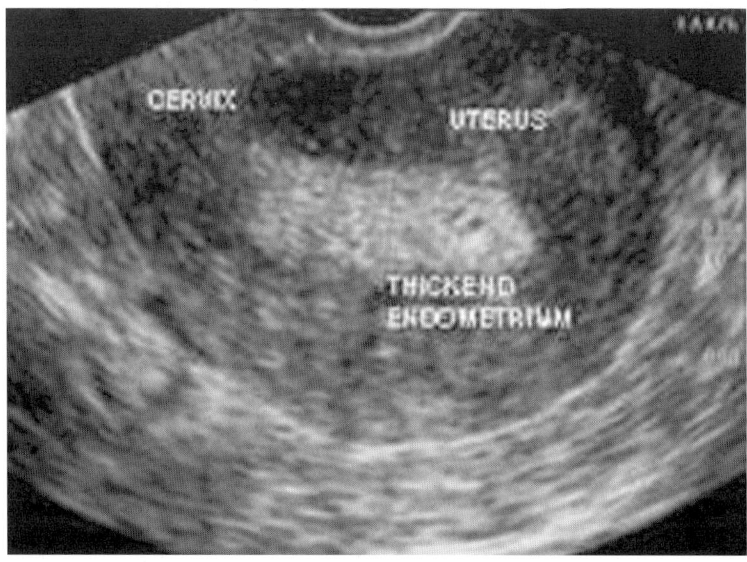

Fig 21.4 Retained placenta.

dates are not valid and the fetus is premature. Under these circumstances, an attempt might be made to stop labor, at least long enough to get steroids on board (if the fetus now seems to be less than 34 weeks).

The epiphyseal centers can also indirectly tell us about the pulmonic maturity of the fetus. Back in 1988, Goldstein et al. [4] from our group published a study to correlate DFEs of 4 mm or more with pulmonic maturity. Patients having amniocenteses for L/S ratios prior to induction or cesarean section had preprocedure ultrasounds to quantify DFEs. In nondiabetics a DFE of 4 mm or more had a 100% correlation with an L/S ratio of >3, a well-established threshold for pulmonic maturity. However, all bets were off for diabetics, since over 20% of the time their L/S ratios were immature in the face of a DFE equal to or greater than >4 mm.

Amniocentesis is not without risk, is uncomfortable, and is often unnecessary in the majority of cases where clinicians feel they need to document fetal pulmonic maturity before inducing labor or performing an elective cesarean section. For this reason, it is surprising that no contemporary investigation has been channeled in this

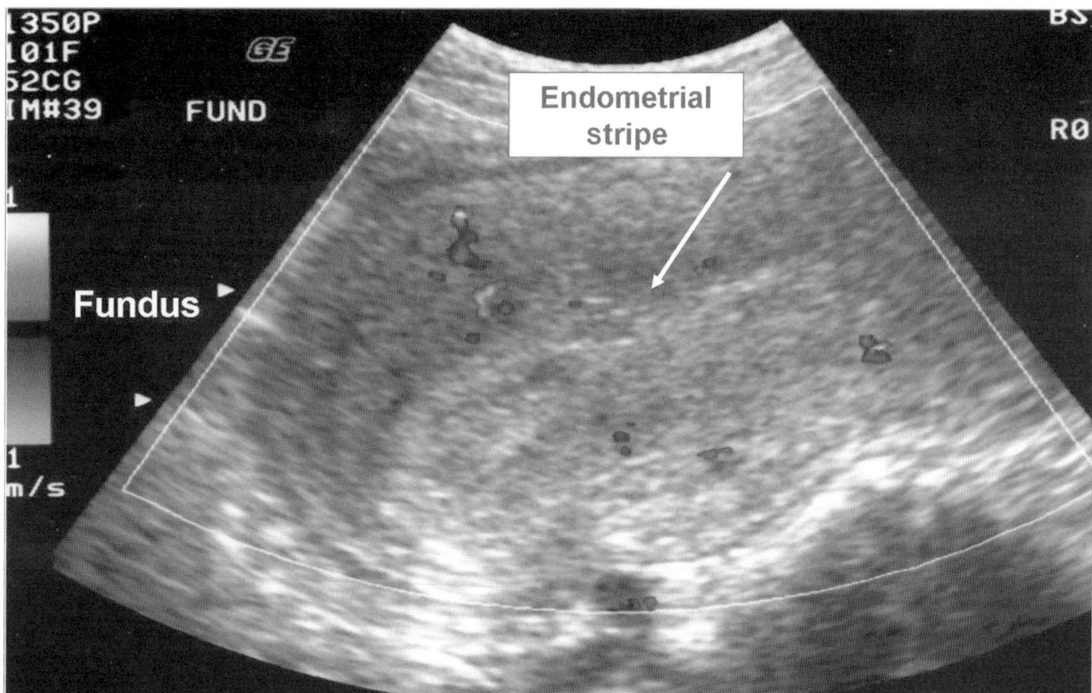

Fig 21.5 Clean uterus.

direction. Our Colorado group has just launched a twenty-first century version of the above study.

Postpartum hemorrhage

This is another area where ultrasound has been particularly useful. Before taking these patients to the operating room for a D and C, a quick transabdominal ultrasound examination will either identify retained tissue in the uterus (Figure 21.4) or a clean cavity (Figure 21.5), which will assure the clinician that the cause of the bleeding is not the presence of retained placental products. If the cavity is empty, an uncomfortable, often anesthesia-requiring, sometimes risky, and totally unnecessary, procedure can be averted. If tissue is found, then gentle removal of the remaining placental tissue can be accomplished under ultrasound guidance quickly and safely.

References

1 Macones GA, Cahill AG, Stamilio DM, et al. Can uterine rupture in patients attempting vaginal birth after cesarean delivery be predicted? Am J Obstet Gynecol 2006; 195: 1148–52.

2 Gotoh H, Masuzaki H, Yoshida A, et al. Predicting incomplete uterine rupture with vaginal sonography during the late second trimester in women with prior Cesarean. Obstet Gynecol 2000; 95: 596–600.

3 Rozenberg P, Goffinet F, Philippe HJ, et al. Ultrasonographic measurement of lower uterine segment to assess risk of defects of scarred uterus. Lancet 1996; 347: 281–4.

4 Goldstein I, Lockwood CJ, Reece EA, et al. Sonographic assessment of the distal femoral and proximal tibial ossification centers in the prediction of pulmonic maturity in normal women and women with diabetes. Am J Obstet Gynecol 1988; 159: 72–6.

22 The Hobbins take on various hot topics

This section contains a mixture of issues, some of which are highly charged, that involve every individual working in the field of obstetrical sonography. My "takes" on each subject will be mine alone and do not necessarily represent the opinions of the publisher, my colleagues, any manufacturer, or either the Democratic or Republican parties. However, I will go on the record that my wife, a nurse-midwife, does agree with me on what is to follow. The first few topics involve day-to-day operation of an ultrasound center.

On the appearance of an ultrasound suite

The tendency today is to "institutionalize" the ultrasound setting—glass partitions between the patients and the office staff; signs saying "do not venture past this point" or "employees only," or "you are expected to pay on site for services rendered" etc. Rarely do the providers, clad in starched white coats, venture out into the waiting area where the patients sit anxiously.

We need to lighten up! Since the overwhelming majority of the time we are not giving bad news, each examination should be a pleasurable experience for both patient *and* provider, and it should start from the time the patient walks through the front door. I think the waiting room should look like a living room, and professionalism should be about how caregivers behave and not just how they look.

I'm constantly amazed at how mechanical and impersonal some receptionists are. These individuals either, on the phone or in person, provide the first impression of any operation (just like a hostess in a restaurant), and, like hostesses, they are often low dollar employees who, not surprisingly, deliver low dollar service to "customers."

Since they are the marquee of a practice, extra effort should be generated to hire an engaging and intelligent individual who seems like the patient's best friend. If these individuals can also multitask, they will be worth their weight in gold.

On how many patients can be comfortably examined per day

This would depend upon whether the patients are at high risk or low risk and what trimester they are in. For example, it is difficult to obsess over a first trimester pregnancy for more than 20 minutes. At the other end of pregnancy, crowding and an abundance of acoustic shadowing interfere with any ability for an exhaustive anatomic search, and very little information can be extracted from a third trimester fetus after 30 minutes. On the other hand, there are so many tasks that need to be completed in a second trimester scan (especially the genetic sonogram) 45 minutes fly by far too quickly.

Throughput is dependent upon the comfort of the operator. However, at a time when we are being pushed to see more patients, either because of a supply and demand mismatch or finances, if operator burnout or repetitive motion injury is the ultimate result, everyone loses—especially the patient.

On the necessity of a patient to have a full bladder

If one is doing a gynecologic scan transabdominally, then it is sometimes convenient to have a small acoustic window

Obstetric Ultrasound: Artistry in Practice. John C. Hobbins. Published 2008 Blackwell Publishing. ISBN 978-1-4051-5815-2.

through which to image the uterus and adnexa. However, in an obstetrical patient, there already is an acoustic window present—the amniotic fluid—and if one wants to thoroughly evaluate the lower uterine segment (for, let's say, a possible placenta previa), then the method of choice is a gentle transvaginal approach with an *empty* bladder.

Recently, I was shown some patient information pamphlets that were meant to be sprinkled around waiting rooms. These bore the official stamp of a large physician organization. In one of these were some sentences designed to prepare patients for an ultrasound scan. It said, "for an ultrasound examination you may be asked to drink 6 glasses of water in a two-hour period." It should have said, "if anyone asks you to accomplish this feat, you should tell that individual to try it him/herself and then to withhold voiding for another hour or two while reading a 3-year-old Parents Magazine in a frigid waiting room." From which planet did this concept originate?

On "waiting room rage"

Most providers occasionally find themselves so occupied with a diagnostic problem that they lose track of time to a point where they are running behind by 30 to 45 minutes. This results in a waiting room full of disgruntled patients. The best way to handle this is to notify those waiting that an unexpected problem has been encountered and everyone is working diligently to get back on track. These messages should be given out frequently and, at least once, by the provider in charge. Nothing bugs me more than to be circling an airport for an hour with nobody telling me why. A simple "from the flight deck: we apologize for the delay, but air traffic control is holding us up because of thunder showers in the area" would suffice to keep me happy.

On proper etiquette for apprising patients of the results of an ultrasound examination

In many ultrasound laboratories, sonographers are interdicted from apprising patients of their findings. Sometimes, it is many minutes before the results are explained on site by the physician, or, occasionally, the patient is not notified until long after she has left the ultrasound facility. Of course, patients fear the worst, and even if the news is bad, they are left to obsess over it for hours/days until the true nature of the problem is conveyed to them.

I realize that many sonographers should not be saddled with the responsibility of explaining the nuances of various findings, but if everything seems normal, why can't this information be passed on to the patient immediately, with the caveat that the formal interpretation will come later? This takes everyone off the hook, and reduces patient anxiety by many angst units. If something is amiss, then the sonologist should be notified immediately so that any delay between the time of acquisition and diagnosis is minimized.

On turf issues in obstetrical ultrasound

Radiologists feel that they are best suited to interpret an obstetrical ultrasound examination because they are super trained in all forms of imagery. Obstetricians cite their ability to apply their knowledge of maternal and fetal physiology to obstetrical ultrasound. Family practitioners say, "Why not us? As those responsible for delivering primary care we are the logical ones to start the diagnostic wheels turning." The emergency room physicians feel that, as point people, they can best answer the first basic questions through ultrasound examinations on site, without waiting hours for these examinations to be conducted and interpreted elsewhere in the hospital.

Frankly, I think that obstetrical ultrasound should not be specialty-specific. However, if the question concerns who can do it the best, the answer is, "the one who is the best trained to do it." In various countries around the world there has been a more formalized approach to accreditation. For example, in Germany, there have been standardization requisites for the training and performance of "Level 1, 2, and 3" examinations. In the USA, organizations such as the American Institute of Ultrasound in Medicine (AIUM), the American College of Radiology (ACR), the American Academy of Family Physicians (AAFP), and the American College of Emergency Physicians (ACEP) have their own accreditation processes. It is interesting that each one only credentials *practices* and not physicians, specifically. However, in order for a practice to be accredited, each physician in the practice must have satisfied specific training and experience requirements.

So, if the training and experience are comparable, we should not care from which discipline the sonologist emerges. It is clear that insurance companies are picking up on this, and some are making practice accreditation the requisite for reimbursement. Here is an example of an attempt by insurance companies to drive the quality of care *upward*.

On advanced practice sonography

The backdrop here is filled with contradictions. I am told that the Centers for Medicare and Medicaid Services (CMS) are considering withholding reimbursement for an ultrasound scan if the physician is not in the room for the duration of the examination. This is happening at a time when the demand for some ultrasound services exceeds the supply. Radiologists are leaving the field faster than newly trained specialists are entering the field, and obstetricians with expertise in ultrasound are not coming out of residencies in large enough numbers to meet the need for these services.

Why not train sonographers, who can scan rings around most sonologists anyway, to take their duties one step further—to acquire the images *and* to do an initial interpretation? In many ways, they already do this. This would free up the physician to handle a higher volume of patients while making the sonographer's job more satisfying. Two recent studies have shown this approach to be effective without affecting the quality of service.

I guess the concept of requiring the physician to hover over the entire examination was conceived to improve patient care. However, this misguided idea will do just the opposite. The sonographer will be rendered superfluous and throughput will be obstructed to the point of constipation.

On the state of ultrasound training today

First, there are a number of trends that are very worrisome for the future of medical education, in general. For a variety of reasons, academic institutions cannot compete well with private practices, especially with regard to salaries, and physicians are leaving universities in droves. At one time, the public thought that if one needed special diagnostic or therapeutic attention, the teaching institution was the place to go. Now there seems to be a feeling that the teaching institution is where only indigents go to be "practiced on" by trainees. Also, in university settings there is often a guarded relationship between hospital administrators and academic physicians. The administrator's concern is to keep the hospital in the black at a time when federal and state support has shrunken appreciably, and the physician's concern is to obtain the best equipment and to retain the highest quality personnel. This save/spend tug-of-war often poisons some once healthy collegial relationships.

Now, in order to woo the public back to the university, one has to offer the niceties that patients think they can only get elsewhere. This is where administrators in large institutions miss the boat. They continue to go "big" when we should go "small." They install systems to mechanize access through telephone multiple-choice trees at a time when we should be emphasizing human-to-human contact. There *is* a way to bring the resident, fellow, medical student or sonography student into the patient's care and still make the patient feel special. However, to accomplish this and other necessary changes, administrators and academicians must work together, rather than at cross purposes.

On "keepsake" videos

The emergence of the private office "Womb with a View" or the shopping mall "Fetal Foto" kiosk (next to the sticky buns) has galvanized the medical profession and has stimulated some of the most entertaining debates at ultrasound conferences and in letters to the editors in medical journals.

Over the last 3 years, I have been assigned the task of arguing both sides of the debate, and, frankly, I have had the most fun arguing the "pro" side.

Here are the main arguments against the practice of nonmedical ultrasound:

1 We do not know that this is safe and, in the USA, the FDA indicates that it is not recommended.

2 False negatives can occur. In other words, a patient may be falsely reassured that her fetus is normal after a pretty picture of a face is generated by a "technician" whose training only involves just that—obtaining a pretty picture. These patients might even skip an indicated ultrasound examination based on this reassuring keepsake experience.

3 False positives can also occur. Patients have been frightened out of their wits after having been told that their fetus "may have a problem" during a scan performed by someone not properly trained in fetal diagnosis.

On the "pro" side: who are we to tell a woman what she can and cannot do, as long as she is properly informed of the above reasons for concern? We frequently proclaim our respect for patient autonomy. Yet, we spend substantial time during office visits telling patients not to smoke, not to drink alcohol or coffee, not to travel, not to have intercourse and, in some instances, not to even get out of bed. No wonder patients are getting the impression that we are overly paternalistic, and, more specifically, are hell bent on spoiling their fun.

The safety card is a difficult one to play since we have said for years that there is no indication that ultrasound is unsafe. We can't have it both ways. Either it is safe or it is not, irrespective of whether or not it is medically indicated. However, the false negatives and false positives cannot be so easily dismissed.

Before moving to my solution to this problem (if it is a problem), no one should be fooled into thinking that the keepsake industry is motivated by altruism. In this land of opportunity this is a way to make a buck, and, although I am mystified by this, many patients will not hesitate to shell out over $200 for a keepsake video (and then later complain about a $15 co-pay for an indicated examination).

If we were to take a few extra minutes at the end of a basic scan to provide a 2D or 3D picture of someone's fetus, there would be no need for patients to continue to stuff the pockets of the shopping mall entrepreneurs.

On the potential for lawsuits

The job of the sonologist/sonographer is to rule out fetal abnormalities. This is why we do a comprehensive fetal survey with every standard ultrasound examination. Occasionally, a fetus will slip through without an anomaly being detected. Unfortunately, in today's society perfection is demanded, and the delivery of an infant with an unexpected anomaly is unacceptable to some parents, and whom better to blame than the person(s) who did not recognize it in utero? This is why prenatal ultrasound has become a medical legal minefield.

Obstetricians already tend to be gun shy, having attained the dubious distinction of being the second most commonly sued group of physicians (neurosurgeons are number one), and this is no longer a phenomenon that is only indigenous to the USA. However, no sonologist is immune, and sonographers, despite their not having the deepest pockets, are now being named as defendants in lawsuits involving ultrasound.

So, should we curl up in a corner sucking our thumbs, or can we do something preemptively to diminish the risk of being sued? First, the vast majority of suits involving obstetrical ultrasound result from errors of omission, not commission, and the way to diminish false negatives is to continue to conduct the fetal survey in a consistent, systematic manner, and to avoid the temptation of cutting corners when under pressure. However, even then, for whatever reason, some anomalies will go unnoticed. Under these circumstances, the provider might have diminished his/her chances of a lawsuit simply by establishing a rapport with the patient during the ultrasound examination.

Our university defense attorneys have consistently informed us that a patient is far more likely to sue if the provider seems cold and uncaring than if he/she is likable and appears to be genuinely interested in the patient's welfare.

This is another reason why full bladders, long waits, lack of communication during the examination, and strict rules against fetal mementos simply do not "cut it."

Lobbying for tort reform—specifically limiting awards for pain and suffering—and cracking down on hired gun "experts" whose strings are being pulled by plaintiffs' attorneys, may possibly discourage unjustified suits. However, the greatest deterrent may result from what happens during the ultrasound examination between the patient and the caregiver.

On the "don't just stand there, do something" mentality that has crept into the practice of obstetrics

We know that the vast majority of women can get through pregnancy and delivery unassisted. However, today, because an occasional patient and/or her fetus can develop potentially serious problems, those of us practicing contemporary obstetrics have a tendency to hover over everyone for the sake of a few. This obsession to not let anything slip by is not just for the patient's welfare, but it also evolved to protect us. This concept also has a tendency to have us pull the trigger at the slightest hint of trouble. One rarely gets sued for doing a cesarean section or early delivery, but many lawsuits are generated from not doing one—ergo, a cesarean section rate in the USA of about 30%.

Now we have dozens of "protocols" so that the practitioner can be guided and protected by practicing according to certain standards. While keeping clinicians on the same page (especially when a single patient's care is in the hands of many providers in a large practice), this cookbook approach can stifle individual thought and leaves little "artistry" in the practice of medicine. It also tends to encourage overtesting.

Ultrasound often can pick out the patient who needs more attention. Better yet, it will also identify the one who should be left alone. A perfect example of this capability to adjust obstetrical management is in patients presenting with preterm contractions. As stated in Chapter 16, four out of five of these patients will not deliver preterm, and a cervical length and/or fetal fibronectin should sort out those who are truly in preterm labor from the majority who are not. Unfortunately, many clinicians ordering or performing these tests will not have the confidence in them to sit on their hands when the tests strongly suggest that the patient is not in labor. Then, what follows is hospitalization for many days accompanied by tocolytics, whose efficacy has been strongly questioned by recent investigation, but whose side effects have never been in question.

The point is that in almost every chapter there are examples of how ultrasound can rule out abnormalities and pregnancy complications far more often than they are ruled in. Yet, we continue to push ahead with more testing, lifestyle restrictions, medications, invasive intervention, etc for patients whose risk for something has already been negated by reassuring diagnostic information.

The solution is simply to trust the ultrasound results.

Parting words

As indicated in the introduction, this book represents an attempt by the author to input, process, filter, and prioritize 35 years worth of information and to pass it on as a condensed and unsanitized product.

It should be obvious that the book does not supply all the answers to vexing obstetrical problems. The field is rapidly evolving, allowing the reader to tap other sources, or wait for another installment. Since the text is sprinkled with opinion, the reader also may disagree with, or have an even better idea, on how to approach a particular facet of investigation or management. I welcome hearing from anyone in this or any other regard. E-mail: John.Hobbins@UCHSC.edu.

Appendix

First trimester

Second trimester

Third trimester

Obstetric Ultrasound: Artistry in Practice. John C. Hobbins. Published 2008 Blackwell Publishing. ISBN 978-1-4051-5815-2.

Table A.1 Crown–rump length.

CRL	MA	CRL	MA	CRL	MA	CRL	MA	CRL	MA	CRL	MA
0.2	5.7	2.2	8.9	4.2	11.1	6.2	12.6	8.2	14.2	10.2	16.1
0.3	5.9	2.3	9.0	4.3	11.2	6.3	12.7	8.3	14.2	10.3	16.2
0.4	6.1	2.4	9.1	4.4	11.2	6.4	12.8	8.4	14.3	10.4	16.3
0.5	6.2	2.5	9.2	4.5	11.3	6.5	12.8	8.5	14.4	10.5	16.4
0.6	6.4	2.6	9.4	4.6	11.4	6.6	12.9	8.6	14.5	10.6	16.5
0.7	6.6	2.7	9.5	4.7	11.5	6.7	13.0	8.7	14.6	10.7	16.6
0.8	6.7	2.8	9.6	4.8	11.6	6.8	13.1	8.8	14.7	10.8	16.7
0.9	6.9	2.9	9.7	4.9	11.7	6.9	13.1	8.9	14.8	10.9	16.8
1.0	7.2	3.0	9.9	5.0	11.7	7.0	13.2	9.0	14.9	11.0	16.9
1.1	7.2	3.1	10.0	5.1	11.8	7.1	13.3	9.1	15.0	11.1	17.0
1.2	7.4	3.2	10.1	5.2	11.9	7.2	13.4	9.2	15.1	11.2	17.1
1.3	7.5	3.3	10.2	5.3	12.0	7.3	13.4	9.3	15.2	11.3	17.2
1.4	7.7	3.4	10.3	5.4	12.0	7.4	13.5	9.4	15.3	11.4	17.3
1.5	7.9	3.5	10.4	5.5	12.1	7.5	13.6	9.5	15.3	11.5	17.4
1.6	8.0	3.6	10.5	5.6	12.2	7.6	13.7	9.6	15.4	11.6	17.5
1.7	8.1	3.7	10.6	5.7	12.3	7.7	13.8	9.7	15.5	11.7	17.6
1.8	8.3	3.8	10.7	5.8	12.3	7.8	13.8	9.8	15.5	11.8	17.7
1.9	8.4	3.9	10.8	5.9	12.4	7.9	13.9	9.9	15.7	11.9	17.8
2.0	8.6	4.0	10.9	6.0	12.5	8.0	14.0	10.0	15.9	12.0	17.9
2.1	8.7	4.1	11.0	6.1	12.6	8.1	14.1	10.1	16.0	12.1	18.0

Predicted menstrual age (MA) in weeks from crown–rump length (CRL) measurements (cm); the 95% confidence interval is ±8% the predicted age.

(From Hadlock FP, Shah YP, Kanon DJ, Lindsey JV. Fetal crown-rump length: re-evaluation to menstrual age (6–18 weeks) with high-resolution real-time US. Radiology 1992; 182: 501–5, with permission from the Radiological Society of North America.)

Table A.2 Gestational sac measurement.

Mean predicted gestational sac (cm)	Gestational age (weeks)	Mean predicted gestational sac (cm)	Gestational age (weeks)
1.0	5.0	3.6	8.8
1.1	5.2	3.7	8.9
1.2	5.3	3.8	9.0
1.3	5.5	3.9	9.2
1.4	5.6	4.0	9.3
1.5	5.8	4.1	9.5
1.6	5.9	4.2	9.6
1.7	6.0	4.3	9.7
1.8	6.2	4.4	9.9
1.9	6.3	4.5	10.0
2.0	6.5	4.6	10.2
2.1	6.6	4.7	10.3
2.2	6.8	4.8	10.5
2.3	6.9	4.9	10.6
2.4	7.0	5.0	10.7
2.5	7.2	5.1	10.9
2.6	7.3	5.2	11.0
2.7	7.5	5.3	11.2
2.8	7.6	5.4	11.3
2.9	7.8	5.5	11.5
3.0	7.9	5.6	11.6
3.1	8.0	5.7	11.7
3.2	8.2	5.8	11.9
3.3	8.3	5.9	12.0
3.4	8.5	6.0	12.2
3.5	8.6		

(From Hellman LM, Kobayashi M, Fillisti L, et al. Growth and development of the human fetus prior to the 20th week of gestation. Am J Obstet Gynecol 1969; 103: 789, with permission from Elsevier.)

Table A.3 Sac size versus human chorionic gonadotropin (hCG) levels for normal pregnancies ($n = 56$).

Mean sac diameter (mm)	hCG level (mIU/mL)		
		95% confidence limits	
	Predicted*	Lower	Upper
5	1,932	1,026	3,636
6	2,165	1,226	4,256
7	2,704	1,465	4,990
8	3,199	1,749	5,852
9	3,785	2,085	6,870
10	4,478	2,483	8,075
11	5,297	2,952	9,508
12	6,267	3,502	11,218
13	7,415	4,145	13,266
14	8,773	4,894	15,726
15	10,379	5,766	18,682
16	12,270	6,776	22,235
17	14,528	7,964	26,501
18	17,188	9,343	31,621
19	20,337	10,951	37,761
20	24,060	12,820	45,130
21	28,464	15,020	53,970
22	33,675	17,560	64,570
23	39,843	20,573	77,164

*$\text{Log(hCG)} = 2.92 + 0.073\ \text{(MSD)}$; $R^2 = 0.93$; $P < 0.001$.

(From Nyberg DA, Filly RA, Filho DL, et al. Abnormal pregnancy: early diagnosis by US and serum chorionic gonadotropin levels. Radiology 1986; 158: 393–6, with permission from the Radiological Society of North America.)

Table A.4 Embryonic trunk circumference.

Trunk circumference (cm)	Gestational age ±2 SD* (weeks)
1.0	7.22 ± 0.5
1.2	7.99 ± 0.4
1.5	8.39 ± 0.3
1.7	8.64 ± 0.3
2.0	8.99 ± 0.2
2.2	9.22 ± 0.2
2.5	9.55 ± 0.2
2.7	9.75 ± 0.2
3.0	10.05 ± 0.2
3.2	10.23 ± 0.2
3.5	10.49 ± 0.2
3.7	10.65 ± 0.2
4.0	10.88 ± 0.2
4.2	11.02 ± 0.2
4.5	11.22 ± 0.2
4.7	11.33 ± 0.2
5.0	11.50 ± 0.2
5.5	11.72 ± 0.3
6.0	11.89 ± 0.5
6.5	12.01 ± 0.7
7.0	12.07 ± 0.9

*Overall 2 SD = ±3 days.

(From Reece EA, Scioscia AL, Green J, et al. Embryonic trunk circumference: a new biometric parameter for estimation of gestational age. Am J Obstet Gynecol 1987; 156: 713–5, with permission from Elsevier.)

Table A.5 Reference values for length of nasal bone.

Gestational age (weeks)	Length of nasal bone (mm)		
	−2 SD	Mean	+2 SD
14	3.3	4.2	5.0
16	3.1	5.2	7.3
18	5.0	6.3	7.6
20	5.7	7.6	9.5
22	6.0	8.2	10.4
24	6.8	9.4	12.0
26	7.2	9.7	12.3
28	7.8	10.7	13.6
30	8.3	11.3	14.4
32	8.0	11.6	15.2
34	7.5	12.3	17.0

(From Guis F, Ville Y, Vincent Y, Doumerc S, et al. Ultrasound evaluation of the length of the fetal nasal bones throughout gestation. Ultrasound Obstet Gynecol 1995; 5: 304–7, with permission from John Wiley and Sons.)

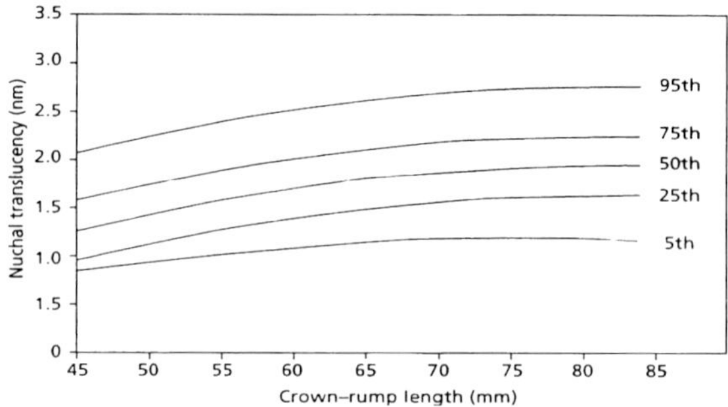

Fig A.1 Nuchal translucency measurements between 11 and 14 weeks' gestation. Nuchal translucency >95th percentile is associated with an increased risk of trisomy 21. (From Nicolaides KH, Sebire NJ, Snijders RJM. The 11–14 Week Scan: The Diagnosis of Fetal Abnormalities. New York: Parthenon Publishing Group; 1999, with permission.)

Table A.6 Prevalence of major cardiac defects by nuchal translucency thickness in chromosomally normal fetuses.

Nuchal translucency	*N*	Major cardiac defects	Prevalence per 1000
<95th percentile	27,332	22	0.8
≥95th percentile: 3.4 mm	1,507	8	5.3
3.5–4.4 mm	208	6	28.9
4.5–5.4 mm	66	6	90.0
≥5.5 mm	41	8	195.1
Total	29,154	50	1.7

(From Hyett J, Perdu M, Sharland G, Snijders R, Nicolaides KH. Using fetal nuchal translucency to screen for major congenital cardiac defects at 10–14 weeks of gestation: a population based cohort study. BMJ 1999; 318: 81–5, with permission from the BMJ Publishing Group, Ltd.)

Table A.7 Biparietal diameter (BPD) and gestational age.

BPD (cm)	Menstrual age (weeks)	BPD (cm)	Menstrual age (weeks)	BPD (cm)	Menstrual age (weeks)	BPD (cm)	Menstrual age (weeks)
2.0	A-8	4.0	18.0	6.0	24.6	8.0	32.5
2.1	12.5	4.1	18.3	6.1	25.0	8.1	32.9
2.2	12.8	4.2	18.6	6.2	25.3	8.2	33.3
2.3	13.1	4.3	18.9	6.3	25.7	8.3	33.8
2.4	13.3	4.4	19.2	6.4	26.1	8.4	34.2
2.5	13.6	4.5	19.5	6.5	26.4	8.5	34.7
2.6	13.9	4.6	19.9	6.6	26.8	8.6	35.1
2.7	14.2	4.7	20.2	6.7	27.2	8.7	35.6
2.8	12.5	4.8	20.5	6.8	27.6	8.8	36.1
2.9	14.7	4.9	20.8	6.9	28.0	8.9	36.5
3.0	15.0	5.0	21.2	7.0	28.3	9.0	37.0
3.1	15.3	5.1	21.5	7.1	28.7	9.1	37.5
3.2	15.6	5.2	21.8	7.2	29.1	9.2	38.0
3.3	15.9	5.3	22.2	7.3	29.5	9.3	38.5
3.4	16.2	5.4	22.5	7.4	29.9	9.4	38.9
3.5	16.5	5.5	22.8	7.5	30.4	9.5	39.4
3.6	16.8	5.6	23.2	7.6	30.8	9.6	39.9
3.7	17.1	5.7	23.5	7.7	31.2	9.7	40.5
3.8	17.4	5.8	23.9	7.8	31.6	9.8	41.0
3.9	17.7	5.9	24.2	7.9	32.0	9.9	41.5
						10.0	42.0

(From Hadlock FP, Deter RL, Harrist RB. Fetal biparietal diameter: a critical re-evaluation of the relation to menstrual age by means of real-time ultrasound. J Ultrasound Med 1982; 1: 97–104, with permission from the American Institute of Ultrasound in Medicine.)

Table A.8 A nomogram of the transverse cerebellar diameter (TCD) (in millimeters).

Gestational age (weeks)	Percentile		
	10th	50th	90th
15	13	14	16
16	14	16	17
17	16	17	18
18	17	18	19
19	18	19	20
20	19	20	21
21	20	21	23
22	22	23	24
23	23	24	26
24	23	26	28
25	25	27	30
26	26	28	32
27	27	30	33
28	28	31	35
29	29	33	38
30	31	35	40
31	33	38	42
32	34	39	43
33	35	40	44
34	38	41	44
35	41	42	45
36	42	43	45
37	43	45	48
38	45	48	50
39	48	52	55
40	52	55	58

(From Goldstein I, Reece EA, Pilu G, et al. Cerebellar measurements with ultrasonography in the evaluation of fetal growth and development. Am J Obstet Gynecol 1987; 156: 1065–9, with permission from Elsevier.)

Table A.9 Reference values for abdominal circumference.

Menstrual age (weeks)	Abdominal circumference (cm)				
	Percentiles				
	3rd	10th	50th	90th	97th
14.0	6.4	6.7	7.3	7.9	8.3
15.0	7.5	7.9	8.6	9.3	9.7
16.0	8.6	9.1	9.9	10.7	11.2
17.0	9.2	10.3	11.2	12.1	12.7
18.0	10.9	11.5	12.5	13.5	14.1
19.0	11.9	12.6	13.7	14.8	15.5
20.0	13.1	13.8	15.0	16.3	17.0
21.0	14.1	14.9	16.2	17.6	18.3
22.0	15.1	16.0	17.4	18.8	19.7
23.0	16.1	17.0	18.5	20.0	20.9
24.0	17.1	18.1	19.7	21.3	22.3
25.0	18.1	19.1	20.8	22.5	23.5
26.0	19.1	20.1	21.9	23.7	24.8
27.0	20.0	21.1	23.0	24.9	26.0
28.0	20.9	22.0	24.0	26.0	27.1
29.0	21.8	23.0	25.1	27.2	28.4
30.0	22.7	23.9	26.1	28.3	29.5
31.0	23.6	24.9	27.1	29.4	30.6
32.0	24.5	25.8	28.1	30.4	31.8
33.0	25.3	26.7	29.1	31.5	32.9
34.0	26.1	27.5	30.0	32.5	33.9
35.0	26.9	28.3	30.9	33.5	34.9
36.0	27.7	29.2	31.8	34.4	35.9
37.0	28.5	30.0	32.7	35.4	37.0
38.0	29.2	30.8	33.6	36.4	38.0
39.0	29.9	31.6	34.4	37.3	38.9
40.0	30.7	32.4	35.3	38.2	39.9

(Adapted from Hadlock FP. Ultrasound evaluation of fetal growth. In: Ultrasonography in Obstetrics and Gynecology. Callen PW (ed). Philadelphia: WB Saunders Company, 2000, with permission from Elsevier.)

Table A.10 Fetal long-bone lengths.

Week number	Humerus percentile			Ulna percentile			Radius percentile			Femur percentile			Tibia percentile			Fibula percentile		
	5th	50th	95th	5th	50th	95th	5th	50th	95th	5th	50th	95th	5th	50th	95th	5th	50th	95th
11	–	6	–	–	5	–	–	5	–	–	6	–	–	4	–	–	2	–
12	3	9	10		8			7			'9			7			5	
13	5	13	20	3	11	18		10		6	12	19	4	10	17		8	
14	5	16	20	4	13	17	8	13	12	5	15	19	2	13	19	6	11	10
15	11	18	26	10	16	22	12	15	19	11	19	26	5	16	27	10	14	18
16	12	21	25	8	19	24	9	18	21	13	22	24	7	19	25	6	17	22
17	19	24	29	11	21	32	11	20	29	20	25	29	15	22	29	7	19	31
18	18	27	30	13	24	30	14	22	26	19	28	31	14	24	29	10	22	28
19	22	29	36	20	26	32	20	24	29	23	31	38	19	27	35	18	24	30
20	23	32	36	21	29	32	21	27	28	22	33	39	19	29	35	18	27	30
21	28	34	40	25	31	36	25	29	32	27	36	45	24	32	39	24	29	34
22	28	36	40	24	33	37	24	31	34	29	39	44	25	34	39	21	31	37
23	32	38	45	27	35	43	26	32	39	35	41	48	30	36	43	23	33	44
24	31	41	46	29	37	41	27	34	38	34	44	49	28	39	45	26	35	41
25	35	43	51	34	39	44	31	36	40	38	46	54	31	41	50	33	37	42
26	36	45	49	34	41	44	30	37	41	39	49	53	33	43	49	32	39	43
27	42	46	51	37	43	48	33	39	45	45	51	57	39	45	51	35	41	47
28	41	48	52	37	44	48	33	40	45	45	53	57	38	47	52	36	43	47
29	44	50	56	40	46	51	36	42	47	49	56	62	40	49	57	40	45	50
30	44	52	56	38	47	54	34	43	49	49	58	62	41	51	56	38	47	52
31	47	53	59	39	49	59	34	44	53	53	60	67	46	52	58	40	48	57
32	47	55	59	40	50	58	37	45	51	53	62	67	46	54	59	40	50	56
33	50	56	62	43	52	60	41	46	51	56	64	71	49	56	62	43	51	59
34	50	57	62	44	53	59	39	47	53	57	65	70	47	57	64	46	52	56
35	52	58	65	47	54	61	38	48	57	61	67	73	48	59	69	51	54	57
36	53	60	63	47	55	61	41	48	54	61	69	74	49	60	68	51	55	56
37	57	61	64	49	56	62	45	9	53	64	71	77	52	61	71	55	56	58
38	55	61	66	48	57	63	45	49	53	62	72	79	54	62	69	54	57	59
39	56	62	69	49	57	66	46	50	54	64	74	83	58	64	69	55	58	62
40	56	63	69	50	58	65	46	50	54	66	75	81	58	65	69	54	59	62

(From Jeanty P. Fetal limb biometry (letter). Radiology 1983; 147: 601–2, with permission from the Radiological Society of North America.)

Table A.11 In utero fetal weight standards.

Menstrual week	Percentiles (g)				
	3rd	10th	50th	90th	97th
10	26	29	35	41	44
11	34	37	45	53	56
12	43	48	58	68	73
13	55	61	73	85	91
14	70	77	93	109	116
15	88	97	117	137	146
16	110	121	146	171	183
17	136	150	181	212	226
18	167	185	223	261	279
19	205	227	273	319	341
20	248	275	331	387	414
21	299	331	399	467	499
22	359	398	478	559	598
23	426	471	568	665	710
24	503	556	670	784	838
25	589	652	785	918	981
26	685	758	913	1068	1141
27	791	876	1055	1234	1319
28	908	1004	1210	1416	1513
29	1034	1145	1379	1613	1724
30	1169	1294	1559	1824	1649
31	1313	1453	1751	2049	2189
32	1465	1621	1953	2285	2441
33	1622	1794	2162	2530	2703
34	1783	1973	2377	2781	2971
35	1946	2154	2595	3036	3244
36	2110	2335	2813	3291	3516
37	2271	2513	3028	3543	3785
38	2427	2686	3236	3786	4045
39	2576	2851	3435	4019	4294
40	2714	3004	3619	4234	4524

(From Hadlock FP, Harrist RB, Martinez-Poyer M. In utero analysis of fetal growth: a sonographic weight standard. Radiology 1991; 181: 129–33, with permission from the Radiological Society of North America.)

Table A.12 Weight (mass) conversion.

	Pounds														
Ounces	**0**	**1**	**2**	**3**	**4**	**5**	**6**	**7**	**8**	**9**	**10**	**11**	**12**	**13**	**14**
0	0	454	907	1361	1814	2268	2722	3175	3629	4082	1536	4990	5443	5897	6350
1	28	482	936	1389	1843	2296	2750	3203	3657	4111	4564	5018	5471	5925	6379
2	57	510	964	1417	1871	2325	2778	3232	3685	4139	4593	5046	5500	2953	6407
3	85	539	992	1446	1899	2353	2807	3260	3714	4167	4621	5075	5528	5982	6435
4	113	567	1021	1474	1928	2381	2835	3289	3742	4196	4649	5103	5557	6010	6464
5	142	595	1049	1503	1956	2410	2863	3317	3770	4224	4678	5131	5585	6038	6492
6	170	624	1077	1531	1984	2438	2892	3345	3799	4252	4706	5160	5613	6067	6520
7	198	652	1106	1559	2013	2466	2920	3374	3821	4281	4734	5188	5642	6095	6549
8	227	680	1134	1588	2041	2495	2948	3402	3856	4309	4763	5216	5670	6123	6577
9	255	709	1162	1616	2070	2523	2977	3430	3884	4337	4791	5245	5698	6152	6605
10	283	737	1191	1644	2098	2551	3005	3459	3912	4366	4819	5273	5727	6180	6634
11	312	765	1219	1673	2126	2580	3033	3487	3941	4394	4848	5301	5755	6209	6662
12	340	794	1247	1701	2155	2608	3062	3515	3969	4423	4876	5330	5783	6237	6600
13	369	822	1276	1729	2183	2637	3090	3544	3997	4451	4904	5358	5812	6265	6719
14	397	850	1304	1758	2211	2665	3118	3572	4026	4479	4933	5386	5840	6294	6747
15	425	879	1332	1786	2240	2693	3147	3600	4054	4508	4961	5415	5868	6322	6776

Note: 1 pound = 453.59237 grams; 1 ounce = 28.349523 grams; 1000 grams = 1 kilogram. Gram equivalents have been rounded to whole numbers by adding 1 when the first decimal place is 5 or greater.

Example: To obtain grams equivalent to 6 pounds, 8 ounces, read "6" on top scale, "8" on side scale; equivalent is 2948 grams.

Table A.13 Fetal foot size throughout gestation.

Gestational age (weeks)	Length (cm)		Percentile		
	Mean	(±) SD	10th	50th	90th
14	1.8	2.5	1.6	18	21
15	1.9	2.3	1.6	19	22
16	2.3	2.3	1.8	22	28
17	2.1	1.3	1.9	22	22
18	2.6	2.5	1.9	27	30
19	3.1	2.6	2.5	30	39
20	3.3	2.5	3.3	33	33
21	3.4	2.6	2.4	24	24
22	3.5	2.8	2.5	36	40
23	4.1	2.6	4.1	41	40
24	4.6	2.5	4.6	46	46
25	4.7	2.1	4.0	47	53
26	4.7	2.5	4.0	47	54
27	5.0	2.6	4.5	50	56
28	5.3	2.8	5.1	53	55
29	5.2	2.9	4.9	54	58
30	6.1	2.8	6.1	61	61
31	5.6	3.5	5.1	56	52
32	5.6	3.5	5.4	57	62
33	5.9	2.9	5.9	59	59
34	6.5	3.1	6.0	65	71
35	7.1	2.9	7.1	71	71

(From Mercer BM, Sklar S, Shariatmader A, et al. Fetal foot length as a predictor of gestational age. Am J Obstet Gynecol 1987; 156: 350–55, with permission from Elsevier.)

Table A.14 Gestational age as obtained from clavicle length.

Clavicle length (mm)	Gestational age (weeks and days) percentile		
	5th	50th	95th
11	8 + 3	13 + 6	17 + 2
12	9 + 1	13 + 4	18 + 1
13	10 + 0	14 + 3	19 + 6
14	11 + 6	15 + 2	20 + 5
15	12 + 5	16 + 1	21 + 4
16	12 + 3	18 + 0	21 + 3
17	13 + 2	18 + 5	22 + 2
18	14 + 1	19 + 4	23 + 0
19	16 + 0	19 + 3	24 + 6
20	16 + 6	20 + 2	25 + 5
21	17 + 4	21 + 1	26 + 4
22	17 + 3	22 + 6	26 + 2
23	18 + 2	23 + 5	27 + 1
24	19 + 1	24 + 4	28 + 0
25	21 + 0	24 + 3	29 + 6
26	21 + 5	25 + 1	30 + 5
27	22 + 4	26 + 0	30 + 3
28	22 + 3	27 + 6	31 + 2
29	23 + 2	28 + 5	32 + 1
30	24 + 0	29 + 4	34 + 4
31	25 + 6	29 + 2	34 + 6
32	26 + 5	30 + 1	35 + 4
33	27 + 4	31 + 0	35 + 3
34	27 + 3	32 + 6	36 + 2
35	28 + 1	33 + 5	37 + 1
36	29 + 0	33 + 3	39 + 0
37	30 + 6	34 + 2	39 + 5
38	31 + 5	35 + 1	40 + 4
39	32 + 4	37 + 0	40 + 3
40	32 + 2	37 + 6	41 + 2
41	33 + 1	38 + 4	42 + 0
42	35 + 0	38 + 3	43 + 6
43	35 + 6	39 + 2	44 + 5
44	36 + 5	40 + 1	45 + 4
45	36 + 3	41 + 6	46 + 3

(From Yarkoni S, Schmidt W, Jeanty P, et al. Clavicular measurements: a new biometric parameter for fetal evaluation. J Ultrasound Med 1985; 4: 467–70, with permission from the American Institute of Ultrasound in Medicine.)

Table A.15 Outer orbital diameter.

Mean gestational age (weeks)	Predicted outer orbital diameter (mm)	Mean gestational age (weeks)	Predicted outer orbital diameter (mm)
11.6	13	24.3	41
11.6	14	24.3	42
12.1	15	24.7	46
12.6	16	25.2	46
12.6	17	25.2	44
13.1	17	25.7	44
13.6	18	26.2	45
13.6	19	26.2	45
14.1	20	26.7	46
14.6	21	27.2	46
14.6	21	27.6	47
15.0	22	28.1	47
15.5	23	28.6	48
15.5	24	29.1	48
16.0	25	29.6	49
16.5	25	30.0	50
16.5	26	30.6	50
17.0	27	31.0	51
17.5	27	31.5	51
17.9	28	32.0	52
18.4	30	32.5	52
18.9	31	33.0	53
19.4	32	33.5	54
19.4	32	34.0	54
19.9	33	34.4	54
20.4	34	35.0	55
20.4	34	35.4	55
10.9	35	35.9	56
21.3	36	36.4	56
21.3	36	36.9	57
21.8	37	37.3	57
22.3	38	37.8	58
22.3	38	38.3	58
22.8	39	38.8	58
23.3	40	39.3	59
23.3	40	39.8	59
23.8	41		

(From Mayden KL, Tortora M, Berkowitz RL, Hobbins JC. Orbital diameters: a new parameter for prenatal diagnosis and dating. Am J Obstet Gynecol 1982; 144: 289–97, with permission from Elsevier.)

Table A.16 Frontothalamic distance by gestational age.

Gestational age (weeks)	Percentile				
	10th	25th	50th	75th	90th
15	24.3	28	28.65	31	33
16	26	27.35	30.5	32.85	34.4
17	29	31.3	33	34.7	35.4
18	32.6	34.3	36	38.1	39.75
19	35	37	38	39.1	40
20	35.7	37.7	39.3	41	42.9
21	38.2	39	40.05	42.15	43.3

(From Bahado-Singh RO, Wyse L, et al. Fetuses with Down syndrome have disproportionately shortened frontal lobe dimensions on ultrasonographic examination. Am J Obstet Gynecol 1992; 167: 1009–14, with permission from Elsevier.)

Table A.17 Standard deviations for various thoracic ratios.

Ratio	Mean predicted value	SD ($n = 543$)
TC:AC*	0.89	0.06
TC:HC*	0.80	0.12
TC:HL	4.31	0.36
TC:FL	4.03	0.33
TL:TC	0.22	0.03
TL:HL*	0.93	0.13
TL:FL	0.87	0.13

*Ratios did not vary significantly with gestational age.

TC, thoracic circumference; AC, abdominal circumference; HC, head circumference; HL, humerus length; FL, femur length; TL, thoracic length.

(From Chitkara U, Rosenberg J, Chervenak FA, et al. Prenatal sonographic assessment of the fetal thorax: normal values. Am J Obstet Gynecol 1987; 156: 1069–74, with permission from Elsevier.)

Table A.18 Fetal thoracic circumference measurements (in centimeters).

Gestational age (weeks)	Number	Predictive percentiles								
		2.5	5	10	25	50	75	90	95	97.5
16	6	5.9	6.4	7.0	8.0	9.1	10.3	11.3	11.9	12.4
17	22	6.8	7.3	7.9	8.9	10.0	11.2	12.2	12.8	13.3
18	31	7.7	8.2	8.8	9.8	11.0	12.1	13.1	13.7	14.2
19	21	8.6	9.1	9.7	10.7	11.9	13.0	14.0	14.6	15.1
20	20	9.5	10.0	10.3	11.7	12.9	13.9	15.0	15.5	16.0
21	30	10.4	11.0	11.3	12.6	13.7	14.8	15.8	16.4	16.9
22	18	11.3	11.9	12.5	13.5	14.6	15.7	16.7	17.3	17.8
23	21	12.2	12.8	13.4	14.4	15.5	16.6	17.6	18.2	18.8
24	27	13.2	13.7	14.3	15.3	16.4	17.5	18.5	19.1	19.7
25	20	14.1	14.6	15.2	16.2	17.3	18.4	19.4	20.0	20.6
26	25	15.0	15.5	16.1	17.1	18.2	19.3	20.3	21.0	21.5
27	24	15.9	16.4	17.0	18.0	19.1	20.2	21.3	21.9	22.4
28	24	16.8	17.3	17.9	18.9	20.0	21.2	22.2	22.8	23.3
29	24	17.7	18.2	18.8	19.8	21.0	22.1	23.1	23.7	24.2
30	27	18.6	19.1	19.7	20.7	21.9	23.0	24.0	24.6	25.1
31	24	19.5	20.0	20.6	21.6	22.8	23.9	24.9	25.5	26.0
32	28	20.4	20.9	21.5	22.6	23.7	24.8	25.8	26.4	26.9
33	27	21.3	21.8	22.5	23.5	24.6	25.7	26.7	27.3	27.8
34	25	22.2	22.8	23.4	24.4	25.5	26.6	27.6	28.2	28.7
35	20	23.1	23.7	24.3	25.3	26.4	27.5	28.5	29.1	29.6
36	23	24.0	24.6	25.2	26.2	27.3	28.4	20.4	30.0	30.6
37	22	24.9	25.5	26.1	27.1	28.2	29.3	30.3	30.9	31.5
38	21	25.9	26.4	27.0	28.0	29.1	30.2	31.2	31.9	32.4
39	7	26.8	27.3	27.9	28.9	30.0	31.1	32.2	32.8	33.3
40	6	27.7	28.2	28.8	29.8	30.9	32.1	33.1	33.7	34.2

(From Chitkara U, Rosenberg J, Chervenak F, et al. Prenatal sonographic assessment of the fetal thorax: normal values. Am J Obstet Gynecol 1987; 156: 1069–74 from Elsevier.)

Table A.19 Normal cardiac dimensions.

	Transverse diameter (mm)			Longitudinal diameter (mm)			Volume (cm^3)		
	5th Percentile	50th Percentile	95th Percentile	5th Percentile	50th Percentile	95th Percentile	5th Percentile	50th Percentile	95th Percentile
Week 12	4	5	6	5	6	7	0.038	0.067	0.0963
Week 13	5	6	7	6	7	9	0.072	0.127	0.182
Week 14	6	7	8	8	9	10	0.128	0.225	0.322
Week 15	7	8	10	9	10	12	0.213	0.374	0.535
Week 16	8	10	11	10	12	14	0.336	0.588	0.84
Week 17	9	11	13	12	14	16	0.504	0.883	1.262
Week 18	10	12	15	13	15	18	0.726	1.271	1.816
Week 19	11	14	16	14	17	20	1.008	1.764	2.52
Week 20	13	15	18	16	19	22	1.356	2.373	3.39
Week 21	14	17	20	18	21	24	1.776	3.106	4.436
Week 22	15	18	21	19	23	26	2.273	3.975	5.677
Week 23	16	20	23	21	24	28	2.851	4.987	7.123
Week 24	18	21	25	22	25	30	3.519	6.155	8.791
Week 25	19	23	27	24	28	32	4.282	7.49	10.698
Week 26	20	24	28	25	30	34	5.15	9.008	12.866
Week 27	22	26	30	27	32	36	6.13	10.723	15.316
Week 28	23	27	32	28	33	38	7.232	12.649	18.066
Week 29	24	29	34	30	35	40	8.458	14.795	21.132
Week 30	25	30	35	31	37	42	9.812	17.163	24.514
Week 31	26	32	37	32	38	44	11.284	19.743	28.202
Week 32	28	33	38	33	40	46	12.857	22.505	32.153
Week 33	29	34	40	34	41	47	14.498	25.388	36.278
Week 34	30	35	41	35	42	49	16.155	28.301	40.447
Week 35	30	37	43	36	43	50	17.75	31.107	44.464
Week 36	31	38	44	37	44	51	19.18	33.626	48.072
Week 37	32	39	45	37	45	52	20.308	35.642	50.976
Week 38	33	39	46	38	46	53	20.966	36.913	52.86
Week 39	33	40	47	38	46	54	20.903	37.156	53.409
Week 40	33	41	48	38	46	55	19.478	35.58	51.682

(From Jeanty P, Romero R, Cantraine F, Cousaert E, Hobbins JC. Fetal cardiac dimensions: a potential tool for the diagnosis of congenital heart defects. J Ultrasound Med 1984; 3: 359–64, with permission from the American Institute of Ultrasound in Medicine.)

Table A.20 Fetal liver length from 20 weeks' gestation to term.

Gestational age (weeks)	Number of measurements	Arithmetic mean (mm)	(=) 2 SD (mm)
20	8	27.3	6.4
21	2	28.0	1.5
22	4	30.6	6.7
23	13	30.9	4.5
24	10	32.9	6.7
25	14	33.6	5.3
26	10	35.7	6.3
27	20	36.6	3.3
28	14	38.4	4.0
29	13	39.1	5.0
30	10	38.7	5.0
31	13	39.6	5.7
32	11	42.7	7.5
33	14	43.8	6.6
34	11	44.8	7.1
35	14	47.8	9.1
36	10	49.0	8.4
37	10	52.0	6.8
38	12	52.9	4.2
39	5	55.4	6.7
40	1	59.0	
41	2	49.3	2.4

Mean length ±2 SD.

(From Vintzileos AM, Neckles S, Campbell WA, et al. Fetal liver ultrasound measurements during normal pregnancy. Obstet Gynecol 1985; 66: 477, with permission from Lippincott, Williams and Wilkins.)

Table A.21 Fetal spleen diameters: sonographic measurements and the clinical implications.

Fetal spleen diameters and the calculated volume and perimeter																
		Diameter (mm)														
		Length			Sagittal			Transverse			Volume (cm^3) perimeter (mm)					
Gestational age (weeks)	Number of Patients	15th	Mean	95th	15th	Mean	95th	15th	Mean	95th	15th	Mean	95th	15th	Mean	95th
8	2	0.7	1.4	2.1	0.3	0.8	1.1	0.4	0.9	1.3		0.7	0.73	2.3	3.5	4.7
19	3	1.2	1.6	2.3	0.4	0.8	1.2	0.4	0.9	1.4	0.4	0.9	1.4	2.7	3.9	5.1
20	3	1.1	1.8	2.6	0.5	0.8	1.2	0.5	1.0	1.5	0.5	1.0	1.5	3.3	4.5	5.7
21	2	1.2	2	2.7	0.5	0.9	1.3	0.6	1.1	1.6	0.8	1.3	1.8	3.5	4.7	5.9
22	3	1.5	2.2	2.9	0.6	1.0	1.3	0.7	1.2	1.6	1.2	1.7	2.2	4.1	5.3	6.5
23	4	1.6	2.3	3.1	0.7	1.0	1.4	0.8	1.2	1.7	1.4	2.0	2.5	4.5	5.7	6.9
24	3	1.9	2.5	3.2	0.7	1.1	1.5	0.8	1.3	1.8	1.6	2.2	2.8	4.9	6.1	7.2
25	3	1.9	2.6	3.3	0.7	1.1	1.5	0.9	1.4	1.9	1.9	2.5	3.1	5.3	6.4	7.7
26	3	2	2.7	3.4	0.8	1.2	1.5	1.0	1.5	1.9	2.1	2.8	3.5	5.5	6.7	7.9
27	5	2.2	2.9	3.7	0.9	1.3	1.7	1.0	1.5	2.0	2.0	3.0	4.1	5.9	7.1	8.3
28	3	2.4	3.1	3.8	1	1.3	1.7	1.1	1.6	2.1	2.2	3.4	4.6	6.2	7.4	8.6
29	3	2.5	3.3	4	1	1.4	1.8	1.2	1.7	2.1	2.4	3.8	5.3	6.5	7.7	8.9
30	4	2.7	3.4	4.1	1.1	1.5	1.9	1.3	1.7	2.2	2.6	4.3	6.1	6.9	8.1	9.3
31	4	3	3.6	4.3	1.2	1.5	1.9	1.3	1.8	2.3	2.9	5.0	7.0	7.3	8.5	9.7
32	3	3.1	3.8	4.5	1.2	1.6	2.0	1.4	1.9	2.4	3.3	5.7	8.1	7.7	8.9	10.1
33	3	3.3	4	4.7	1.3	1.6	2.0	1.5	2.0	2.4	3.8	6.6	9.2	8.1	9.3	10.5
34	4	3.5	4.3	5	1.3	1.7	2.1	1.6	2.0	2.5	4.5	7.6	10.7	8.6	9.8	11.0
35	4	3.8	4.5	5.2	1.4	1.8	2.2	1.6	2.1	2.6	5.2	8.8	12.3	9.1	10.3	11.5
36	5	4.1	4.8	5.5	1.5	1.9	2.2	1.7	2.2	2.7	6.1	10.1	14.1	9.7	10.9	12.1
37	6	4.4	5.1	5.8	1.5	1.9	2.3	1.8	2.3	2.7	7.3	11.8	16.2	10.4	11.6	12.8
38	3	4.7	5.4	6.2	1.6	2.0	2.3	1.8	2.3	2.8	8.6	13.6	18.6	11.1	12.3	13.4
39	3	5.1	5.8	6.5	1.7	2.0	2.4	1.9	2.4	2.9	10.1	15.6	21.1	11.8	13.0	14.2
40	3	5.5	6.2	7	1.7	2.1	2.4	2.0	2.5	2.9	11.8	17.9	24.1	12.7	13.8	15.1

(From Schmidt E, Yarkoni S, Jeanty P, et al. Sonographic measurements of the fetal spleen: clinical implications. J Ultrasound Med 1985; 4: 667–72, with permission from the American Institute of Ultrasound in Medicine.)

Table A.22 Mean fetal kidney circumference/abdominal circumference ratios and the standard deviations.

	Gestational age (weeks)					
	<16 ($n = 9$)	17–20 ($n = 18$)	21–25 ($n = 7$)	26–30 ($n = 11$)	31–35 ($n = 19$)	36–40 ($n = 25$)
Mean	0.28	0.30	0.30	0.29	0.28	0.27
SD	0.02	0.03	0.02	0.02	0.03	0.04

(Adapted from Grannum PAT, Bracken M, Silverman R, et al. Assessment of fetal kidney size in normal gestation by comparison of kidney circumference to abdominal circumference (KC/AC) ratio. Am J Obstet Gynecol 1980; 136: 2, with permission from Elsevier.)

Table A.23 Normal anterior–posterior diameter of the fetal kidneys at different gestational ages.

Menstrual age (weeks)	(−) 2 SD ± (mm)	Predicted value (mm)	(+) 2 SD ± (mm)
22	8.9	11.3	13.7
23	9.3	11.7	14.1
24	9.7	12.1	14.5
25	10.2	12.6	15.0
26	10.7	13.1	15.5
27	11.3	13.7	16.1
28	11.9	14.3	16.7
29	12.5	15.0	17.4
30	13.2	15.6	18.0
31	14.0	16.4	18.8
32	14.8	17.2	19.6
33	15.6	18.0	20.4
34	16.5	18.9	21.3
35	17.5	19.9	22.3
36	18.5	20.9	23.3
37	19.5	21.9	24.4
38	20.7	23.1	25.5
39	21.8	24.3	26.7
40	23.1	25.5	27.9

Length = 8.457278951 + 0.00026630314 (menstrual age)^3; SD = 1.209.
(From Bertagnoli L, Lalatta F, Gallicchio R, et al. Quantitative characterization of growth of the fetal kidney. J Clin Ultrasound 1983; 11: 349–56, with permission from John Wiley and Sons.)

Table A.24 Amniotic fluid index values in normal pregnancy.

	Amniotic fluid index percentile values (mm)				
Week	3rd	5th	50th	95th	97th
16	73	79	121	185	201
17	77	83	127	194	211
18	80	87	133	202	220
19	83	90	137	207	225
20	86	93	141	212	230
21	88	95	143	214	233
22	89	97	145	216	235
23	90	98	146	218	237
24	90	98	147	219	238
25	89	97	147	221	240
26	89	97	147	223	242
27	85	95	146	226	245
28	86	94	146	228	249
29	84	92	145	231	254
30	82	90	145	234	258
31	79	88	144	238	263
32	77	86	144	242	269
33	74	83	143	245	274
34	72	81	142	248	278
35	70	79	140	249	279
36	68	77	138	249	279
37	66	75	135	244	275
38	65	73	132	239	269
39	64	72	127	226	255
40	63	71	123	214	240
41	63	70	116	194	216
42	63	69	110	175	192

(Adapted from Moore TR, Coyle JE. The amniotic fluid index in normal human pregnancy. Am J Obstet Gynecol 1990; 162: 1168, with permission from Elsevier.)

Table A.25 Amniotic fluid volume assessment (mean values) using the four-quadrant technique.

Gestational age (weeks)	Number of patients	Amniotic fluid volume (cm)
36	19	12.8 ± 4.8
37	63	13.1 ± 4.3
38	83	13.4 ± 4.7
39	55	12.4 ± 4.9
40	33	12.4 ± 4.6
41	68	8.8 ± 4.5
42	32	8.5 ± 4.7

(From Phelan JP, Smith SV, Broussard P, et al. Amniotic fluid volume assessment using the four-quadrant technique at 36–42 weeks' gestation. J Reprod Med 1987; 32: 540–42, with permission from the Journal of Reproductive Medicine.)

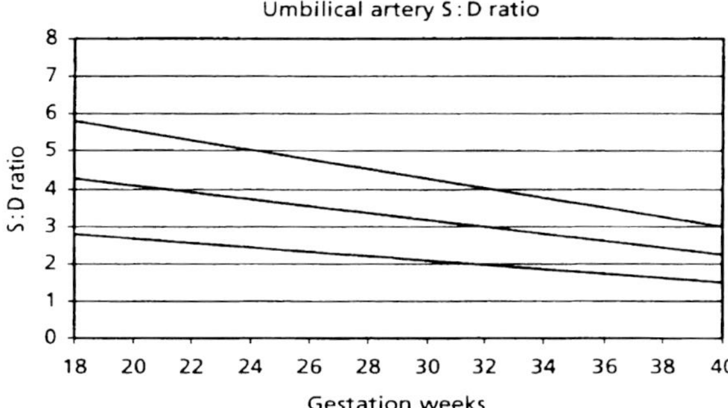

Fig A.2 Umbilical artery systolic:diastolic ratio throughout gestation. (From Ferrazzi E, Gementi P, Bellotti M, et al. Doppler velocimetry: critical analysis, cerebral, and aortic reference values. Eur J Obstet Gynaecol 1991; 38: 189–96, with permission from Elsevier.)

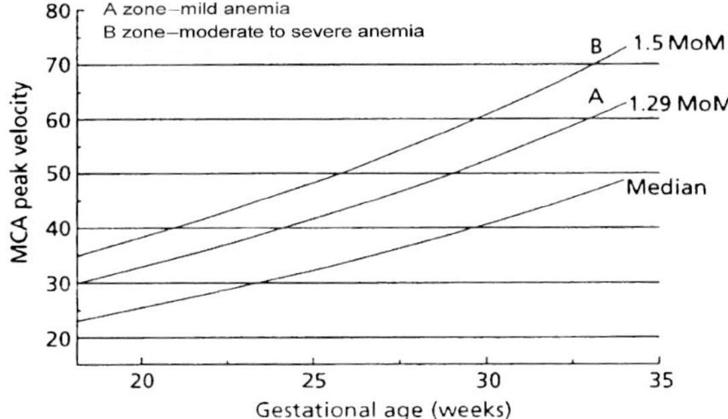

Fig A.3 Middle cerebral artery (MCA) Doppler peak velocities. Peak MCA Doppler velocity >1.5 MoM for gestational age predictive of fetal anemia. (From Moise KJ. Modern management of Rhesus alloimmunization in pregnancy. Obstet Gynecol 2002; 100: 600, with permission from Lippincott, Williams and Wilkins.)

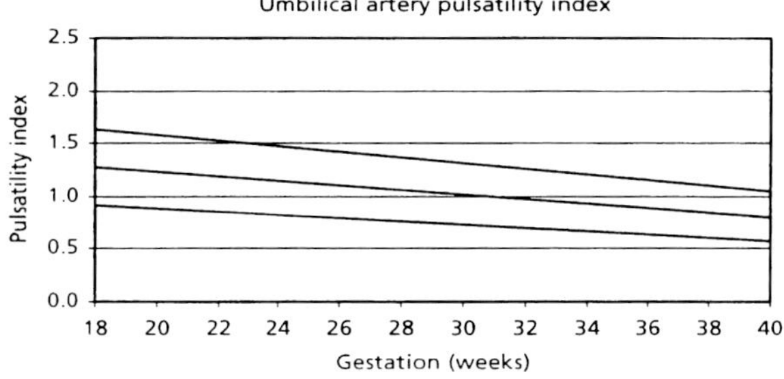

Fig A.4 Umbilical artery pulsatility index throughout gestation. (From Ferrazzi E, Gementi P, Bellotti M, et al. Doppler velocimetry: critical analysis of umbilical, cerebral, and aortic reference values. Eur J Obstet Gynaecol 1991; 38: 189–96, with permission from Elsevier.)

Table A.26 Reference values for umbilical artery Doppler resistive index and systolic:diastolic ratio.

	Percentiles					
	5th		50th		95th	
Gestational age (weeks)	Resistive index	Systolic: diastolic ratio	Resistive index	Systolic: diastolic ratio	Resistive index	Systolic: diastolic ratio
16	0.70	3.39	0.80	5.12	0.90	10.50
17	0.69	3.27	0.79	4.86	0.89	9.46
18	0.68	3.16	0.78	4.63	0.88	8.61
19	0.67	3.06	0.77	4.41	0.87	7.90
20	0.66	2.97	0.76	4.22	0.86	7.30
21	0.65	2.88	0.75	4.04	0.85	6.78
22	0.64	2.79	0.74	3.88	0.84	6.33
23	0.63	2.71	0.73	3.73	0.83	5.94
24	0.62	2.64	0.72	6.59	0.82	5.59
25	0.61	2.57	0.71	3.46	0.81	5.28
26	0.60	2.50	0.70	3.34	0.80	5.01
27	0.59	2.44	0.69	3.22	0.79	4.76
28	0.58	2.38	0.68	3.12	0.78	4.53
29	0.57	2.32	0.67	3.02	0.77	4.33
30	0.56	2.26	0.66	2.93	0.76	4.14
31	0.55	2.21	0.65	2.84	0.75	3.97
32	0.54	2.16	0.64	2.76	0.74	3.81
33	0.53	2.11	0.63	2.68	0.73	3.66
34	0.52	2.07	0.62	2.61	0.72	3.53
35	0.51	2.03	0.61	2.54	0.71	3.40
36	0.50	1.98	0.60	2.47	0.70	3.29
37	0.49	1.94	0.59	2.41	0.69	3.18
38	0.47	1.90	0.57	2.35	0.67	3.08
39	0.46	1.87	0.56	2.30	0.66	2.98
40	0.45	1.83	0.55	2.24	0.65	2.89
41	0.44	1.80	0.54	2.19	0.64	2.81
42	0.43	1.76	0.53	2.14	0.63	2.73

Note: Resistive index $= 0.97199 - 0.01045 \times$ gestational age (SD $= 0.06078$); systolic:diastolic ratio $= 11$ (1 − resistive index).

(From Kofinas AD, Espeland MA, Penry M, et al. Uteroplacental Doppler flow velocity waveform indices in normal pregnancy: a statistical exercise and the development of appropriate reference values. Am J Perinatol 1992; 9: 94–101, with permission from Thieme.)

Table A.27 Clinical parameters in estimation of gestational age.

Priority for estimating gestational age	*Estimated range for 95% cases
In vitro fertilization	Less than 1 day
Ovulation induction	3–4 days
Recorded basal body temperature	4–5 days
Ultrasound crown–rump length (CRL)	(±) .7 weeks
First trimester physical examination (normal uterus)	(±) 1 week
Ultrasound BPD prior to 20 weeks	(±) 1 week
Ultrasound gestational sac volume	(±) 1.5 weeks
Ultrasound BPD from 20–26 weeks	(±) 1.6 weeks
LNMP from recorded dates (good history)	(±) 2-3 weeks
Ultrasound BPD 26–30 weeks	(±) 2-3 weeks
LNMP from memory (good history)	3–4 weeks
Ultrasound BPD after 30 weeks	3–4 weeks
Fundal height measurement	4–6 weeks
LNMP from memory (not good history)	4–6 weeks
Fetal heart tones first heard	4–6 weeks
Quickening	4–6 weeks

A "good" history requires knowledge of both LNMP and previous period with regular periods and no use of birth control pills for at least 6 months prior to the LNMP.

*Rule is to always use a more reliable indicator in preference to a less reliable one.

(Courtesy James D. Bowie, MD.)

Index